Nursing
TimeSavers

Neurologic
Disorders

Nursing
TimeSavers

Neurologic
Disorders

Springhouse Corporation
Springhouse, Pennsylvania

Staff

Executive Director, Editorial
Stanley Loeb

Senior Publisher
Matthew Cahill

Art Director
John Hubbard

Clinical Manager
Cindy Tryniszewski, RN, MSN

Senior Editor
Michael Shaw

Clinical Editors
Kathy Craig, RN, BA; Tina Dietrich, RN, BSN, CCRN; Mary Chapman Gyetvan, RN, MSN; Mary Jane McDevitt, RN, BS

Editors
Mary Lou Bertucci, J. Allen Canale, Neal Fandek, Traci A. Ginnona, Judd L. Howard, Richard Koreto, Ann Lenkiewicz, Art Ofner

Copy Editors
Cynthia C. Breuninger (supervisor), Priscilla DeWitt, Jennifer George Mintzer, Nancy Papsin, Doris Weinstock

Designers
Stephanie Peters (associate art director), Matie Patterson (senior designer), Kaaren Mitchel, Amy Smith

Illustrators
Kevin Curry, Dan Fione, Robert Jackson, Judy Newhouse

Manufacturing
Deborah Meiris (director), Pat Dorshaw (manager), Anna Brindisi, Kate Davis, T.A. Landis

Editorial Project Coordination
Patricia McCloskey

Editorial Assistants
Maree DeRosa, Beverly Lane, Mary Madden

Indexer
Barbara Hodgson

Printed in the United States of America.
NTS3-010294

Library of Congress Cataloging-in-Publication Data
Neurologic disorders.
   p. cm. — (Nursing timesavers)
   Includes bibliographical references and index.
   1. Neurological Nursing   I. Springhouse Corporation. II. Series.
   [DNLM: 1. Central Nervous System Diseases—nursing. WY 160 N49426 1994]
RC350.5.N482 1994
610.73'68—dc20
DNLM/DLC   93-43682
ISBN 0-87434-686-X   CIP

Contents

Contributors and consultants

Contributors

Ellie Z. Franges, RN, MSN, CNRN, CCRN
Director, Patient Care Services,
Neurosurgery Intensive Care Unit
Lehigh Valley Hospital
Allentown, Pa.

Jim Herbert, RN, MSN, FNP
Family Nurse Practitioner
Mary Imogene Bassett Hospital
Cooperstown, N.Y.

Consultants

Kathleen Coughlin Bradley, RN
Coordinator, Outpatient Services
Comprehensive Headache Center at
Germantown Hospital
Philadelphia

Daniel R. Brennan, RN, MSN, CS
Clinical Nurse Specialist
Department of Neurology
University of Pennsylvania Medical
Center
Philadelphia

Marlene M. Ciranowicz, RN, MSN, CDE
Independent Nurse Consultant
Dresher, Pa.

Elizabeth A. Hoffman, RN, MSN, CCRN, ONC
Nursing Care Coordinator
Neurosurgery Intensive Care Unit
Thomas Jefferson University Hospital
Philadelphia

Patricia A. Kane-Carlsen, RN, MSN, CS
Nurse Consultant
Coppell, Tex.

Steven B. Meisel, PharmD
Assistant Director of Pharmacy
Fairview Southdale Hospital
Minneapolis

Jacqueline Sullivan, RN, MSN, CCRN, CNRN
Clinical Nurse Specialist, Neurosurgery
Intensive Care Unit
Clinical Assistant Professor
Thomas Jefferson University Hospital
Philadelphia

Barbara J. Taptich, RN, MA
Director, Heart Institute
St. Francis Medical Center
Trenton, N.J.

Foreword

In recent years, nursing care of neurologic patients has changed dramatically. Consider the manifold advances in diagnostic tests and monitoring techniques, with magnetic resonance imaging, fiberoptic intracranial pressure monitoring, and jugular venous oxygen saturation monitoring all achieving greater accuracy and effectiveness. Consider, too, how varied and complex the demands of neurologic care have become. During a given day, you may be called on to:
• assess the neuromuscular condition of a patient with spinal cord injury or peripheral nerve damage
• monitor level of consciousness in a patient with an evolving cerebrovascular accident
• interpret diagnostic test findings in a patient with altered cerebral perfusion
• respond rapidly to sharply increased intracranial pressure
• teach bladder retraining techniques to a patient with multiple sclerosis
• explain the need for plasmapheresis to a patient with myasthenia gravis
• teach family members how to ensure the safety of a relative with Alzheimer's disease.

Successfully fulfilling such complex responsibilities requires thorough preparation and sound clinical skills. And, with today's fast-paced delivery of health care, it requires that you quickly learn and refine these skills.

Neurologic Disorders, the latest book in the Nursing TimeSavers series, can help you meet today's challenges. Concise and easy to use, this compact reference provides you with up-to-date clinical information on caring for neurologic patients. It was developed by nursing professionals — all with years of bedside know-how — who understand the demands and time constraints you encounter every day.

Chapter 1 explains how to use the nursing process to provide expert care. You'll learn how to identify patient problems, develop a plan of care, set outcomes for the patient, determine the necessary interventions, and evaluate whether outcomes have been achieved. You'll also find concise coverage of key nursing diagnoses used in neurologic care.

Chapter 2 provides guidelines for assessing your patient's chief complaint. For instance, if your patient says, "My head hurts" or "I feel dizzy most of the time," turn to this chapter for a list of questions to ask and techniques to perform. This chapter also covers other common signs and symptoms of neurologic dysfunction — neck and back pain, vision loss, sensory disturbances, weakness, memory loss, decreased level of consciousness, and confusion.

In Chapter 3, you'll find step-by-step instructions for monitoring your patient's condition. You'll find guidelines for monitoring intracranial pressure, cerebral blood flow, jugular venous oxygen saturation, and regional cerebral oxygen saturation.

Chapters 4 through 10 cover the most common neurologic disorders: meningitis, Alzheimer's disease, seizure disorders, Parkinson's disease, multiple sclerosis, head, neck, and spinal injuries, and many others. To save you time, each disorder is organized according to the nursing process with five easy-to-spot text headings:

• *Assessment.* This section tells you what health history data, physical examination findings, and diagnostic test results to expect.

• *Nursing diagnosis.* In this section, you'll find the most common nursing diagnoses and related etiologies for each disorder.

• *Planning.* This section provides a list of expected patient outcomes for each nursing diagnosis. This feature will ensure that your documentation includes accurate outcome statements.

• *Implementation.* In this section, you'll find complete, step-by-step nursing interventions as well as guidelines for patient teaching.

• *Evaluation.* This section provides criteria to judge the effectiveness of your nursing care and gauge your patient's progress toward meeting expected outcomes.

Throughout the book, you'll see special graphic devices called logos that direct you to important and timesaving information. The *FactFinder* logo, for instance, highlights key points about a disorder, covering such topics as risk factors, demographics, and prognosis. The *Timesaving tip* logo alerts you to ways to save time as you proceed with your nursing care. The *Assessment TimeSaver* logo helps you organize and expedite the initial step of the nursing process. The *Treatments* logo summarizes the latest medical therapies for each disorder. The *Teaching TimeSaver* logo provides suggestions and guidelines for teaching patients. And the *Discharge TimeSaver* logo signals a checklist of teaching topics, referrals, and follow-up appointments to promote your patient's well-being after hospitalization.

Additionally, *Neurologic Disorders* includes valuable appendices on common neurologic treatments and drugs. The first appendix outlines current procedures for managing neurologic disorders, complete with concise descriptions, indications, and complications. The second appendix covers common neurologic drugs, including their generic and trade names, pharmacologic and therapeutic classifications, indications and dosages, and adverse reactions. Common and life-threatening adverse reactions are clearly marked.

By providing current clinical information in a focused, quick-reference format, *Neurologic Disorders* can save you time and help you provide better care for your neurologic patients. Become familiar with this tool and use it at home or at work. A better understanding of neurologic care will enhance your confidence and increase your chances for success in today's fast-changing world of health care.

Jacqueline Sullivan, RN, MSN, CCRN, CNRN
Clinical Nurse Specialist, Neurosurgery Intensive Care Unit
Clinical Assistant Professor
Thomas Jefferson University Hospital
Philadelphia

CHAPTER 1

Applying the nursing process to neurologic care

For many nurses, neurologic care poses a formidable challenge. Neurologic assessment, for instance, can take longer than most other assessments and requires sophisticated skills. What's more, some significant neurologic changes are subtle and difficult to detect, requiring meticulous testing to elicit them. Successfully meeting challenges like these requires thorough preparation, sound clinical skills and, above all, a systematic approach to nursing action. By using the nursing process to structure your neurologic care, you can provide care expertly and thoroughly. And you'll save time.

You'll use the nursing process to:
• identify patient problems you can treat
• identify patient problems you can help prevent
• develop a plan that addresses the patient's actual and potential problems
• determine what kind of assistance the patient needs and who can best provide it
• select goals for the patient and determine whether they've been achieved
• accurately document your contribution to achieving patient outcomes.

The nursing process consists of a series of steps. Understanding each of them — assessment, nursing diagnosis, planning, implementation, and evaluation — will help you address the complex needs of patients with neurologic disorders. Keep in mind, however, that these steps are dynamic and flexible; they often overlap.

Assessment

Assessment, the first step of the nursing process, is critical. That's because the quality of assessment data will determine the success of subsequent nursing process steps. A complete nursing assessment usually includes taking a health history, performing a physical examination, and reviewing the results of diagnostic tests.

You can identify neurologic problems while performing a complete assessment or while investigating a complaint. You can evaluate overall neurologic function and detect abnormalities as you assess mental status, the cranial nerves, sensorimotor function, and reflexes.

Health history
During the health history, you'll explore the patient's chief complaint and other symptoms, assess the impact of the illness or complaint on him and his family, and begin to develop and implement a plan of care. You'll also gather information to guide diagnosis and treatment.

Include the patient's family members or close friends when taking the history. Don't assume that the patient remembers accurately; corroborate the information you obtain with others to get a better picture.

Chief complaint
Ask the patient why he's seeking care. Document the chief complaint in the patient's own words. Ask about its onset, frequency, and precipitating, alleviating, and influencing factors. Ask the patient if he has noticed any associated signs and symptoms or if he has experienced adverse effects from any treatment.

Common neurologic complaints include headache, sensory disturbances, neck or back pain, sudden vision loss, dizziness, hearing loss, motor disturbances (including weakness, paresis, and paralysis), memory loss, altered level of consciousness (LOC), and confusion. For further information, see Chapter 2, Exploring chief complaints.

Ask the following questions to help the patient elaborate on his present illness or complaint:

• Does he have headaches? If so, how often and when?
• Does he ever feel dizzy?
• Does he ever have a tingling or prickling sensation or numbness anywhere in his body?
• Has he ever had seizures or tremors? Weakness or paralysis in his arms or legs?
• Does he have trouble walking?
• Does he have any difficulty swallowing?
• Does he have any difficulty urinating?
• How is his memory and ability to concentrate?
• Does he ever have trouble speaking or understanding something someone says to him?
• Does he have trouble reading or writing?

Illnesses

Find out if the patient has any disorders that can affect the neurologic system or influence recovery, such as lupus erythematosus, sarcoidosis, metastatic cancer, tuberculosis, or human immunodeficiency virus infection. Explore all of the patient's previous major illnesses, recurrent minor illnesses, accidents or injuries, surgical procedures, and allergies.

Ask the patient if he's taking any prescription or over-the-counter drugs. If so, document the name and dosage of each drug, the duration of therapy, and the reason for it. If the patient can't remember which medications he's taking, find out if he has brought any with him. If he has, examine the label and contents.

Family history

Information about the patient's family may help uncover hereditary disorders. Ask him if anyone in his family has had diabetes, cardiac or renal disease, hypertension, cancer, bleeding disorders, mental disorders, seizures, or a cerebrovascular accident (CVA).

Lifestyle factors

Assess the patient's cultural and social background. Consider the following questions:

• Does the patient live alone or with others?
• Does he have any hobbies?
• Does he view his illness as a stigma?
• What is his religion? Does he observe religious conventions and practices?
• What is his education level and occupation?
• Is his employment history stable or erratic?
• Has his illness or complaint affected family relationships? Must family members take on responsibilities that he once handled?
• Does he receive adequate support from family members?
• Does he use cigarettes, alcohol, or illicit drugs? If the patient drinks alcohol, determine the number of drinks he has daily and the type of alcohol. Also ask him about his lifetime drinking pattern. Chronic alcohol use can result in cerebellar degeneration, peripheral neuropathy, seizures, and dementia.

Coping patterns

Assess the patient's ability to cope with stress. Consider the following questions:
• What types of activities help him cope?
• Do his current coping strategies help or hinder his progress?
• Are there any indications that he is having difficulty coming to terms with his illness or complaint?

Use your assessment of the patient's coping mechanisms to determine his learning needs. Does he seem ready to accept change? How important is good health to him? Is he willing to work to regain it? If he isn't ready or willing to accept change, he's unlikely to respond to teaching.

Physical examination

Your next step is to perform a physical examination, including a complete neurologic assessment. During the neurologic screening, you'll assess five areas: mental status, cranial nerves, sensory system, motor system, and reflexes.

A complete neurologic examination is complex and time-consuming, often taking several hours. If time and the patient's condition are critical, you may perform an abbreviated assessment that focuses on the following key indicators of neurologic function:
• rapid LOC assessment in a head trauma patient
• assessment of sensorimotor function in a patient who has lumbar spinal fusion with no cranial involvement
• assessment of sensorimotor function in a spinal cord-injured patient with no cranial involvement.

In other instances, you may perform a neurocheck — a brief neurologic assessment of the following key indicators:

• LOC
• pupil size and response
• verbal responsiveness
• extremity strength and movement
• vital signs.

After you've established baseline values for these indicators, you can reevaluate them regularly to reveal trends in a patient's neurologic function and help detect complications.

Assessing overall appearance

Observe the patient's clothing, grooming, and personal hygiene. Are his clothes appropriate for the setting and the weather? For example, a patient with organic mental syndrome may wear multiple layers of clothing. Someone suffering from dementia may exhibit poor hygiene and grooming.

Observe the patient's posture and movements. Look for a stiff posture and lack of movement — possible signs of Parkinson's disease or advanced dementia. Also note restlessness, pacing, or agitation.

Observe the patient's facial expressions. Are they consistent with his mood and conversation?

Timesaving tip: Save time by combining assessment steps. For example, you can take note of the patient's general appearance and cerebral function (LOC, mental status, and language) while obtaining his medical history.

Checking vital signs

The central nervous system (CNS), primarily by way of the brain stem and autonomic nervous system (ANS), controls the body's vital functions, which include:
• body temperature
• heart rate and rhythm
• respiratory rate, depth, and pattern
• blood pressure.

These vital control centers lie deep within the cerebral hemispheres and in the brain stem. Because of this, changes in vital signs aren't usually early indicators of CNS deterioration. When evaluating the significance of vital sign changes, consider each sign individually as well as in relation to the others.

Temperature

Damage to the hypothalamus or upper brain stem can impair the body's ability to maintain a constant temperature, resulting in profound hypothermia (temperature below 94° F, or 34.4° C) or hyperthermia (temperature above 106° F, or 41.1° C). Such damage can result from petechial hemorrhages in the hypothalamus or brain stem, trauma (causing pressure, twisting, or traction), or destructive lesions.

Heart rate

Because the ANS controls heart rate and rhythm, pressure on the brain stem and cranial nerves slows the pulse rate by stimulating the vagus nerve. In patients with increasing intracranial pressure (ICP), bradycardia is a late sign and usually accompanies rising systolic pressure, widening pulse pressure, and a bounding pulse. Cervical spine injuries can also cause bradycardia.

In a patient with acutely increased ICP or a brain injury, tachycardia signals decompensation (a condition in which the body can no longer compensate for elevated ICP), which rapidly leads to death.

Respiration

Respiratory centers in the medulla and pons control the rate, depth, and pattern of respiration. Neurologic dysfunction, particularly involving

the brain stem or both cerebral hemispheres, may alter respiration.

One of the first signs of a cerebral or upper brain stem disorder is Cheyne-Stokes respiration, a breathing pattern characterized by a period of apnea lasting 10 to 60 seconds followed by gradually increasing respiratory rate and depth. However, this breathing pattern may occur normally in an elderly patient during sleep, probably the result of generalized brain atrophy from aging, and in children.

Blood pressure

Pressor receptors in the medulla oblongata of the brain stem constantly monitor blood pressure. In a patient with no history of hypertension, rising blood pressure may signal rising ICP. If ICP continues to increase, pulse pressure widens as systolic pressure climbs and diastolic pressure remains stable or falls. In the late stages of acutely elevated ICP, blood pressure plummets as cerebral perfusion fails, resulting in death.

Although rare, hypotension accompanying a brain injury is an ominous sign. In addition, cervical spine injuries may interrupt sympathetic nervous system pathways, causing peripheral vasodilation and hypotension.

Assessing mental status

Begin your evaluation of the patient's mental status when listening to his answers during the health history. Consider such factors as recent and remote memory, attention span, and coherence of thoughts. If confusion or deteriorating mental status is the chief complaint, or if the patient has obvious neurologic deficits, you'll need a more detailed assessment of his mental status during your physical examination.

Assessment TimeSaver

Mental status screening questions

To quickly screen patients for disordered thought processes, ask the questions listed below. An incorrect answer to any question may indicate a need for a complete mental status examination.

Question	Function screened
What is your name?	Orientation to person
What is your mother's name?	Orientation to other people
What is today's date?	Orientation to time
What year is it?	Orientation to time
Where are you now?	Orientation to place
How old are you?	Memory
Where were you born?	Remote memory
What did you have for breakfast?	Recent memory
Who is the U.S. president?	General knowledge
Can you count backward from 20 to 1?	Attention span and calculation skills
Why are you here?	Recent memory

You may perform an abbreviated version of the complete mental status examination to determine the need for further evaluation. A brief screening can prove useful if the patient's responses to interview questions seem unreliable or indicate a possible memory or cognitive disturbance. (See *Mental status screening questions.*)

Level of consciousness
Change in a patient's LOC is the earliest and most sensitive indicator of a change in his neurologic status. To describe the patient's LOC, you may use the following terms:
• *Alert.* The patient is awake and responds fully and appropriately to all stimuli.

• *Lethargic.* The patient is drowsy and indifferent, and his verbal responses to stimuli are delayed. He reacts to stimuli but falls asleep when stimulation stops.
• *Obtunded.* The patient is even more lethargic and sleeps unless aroused.
• *Stuporous.* The patient can be aroused from sleep only by vigorous stimulation.
• *Comatose.* The patient has lost consciousness and no longer interacts with the environment.

However, most clinicians don't use these terms because of their subjectivity and potential for variable interpretation, preferring the Glasgow Coma Scale. This scale presents data more objectively and interprets them more consistently than brief screen-

Interpretation

Determining LOC using the Glasgow Coma Scale

The Glasgow Coma Scale provides an objective way to evaluate a patient's level of consciousness (LOC) and to detect changes from his baseline status. To use this scale, evaluate and score your patient's best eye-opening response, verbal response, and motor response. A total score of 15 indicates that he is alert; is oriented to person, place, and time; and can follow simple commands. A comatose patient will score 7 points or less. A score of 3 indicates deep coma with a poor prognosis, or even death.

Test	Reaction	Score
Eye-opening response	Open spontaneously	4
	Open to verbal command	3
	Open to pain	2
	No response	1
Verbal response	Oriented and converses	5
	Disoriented and converses	4
	Uses inappropriate words	3
	Makes incomprehensible sounds	2
	No response	1
Motor response	Obeys verbal command	6
	Localizes painful stimulus	5
	Flexion — withdrawal	4
	Flexion — abnormal (decorticate rigidity)	3
	Extension (decerebrate rigidity)	2
	No response	1

ings. (See *Determining LOC using the Glasgow Coma Scale.*)

Begin by quickly observing the patient's behavior. If the patient is dozing or asleep, attempt to arouse him by providing an appropriate auditory, tactile, or painful stimulus. Always start with a mild stimulus, and increase its intensity as necessary.

Timesaving tip: Be sure to stimulate the patient sufficiently to get a rapid and precise picture of his neurologic status. Being too gentle when attempting to stimulate a patient may prevent you from obtaining an accurate response and waste time.

Speech
Note how well the patient expresses himself and how well he comprehends your speech. Note the volume and clarity of his voice, and the pace and spontaneity of his speech. To test

for dysarthria or garbled speech, ask him to repeat the phrase "No ifs, ands, or buts."

Timesaving tip: To save time, assess his comprehension by determining if he can follow instructions during your examination.

Note whether the patient has aphasia, a speech impairment that usually results from an injury to the cerebral cortex, which may result from a CVA or brain tumor. Types of aphasia include the following:

• *Expressive (Broca's) aphasia.* In this disorder, you'll note impaired fluency and word-finding ability. The patient may use single words without articles or prepositions. His ability to repeat words and to write may also be impaired. This type of aphasia results from damage to the frontal lobe.

• *Receptive (Wernicke's) aphasia.* A patient with this disorder can't understand written words or speech. He may invent words (neologisms). Receptive aphasia results from damage to the temporal or parietal lobe.

• *Global aphasia.* Damage to both the anterior and posterior cortex results in the loss of expressive and receptive speech.

Cognitive function
Assess orientation, memory, attention span and calculation, thought content, abstract thought, judgment, insight, and emotional status.

• *Orientation.* Test orientation to time by asking the patient the time of day, day of the week, date (month and year), and season. If mental status becomes impaired, orientation to time usually vanishes before orientation to place and person. When evaluating orientation to time, be sure to consider the patient's environment and physical condition. A patient who has been in the intensive care unit for a

few days probably won't be oriented to time.

Test orientation to place by asking the patient to tell you where he is. Also ask for his home address, including the house number, street, city, and state.

Test orientation to person by asking the patient his name. Typically, this is the last type of orientation a patient loses. Then ask the names of family members and friends.

• *Memory.* To test short-term memory, ask the patient why he has been hospitalized. Make sure that you can verify his answer. Next, have him repeat a series of five nonconsecutive numbers. The patient with an intact short-term memory and a good attention span can repeat a series of five to seven numbers.

Test the patient's remote memory by asking his date and place of birth or the names of relatives. Again, be sure to verify the accuracy of the information.

• *Attention span and calculation.* Evaluate the patient's ability to maintain his attention throughout the mental status exam. To formally test attention span and calculation, ask the patient to count backward from 100 by 7s until he reaches 0. He should be able to complete this task in 90 seconds with fewer than four errors. Keep in mind that anxiety and mathematical ability may affect the patient's performance.

If the patient has difficulty with numerical computation, ask him to spell the word "world" backward.

• *Thought content.* Assessing thought content includes evaluating the clarity and cohesiveness of ideas. Note whether the patient's conversation has smooth, logical transitions between ideas. Does he have hallucinations (sensory perceptions that lack appropriate external stimuli) or delusions (beliefs not supported by reality)? Disordered thought patterns may indicate delirium or psychosis.

• *Abstract thought.* Test the patient's ability to think abstractly by asking him to interpret a common proverb, such as "A stitch in time saves nine" or "A rolling stone gathers no moss." A patient with dementia may interpret the proverb literally, failing to comprehend its figurative meaning. Keep in mind that if English isn't the patient's first language, he may have difficulty interpreting a proverb.

• *Judgment.* Describe a hypothetical situation and ask the patient to tell you how he would respond. For example, ask what he'd do if he were in a public building and heard the fire alarm sound. Evaluate the appropriateness of his answer.

• *Insight.* Assess the patient's ability to understand the implications of his situation and to recognize any abnormalities in his perceptions, judgments, and thought content. When you ask why he has sought health care, a patient who lacks insight may tell you that nothing is wrong with him. A cognitively impaired elderly patient may lack insight into the risks of living alone and make decisions that put him at further risk.

• *Emotional status.* Evaluate the patient's emotional state throughout the interview by noting his mood, emotional lability, and the appropriateness of his emotional responses. Also assess mood by asking him how he feels about himself and how he looks at the future.

If the patient is depressed, ask when his depression began. What caused it? Has he experienced insomnia, anorexia, or fatigue? Also ask about suicidal ideation. Keep in mind that an elderly person may exhibit depression by decreased function or increased agitation, rather than the usual sad affect.

Assessing the cranial nerves

The 12 pairs of cranial nerves transmit motor and sensory messages between the brain and the head and neck. The cranial nerves are designated by both a name and a Roman numeral. The names of the nerves indicate their function. The Roman numerals indicate the order in which the nerves are found in the brain, from the top (cephalad) to the bottom (caudad) of the brain stem. (See *Origin and function of cranial nerves,* page 10, and *Abnormal findings in cranial nerve assessment,* pages 11 and 12.)

Assessing the sensory system

Your examination of the patient's sensory system includes testing his ability to feel pain and light touch. You'll also evaluate the patient's vibratory sense, position sense, and discriminative sensations.

Pain

To test for pain, use the same technique that you used to evaluate the sensory component of the trigeminal nerve. Ask the patient to close his eyes. Then touch the major dermatomes of the trunk and limbs with a sterile needle or the clean tip of a safety pin. Ask him to indicate whether he feels a sharp or dull sensation.

If he has diminished pain sensation (hypesthesia) or no pain sensation (anesthesia), determine the borders of the area of sensory deficit by applying pinpricks at short intervals, starting in the area of anesthesia and working outward until he can perceive the stimulus.

(Text continues on page 12.)

Origin and function of cranial nerves

This illustration shows the origin of each cranial nerve (CN) and describes its type (motor, sensory, or both) and function.

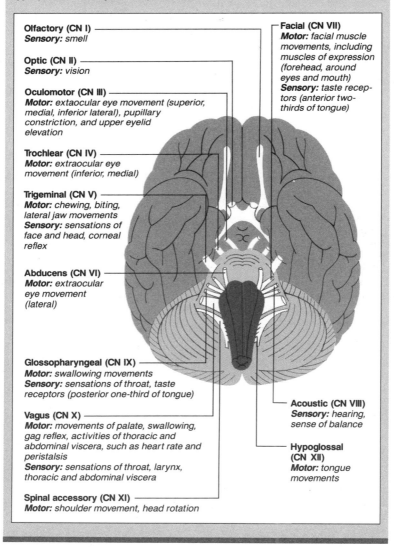

Olfactory (CN I)
Sensory: smell

Optic (CN II)
Sensory: vision

Oculomotor (CN III)
Motor: extaocular eye movement (superior, medial, inferior lateral), pupillary constriction, and upper eyelid elevation

Trochlear (CN IV)
Motor: extraocular eye movement (inferior, medial)

Trigeminal (CN V)
Motor: chewing, biting, lateral jaw movements
Sensory: sensations of face and head, corneal reflex

Abducens (CN VI)
Motor: extraocular eye movement (lateral)

Glossopharyngeal (CN IX)
Motor: swallowing movements
Sensory: sensations of throat, taste receptors (posterior one-third of tongue)

Vagus (CN X)
Motor: movements of palate, swallowing, gag reflex, activities of thoracic and abdominal viscera, such as heart rate and peristalsis
Sensory: sensations of throat, larynx, thoracic and abdominal viscera

Spinal accessory (CN XI)
Motor: shoulder movement, head rotation

Facial (CN VII)
Motor: facial muscle movements, including muscles of expression (forehead, around eyes and mouth)
Sensory: taste receptors (anterior two-thirds of tongue)

Acoustic (CN VIII)
Sensory: hearing, sense of balance

Hypoglossal (CN XII)
Motor: tongue movements

Abnormal findings in cranial nerve assessment

Damage to the cranial nerves may cause numerous abnormalities, including olfactory, visual, auditory, and muscular problems. Vertigo and dysphagia also indicate cranial nerve damage.

Olfactory (CN I)
If the patient can't detect odors with both nostrils (anosmia), he may have a disorder of the olfactory nerve. This symptom can result from a lesion in the olfactory tract caused by an intracranial mass, a hemorrhage, or a facial bone fracture. A complaint about food taste may also signal olfactory nerve damage because anosmia also impairs the sense of taste.

Optic (CN II) and oculomotor (CN III)
Visual fields may be impaired by lesions, such as tumors or infarcts of the optic nerve, the optic chiasm, or the optic tract.

If the patient's pupillary response to light is impaired, he may have damage to both the optic and oculomotor nerves. Increased intracranial pressure (ICP) can cause bilateral dilation of the pupils.

A drooping eyelid on one side, or *ptosis,* results from a defect of the oculomotor nerve. It is detected more readily when the patient is sitting up. The pupil may also be dilated on the affected side.

Oculomotor (CN III), trochlear (CN IV), and abducens (CN VI)
Weakness or paralysis of eye muscles or eyelids can result from cranial nerve damage. Increased ICP and in-

tracranial lesions can affect the motor nuclei of the oculomotor, trochlear, and abducens nerves.

In *nystagmus,* the patient's eyes drift slowly in one direction and then jerk back in the other direction. Nystagmus is associated with nerve damage in a number of sites, most commonly the peripheral labyrinth (inner ear), the brain stem (CN III, IV, and VI), and the cerebellum. It may also be caused by drug toxicity, as from the anticonvulsant phenytoin.

Trigeminal (CN V)
If the patient responds inadequately to sensory stimuli of the skin (forehead, cheek, jaw) or eye, the trigeminal nerve may be damaged. Lesions of the sensory component of the nerve may cause decreased skin perception of pain, temperature, and light touch. *Trigeminal neuralgia,* or tic douloureux, causes severe, lancinating pain over one or more of the facial dermatomes.

Facial (CN VII)
Unilateral facial weakness can reflect an upper motor neuron problem, such as a cerebrovascular accident or a tumor that has damaged neurons in the facial control area of the motor strip in the cerebral cortex. If the weakness originates in the cerebral cortex, the patient will retain the ability to wrinkle his forehead. However, if the facial nerve itself is damaged, the weakness will extend to the forehead, and the eye on the affected side won't close.

(continued)

Abnormal findings in cranial nerve assessment *(continued)*

Acoustic (CN VIII)
Sensorineural hearing loss can result from lesions of the cochlear branch of the acoustic nerve or from lesions in any part of the nerve's pathway to the brain stem. A patient with this type of hearing loss may have trouble hearing high-pitched sounds, or he may lose all hearing in the affected ear. Sensorineural hearing loss can occur in one or both ears.

The illusion of movement, or vertigo, can result from a disturbance of the vestibular centers. If the patient has a peripheral lesion in the labyrinth system, vertigo and nystagmus will occur 10 to 20 seconds after he changes position, but the symptoms will diminish with repeated position changes. If the vertigo originates in the brain, there is no latent period and the symptoms will not diminish with repeated position changes.

Glossopharyngeal (CN IX) and vagus (CN X)
Damage to the glossopharyngeal and vagus nerves may cause dysphagia. A diminished gag reflex may be normal. In multi-infarct dementia and bilateral cortical or subcortical disease, the gag reflex may increase.

Spinal accessory (CN XI)
Unilateral weakness, atrophy, or paralysis of the muscles innervated by the spinal accessory nerve suggests a peripheral nerve lesion. Signs include shoulder asymmetry or a scapula that appears displaced toward the affected side.

Hypoglossal (CN XII)
Unilateral flaccid paralysis of the tongue, atrophy of the affected side, and deviation of the tongue result from a peripheral nerve lesion. Unilateral spastic paralysis of the tongue produces poorly articulated, difficult speech (dysarthria) characterized by an explosive production of words, with the tongue deviating toward the unaffected side.

You can test most of the major dermatomes by applying the sterile needle or pin to the patient's shoulders, the inside and outside of the upper and lower arms, the thumbs, the fifth fingers, the anterior chest, the anterior and posterior thighs, the inside and outside of the thighs and lower legs, and the great toes. Be sure to test for pain sensation on the tips of fingers and toes. The patient with peripheral neuropathy develops hypesthesia first in the most distal aspects of the extremities. (See *Mapping sensory function by dermatomes,* pages 14 and 15.)

Light touch
Touch the major dermatomes with a wisp of cotton. Don't swab or sweep with the cotton because you might miss an area of sensory loss. If you do detect a sensory deficit, determine the borders of the area.

Some patients with peripheral neuropathy retain their light-touch sensation after they've lost their pain sensation. However, pain, temperature, light touch, tickle, and itch sensations are all transmitted up the spinal cord by the same sensory pathways. Therefore, when one sensation is affected, the others may be as well.

Vibratory sense
First, ask the patient to close his eyes. Then strike the tines of a tuning fork against your hand, and apply the base of the vibrating fork to the interphalangeal joint of the patient's great toe. Make sure you hold the fork on the stem; holding the tines will dampen the vibration.

Timesaving tip: When you test for vibratory sense, don't ask the patient, "Do you feel the vibration?" A patient may lose his vibratory sense but retain light-touch sensation. When such a patient feels the tuning fork on his skin, he may tell you he feels the vibration. Instead ask, "What do you feel?" Typically, he should report a vibration or buzzing.

If the patient doesn't feel the vibration over the interphalangeal joint, move to the medial malleolus of the ankle. If he still doesn't feel it, apply the vibrating fork to the anterior tibia. Move the fork proximally until he can feel the vibration. Then note where he felt it. Repeat the test on the other leg.

Also assess for vibratory sense on the arms. Start at the distal interphalangeal joint of the index finger and move proximally as necessary.

Position sense
A patient needs intact position sense, known as proprioception, together with intact vestibular and cerebellar function to maintain balance. When testing the patient's position sense,

you'll evaluate both his arms and his legs.
• *Arms.* Ask the patient to close his eyes; then grasp the sides of his index finger. Move the finger up or down, and ask the patient to tell you the direction in which you moved it. If the patient doesn't answer correctly, repeat the test at his wrist. If he still doesn't answer correctly, test his elbow and, if necessary, his shoulder. Note where he's able to perceive a position change. Perform this test on each arm.
• *Legs.* Grasp the sides of the great toe, move it up and down, and ask the patient to tell you the direction of the movement. If necessary, proceed to the ankles, the knees, and the hips until the patient gives you a correct response. Always grasp the sides of the body part, not the top and bottom. If you grasp the top and bottom of the toe, for instance, the pressure you apply may signal the position to the patient even though he has diminished position sense.

The same sensory pathway transmits position and vibratory sensations. Thus, peripheral neuropathy may diminish both, even though the patient's ability to feel pain, temperature, and light touch remain intact. In some disorders, vibratory sense may diminish sooner than position sense.

Discriminative sensations
If peripheral sensations are intact, test the more finely tuned integrative functions of the cerebral cortex. Begin by evaluating stereognosis, the ability to perceive the shape, size, weight, texture, and form of an object by touching and manipulating it. Ask the patient to close his eyes and open his hand. Then place a small, common object, such as a coin or key, in his palm and ask him to identify it.

(Text continues on page 16.)

Mapping sensory function by dermatomes

The body is divided into dermatomes, each of which represents an area of the skin supplied with afferent (sensory) nerve fibers that transmit pain, temperature, and touch from an individual spinal root — cervical (C), thoracic (T), lumbar (L), or sacral (S). These illustrations show the dermatomes of the body.

As you assess the patient's sensory function, use this chart as a reference to document the specific area tested, as well as the test results.

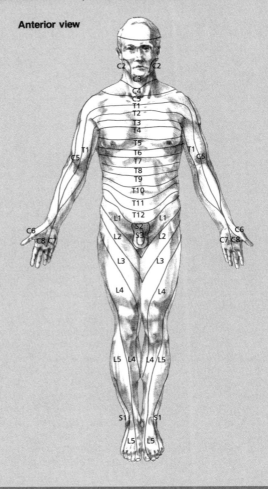

Anterior view

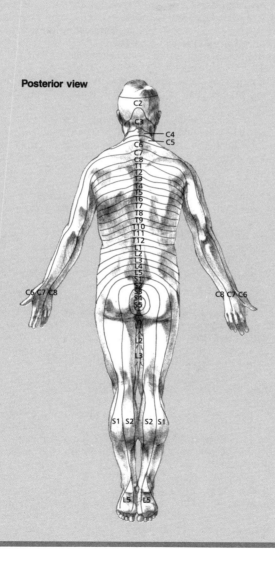

Posterior view

If he can't identify the object or perform the fine motor movements necessary to identify a small object, test graphesthesia, the ability to identify letters written on the palms, back, or other body surfaces. Have the patient hold out his hand. Then trace a large number on his palm using the eraser of a pencil. Ask him to identify the number.

Successful completion of these tests indicates that the sensory cortex can integrate sensory input. An inability to recognize objects by touch, called tactile agnosia, may indicate a parietal lobe lesion.

Next, test point localization by asking the patient to close his eyes while you touch one of his limbs and ask him to point to the spot you touched. His inability to do so may indicate a lesion in the sensory cortex.

Finally, test extinction by touching the patient simultaneously in the same area on both sides of his body. He should be able to feel the touches on both sides. If he feels the touch on only one side, he may have a cortical lesion on the other side.

Assessing the motor system

Assessment of the motor system includes inspecting the muscles and testing muscle tone and muscle strength. You'll also evaluate cerebellar function because the cerebellum plays a role in smooth-muscle movements, balance, and gait. (See *Assessing motor responses to pain.*)

Inspecting the muscles

Observe the symmetry of large muscle masses on each side of the body, noting any atrophy. In some cases, you may need to measure muscle mass to make a comparison. To do so, wrap a tape measure around the widest circumference of the muscle on each side. Muscle atrophy may re-

sult from decreased neural input, as occurs in paraplegia.

Look too for any abnormal muscle movements, such as tics, tremors, or fasciculations.

Timesaving tip: When time is critical, inspect the patient's muscles and look for abnormal muscle movement at the same time that you're testing muscle tone and strength.

Testing muscle tone

Muscle tone represents the muscles' resistance to passive stretching. To test muscle tone, move the patient's joints through passive range-of-motion (ROM) exercises. The systematic assessment proceeds from the fingers, wrist, elbow, and shoulder (upper extremities) to the ankle, knee, and hip (lower extremities).

Muscle tone abnormalities are described in terms of rigidity, flaccidity, and spasticity. In rigidity, the patient has heightened muscle tone; in flaccidity, diminished muscle tone. Both may result from a motor neuron lesion. Upper motor neuron lesions usually result in spasticity, whereas lower motor neuron lesions usually result in flaccidity. Spasticity, a state of increased muscle tone with exaggerated deep tendon reflexes, may occur secondary to injuries to the cerebral cortex or spinal cord.

Testing muscle strength

Evaluate general muscle strength by observing the patient's gait and motor activities. To test specific muscle groups, have the patient use the muscles against your resistance, as described below. Always compare the strength of muscle groups bilaterally.

Begin by testing the strength of the major muscle groups. Document muscle strength according to your hospital's policy or by using a grad-

Assessing motor responses to pain

When you apply a painful stimulus to your unconscious patient's supraorbital notch, his motor response can indicate his neurologic status. Normally, he will reach above shoulder level toward the pain stimulus. Remember, a focal motor deficit, such as hemiplegia, may prevent a bilateral response.

As the patient's brain stem function deteriorates, he may respond by assuming one of the following positions. Each posture suggests advanced deterioration.

Decorticate (flexor) posturing
The patient flexes one or both arms on his chest and may extend his legs stiffly.

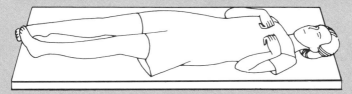

Decerebrate (extensor) posturing
The patient stiffly extends one or both arms and, possibly, his legs.

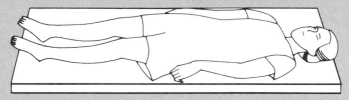

Flaccid posturing
The patient displays no motor response in any extremity.

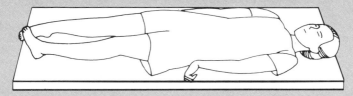

Grading muscle strength

To grade the patient's muscle strength, use the scale below.
• **5/5:** Normal movement against gravity and resistance; normal muscle strength.
• **4/5:** Full range of motion against moderate resistance and gravity; slight weakness.
• **3/5:** Full range of motion against gravity only, not against resistance; moderate weakness.
• **2/5:** Full range of motion, but not against gravity (can roll but can't lift); severe weakness.
• **1/5:** Weak muscle contraction but extremity can't move; very severe weakness.
• **0/5:** No visible or palpable muscle contraction or movement of extremity; complete paralysis.

ing system. For example, you can grade muscle strength on a scale of 0 to 5, with 0 indicating no strength and 5 indicating maximum strength. You can document your findings as a fraction, with the patient's score as the numerator and the maximum strength as the denominator, for example, 2/5 or 5/5. (See *Grading muscle strength.*)
• *Arms.* To test shoulder girdle strength, instruct the patient to extend his arms with his palms up and to maintain this position for 30 seconds. If he has shoulder girdle weakness in one arm, he may be unable to lift or he may be unable to lift it as high as he can lift the other arm. If he does lift both arms equally, look for pronation of the hand and downward drift

of the arm on the weaker side. If he can maintain his arms outstretched, further test his strength by placing your hands on his forearms and pressing down as he resists.

To test wrist flexion, ask the patient to flex his wrist against your resistance. Test wrist extension by asking him to extend his wrist as you push down. Test handgrip by asking the patient to squeeze your fingers as hard as he can. To check finger abduction, ask him to spread his fingers; then try to force them together.
• *Legs.* Begin by asking the patient to lift both legs off the bed simultaneously. If he's hemiplegic, he may not be able to lift the affected leg, to lift it as high, or to hold it up. To check quadriceps strength, ask him to lift both legs simultaneously as you press down on his anterior thighs.

Next, ask him to flex his legs at the knees and put his feet flat on the bed. To check lower leg strength, try to pull his lower leg forward as he resists. Then try to push his lower leg backward as he tries to extend his knee.

You'll also have to evaluate biceps, triceps, and ankle strength. (See *Testing muscle strength,* pages 19 and 20.)

Cerebellar testing
Before you test cerebellar function, observe the patient's general balance and coordination. Can he sit upright without support? Can he sit on the edge of the bed? Stand at the bedside? Remember that the ability to sit on the edge of the bed and to stand may be diminished by weakness unrelated to cerebellar dysfunction.

To assess the patient's cerebellar function, you'll evaluate his whole-body and extremity coordination, and his point-to-point and rapid skilled movement. (See *Assessing cerebellar function,* pages 21 and 22.)

Testing muscle strength

To evaluate the motor system, you'll test the strength of the major muscle groups of the patient's arms and legs, including biceps strength, triceps strength, and ankle strength (plantar flexion and dorsiflexion).

Biceps strength
To test biceps strength, ask the patient to hold his arm up in front of him with his elbow flexed and to maintain this position while you try to move his arm. Then pull down on the flexor surface of his forearm as he resists. Repeat this test on the other arm.

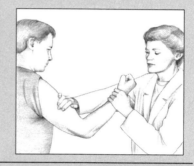

Triceps strength
To test triceps strength, ask the patient to hold his arm up in front of him with his elbow flexed and to maintain this position while you try to move his arm. Then push against the extensor surfaces of his forearm as he tries to straighten his arm. Repeat this test on the other arm.

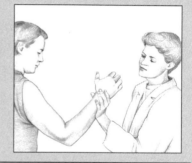

Ankle strength: Plantar flexion
Evaluate ankle strength by asking the patient to push his foot down (plantar flexion) as you resist.

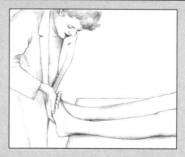

(continued)

Testing muscle strength *(continued)*

Ankle strength: Dorsiflexion
To test dorsiflexion, ask the patient to push his foot up as you press down on the dorsum of his foot.

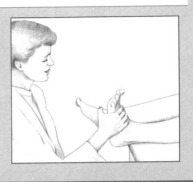

• *Whole-body coordination.* Observe the patient as he walks across the room, turns, and walks back. Note any imbalance or abnormalities in his gait. He should be able to maintain his posture, his arms swinging in tandem with his leg movements. His movements should be smooth and rhythmic, without hesitation or jerkiness. A patient with cerebellar dysfunction will exhibit a wide-based, unsteady gait. Deviation to one side may indicate a cerebellar lesion on that side.

Patients with cerebellar dysfunction have difficulty maintaining balance with their eyes closed because they cannot use the internal cues that orient them to the upright position.

You can also test whole-body coordination by asking the patient to do deep knee bends or to hop first on one foot and then the other. Keep in mind that this may be difficult for patients with arthritis or other musculoskeletal disorders.

• *Extremity coordination.* To evaluate the patient's extremity coordination, you'll test point-to-point movements, and rapid skilled and rapid alternating movements. During these tests, you will observe the patient's ability to perform precise movements with his fingers and hands, noting speed and accuracy.

Expect the patient to be more accurate with his dominant hand. A patient with cerebellar dysfunction will overshoot his target, and his movements will be jerky.

As another test of extremity coordination, ask the patient to touch the heel of his right foot to his left shin and to run his heel down his shin. Then have him repeat the maneuver with his left foot. If he has cerebellar dysfunction, he'll have difficulty placing his heel on his shin and maintaining the position. Plus, his movements will be jerky.

To test rapid alternating movements, have the patient sit with his palms down on his thighs. Next, tell him to turn his palms first up and then down. Instruct him to gradually increase his speed. Then have the pa-

Assessing cerebellar function

To evaluate cerebellar function, you'll test the patient's balance and coordination while he performs heel-to-toe walking, the Romberg test, point-to-point movements, and rapid skilled movements.

Heel-to-toe walking
Ask the patient to walk heel to toe and observe his balance. Although he may be slightly unsteady, he should be able to maintain his balance while walking forward.

Romberg test
Ask the patient to stand with his feet together, his eyes open, and his arms at his side. Observe his balance, and then ask him to close his eyes. Hold your outstretched arms on either side of him so that you can support him if he sways to one side. Note whether he loses his balance or sways. If he falls to one side, the Romberg test is positive.

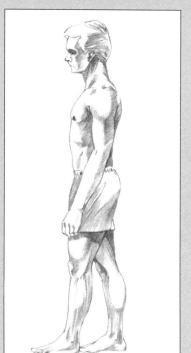
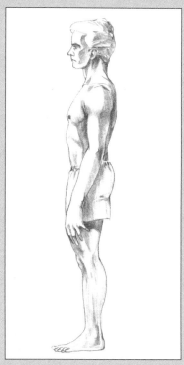

(continued)

Assessing cerebellar function *(continued)*

Point-to-point movements
Have the patient sit about 2′ (0.5 m) away from you. Hold your index finger up, and ask him to touch the tip of his index finger to the tip of yours and then to touch his nose. Next, move your finger to another position and ask him to repeat the maneuver. Have him increase his speed gradually as you repeat the test. Then test his other hand.

Rapid skilled movements
Ask the patient to touch the thumb of his right hand to his right index finger and then to each of his remaining fingers. Then instruct him to increase his speed. Observe his movements for smoothness and accuracy. Repeat the test on his left hand.

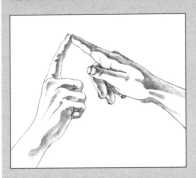
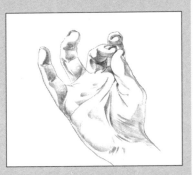

tient lie supine. Stand at the foot of the bed and hold your palms near his soles. Instruct him to alternately tap the sole of his right foot and then his left foot against your palms. Tell him to increase his speed as you observe his coordination. A patient with cerebellar dysfunction exhibits dysdiadochokinesia (an inability to perform coordinated alternating movements).

Assessing the reflexes
Evaluating your patient's reflexes includes testing deep tendon and superficial reflexes as well as observing for primitive reflexes.

Deep tendon reflexes
Before you test a deep tendon reflex, make sure the limb is relaxed and the joint is in the midpoint in the range of motion; for instance, the knee or elbow should be flexed at a 45-degree angle. Then distract the patient by asking him to focus on an object across the room. If he focuses on his performance, the cerebral cortex may dampen his response.

When testing deep tendon reflexes, always move from head to toe and be sure to compare reflexes bilaterally. To elicit the reflex, tap the tendon lightly but firmly with the reflex hammer. Then grade the briskness of the response on a scale of 0 (no response) to 4+ (hyperactive).

Deep tendon reflexes should be symmetrical. A markedly brisk hyperreflexic response indicates an upper motor neuron lesion. Such lesions can also cause clonus at the ankle — a repetitive movement, alternating between dorsiflexion and plantar flexion. Diminished or absent deep tendon reflexes indicate damage to the lower motor neurons. (See *Grading deep tendon reflexes,* at right, and *Assessing deep tendon reflexes,* pages 24 and 25.)

Superficial reflexes

These reflexes include the plantar, abdominal, and cremasteric reflexes. To elicit these reflexes, you'll stimulate the patient's skin or mucous membranes. To document your findings, use a plus sign (+) to indicate that a reflex is present and a minus sign (-) to indicate that it's absent. (See *Assessing superficial reflexes,* page 26.)

Primitive reflexes

Although normal in infants, primitive reflexes are abnormal in adults. Primitive reflexes are also called frontal release signs. These signs indicate the presence of diffuse cortical damage. They include the grasp, snout, sucking, and glabellar reflexes. (See *Assessing primitive reflexes,* pages 27 and 28.)

Diagnostic tests

Together with the health history and physical examination, diagnostic tests form a profile of your patient's condition. The list below reviews diagnostic tests commonly ordered for patients with known or suspected neurologic problems.

• Skull X-rays diagnose skull fractures and the bony changes associat-

Grading deep tendon reflexes

When testing the patient's deep tendon reflexes, use the following grading scale:

  0 absent

  + present but diminished

  + + normal

  + + + increased but not necessarily abnormal

  + + + + hyperactive, clonic.

Record the patient's reflex scores by drawing a stick figure and entering the scores at the proper location. The figure below indicates normal deep tendon reflex activity.

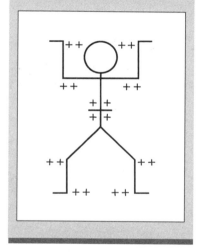

ed with Paget's disease, hyperostosis, and osteolytic disease. Calcifications seen in the brain may indicate an intracranial mass, although their pathologic significance can't be identified by X-ray alone. Alterations in bony contours, sutures, and bony cavities

(Text continues on page 27.)

Assessing deep tendon reflexes

During your neurologic examination, you'll evaluate your patient's deep tendon reflexes. You'll test the biceps, triceps, brachioradialis, patellar (quadriceps), and achilles reflexes.

Biceps reflex
Position the patient's arm so that his elbow is flexed at a 45-degree angle and his arm is relaxed. Place your thumb or index finger over the biceps tendon and your remaining fingers loosely over the triceps muscle. Strike your thumb or index finger with the pointed tip of the reflex hammer, and watch and feel for contraction of the biceps muscle and flexion of the forearm.

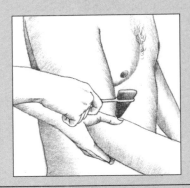

Triceps reflex
Have the patient abduct his arm and place his forearm across his chest. Strike the triceps tendon about 2" (5 cm) above the olecranon process on the extensor surface of the upper arm. Watch for contraction of the triceps muscle and extension of the forearm.

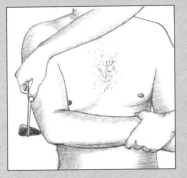

If you don't elicit the triceps reflex, try this alternative technique: Ask the patient to abduct his arm at the shoulder. If you're right-handed, support his upper arm with your left arm. Ask him to let his arm hang loosely over yours. With the hammer in your right hand, strike the triceps tendon briskly, using either the blunt or the pointed end. Again, watch for contraction of the triceps muscle and extension of the forearm at the elbow.

Assessing deep tendon reflexes *(continued)*

Brachioradialis reflex
Instruct the patient to partially flex his elbow with his palm down while you support his lower arm. Alternatively, you can instruct the patient to rest the ulnar surface of his hand on his knee with his elbow partially flexed. With the tip of the hammer, strike the radius about 2" (5 cm) proximal to the styloid process of the radius. Watch for supination of the hand and flexion of the forearm at the elbow.

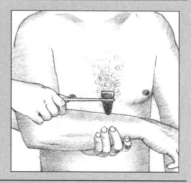

Patellar reflex
Have the patient sit on the side of the bed with his legs dangling freely. If he can't sit up, flex his knee at a 45-degree angle and place your nondominant hand behind it for support. Strike the patellar tendon just below the patella, and look for contraction of the quadriceps muscle in the anterior thigh and for extension of the leg.

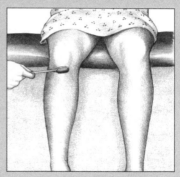

Achilles reflex
Slightly flex the foot and support the plantar surface. Using the pointed end of the reflex hammer, strike the Achilles tendon. Watch for plantar flexion of the foot at the ankle. If the patient is bedridden, position him with his hip externally rotated and his foot resting on his other knee. Slightly flex the foot at the ankle and strike the tendon briskly.

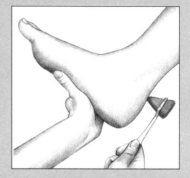

Assessing superficial reflexes

To assess the superficial reflexes, you'll test the plantar and abdominal reflexes as shown below. In male patients, you'll also test the cremasteric reflex: Using an applicator stick, lightly stroke the patient's inner thigh and watch for contraction of the cremaster muscle in the scrotum and prompt elevation of the testicle on the side of the stimulus. The cremasteric reflex may be absent in upper or lower motor neuron disorders.

Plantar reflex

Slowly stroke the lateral side of the patient's sole from the heel to the great toe, using an applicator stick, a tongue blade, or a key. The normal response is plantar flexion of the toes. In an elderly patient, this response may be diminished because of arthritic deformities of the toe or foot.

Patients with disorders of the pyramidal tract may respond to the stimulus by dorsiflexion of the great toe (Babinski's reflex). In some patients, other toes extend and abduct; you may even see dorsiflexion of the ankle, knee, and hip.

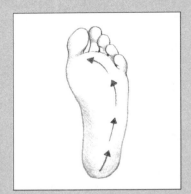

Abdominal reflex

Place the patient in the supine position with his arms at his sides and his knees slightly flexed.

Using the tip of the reflex hammer, a key, or an applicator stick, stroke both sides of the abdomen above and below the umbilicus, moving from the periphery toward the midline. After each stroke, watch for abdominal muscle contraction and movement of the umbilicus toward the stimulus.

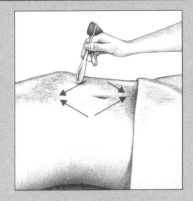

Assessing primitive reflexes

During your assessment of primitive reflexes, you'll test for the grasp reflex, the snout reflex, the sucking reflex, and the glabellar reflex.

Grasp reflex
Apply gentle pressure to the patient's palm with your fingers. Avoid finger injury or pain by crossing your middle and index fingers before placing them in his palm. If he grasps your fingers between his thumb and index finger and does not release his grasp on command, suspect cortical damage (especially frontal lobe involvement).

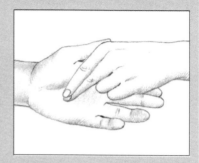

Snout reflex
Tap lightly on the patient's upper lip. Lip pursing, known as the snout reflex, indicates frontal lobe damage.

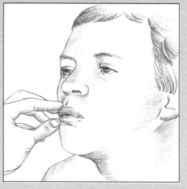

(continued)

may result from increased ICP or displacement of cranial contents by a mass.
• Spinal X-rays show the structure of a patient's vertebrae, the intervertebral disk spaces, the vertebral foramina, and the width of the spinal canal. They can aid the diagnosis of fractured vertebrae, herniated disks, bone spurs, spinal cord masses, and structural abnormalities, such as scoliosis and kyphosis.
• A computed tomography (CT) scan produces a computer image of the brain, showing the precise location and extent of intracranial abnormalities. Cranial contents, such as bone, blood vessels, and brain tissue, have different densities and absorb varying amounts of radiation during the scan.

Assessing primitive reflexes *(continued)*

Sucking reflex
Observe the patient while you are feeding him, suctioning him, or stimulating his mouth with a mouth swab. If he begins sucking, you've elicited the sucking reflex — an indication of cortical damage typically seen in patients with advanced dementia. This reflex can also be elicited by lightly stroking the patient's cheek (similar to the rooting reflex, which is normal in neonates).

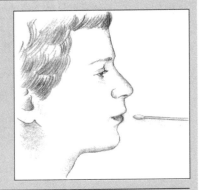

Glabellar reflex
Gently and repeatedly tap the patient's forehead in the midline, just above the bridge of his nose, with your index finger. Normally, this elicits rhythmic contraction of the eyelids, which disappears in a few seconds. Persistent closure of the eyes and blepharospasm in response to each stimulus may indicate Parkinson's or Alzheimer's disease, or frontal lobe infarction or tumors.

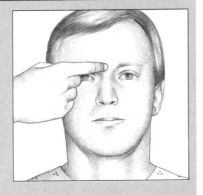

Contents of greatest density (bone) appear white, and those of lesser density (such as air) appear darker. The quality of the scan can be enhanced by injecting an iodine-based contrast dye.
• In lumbar puncture, a small amount of cerebrospinal fluid (CSF) is withdrawn and analyzed for the presence of white blood cells, glucose, protein, and electrolytes. The presence of red blood cells or bacteria may indicate an abnormality. The lumbar puncture is used to detect subarachnoid hemorrhage, infectious encephalopathy, demyelinating disorders (such as multiple sclerosis [MS]), Guillain-Barré syndrome, and tumors of the spinal cord or cerebrum. (See *Interpreting findings in CSF studies.*)

Interpreting findings in CSF studies

Normal findings	Abnormal findings	Possible causes of abnormal findings
Pressure: 60 to 180 mm H_2O	Above-normal level	Intracranial abscess or tumor, cerebral infarct, subarachnoid hemorrhage, acute bacterial meningitis
Color: clear, colorless	Cloudy (caused by increased leukocytes and proteins), xanthochromic (bloody)	Infection, such as meningitis; subarachnoid, intracerebral, or intraventricular hemorrhage; spinal cord obstruction; traumatic lumbar puncture (usually noted only in initial specimen)
Glucose: 50 to 80 mg/ dl (or two-thirds of blood glucose level)	Above-normal level	Systemic hyperglycemia (no neurologic significance)
	Below-normal level	Bacterial, tubercular, or fungal meningitis; some viral central nervous system (CNS) infections (herpes); meningeal neoplasm; meningeal sarcoidosis; postsubarachnoid hemorrhage; brain abscess
Protein: 15 to 45 mg/dl	Above-normal level	Peripheral neuropathy involving nerve roots, brain tumor, encapsulated brain abscess, bacterial meningitis, viral CNS infections, degenerative CNS diseases (multiple sclerosis, neurosyphilis), Guillain-Barré syndrome, subarachnoid hemorrhage, blood in cerebrospinal fluid (CSF) from traumatic lumbar puncture
	Below-normal level	Rapid CSF production
Gamma globulin: 3% to 12% of total protein	Above-normal level	Herpes encephalitis, Guillain-Barré syndrome, neurosyphilis
Red blood cells: None	Presence	Hemorrhage (subarachnoid, intracerebral), bleeding into ventricular system, CNS trauma, traumatic lumbar puncture
White blood cells: 0 to 5/mm^3	Increase (more than 10/mm^3)	Meningitis, CNS infections, infectious mononucleosis, subarachnoid hemorrhage, thrombosis

• In magnetic resonance imaging (MRI), a magnetic field is created around the patient. Radio frequency pulses are applied to the brain, causing groups of atomic nuclei within it to resonate. Energy signals resulting from this process are analyzed by a computer and copied onto film.

MRI offers several advantages over CT scanning. It doesn't expose the patient to radiation, and it offers better contrast images of soft tissues.

MRI can also differentiate between the brain's gray and white matter and is therefore better than the CT scan in diagnosing demyelinating disorders, tumors, vascular infarctions, arteriovenous malformations, and aneurysms.

• In positron emission tomography (PET) scanning, molecules in the brain are labeled with a radioisotope and followed by radiation-sensitive detectors in the scanner. The scanner follows the activity of the radioisotope within the patient's brain cells and provides information about protein synthesis and energy production within the brain. By identifying chemical tissue changes, such as the use of glucose by tumor cells, PET scans can help evaluate the effectiveness of antineoplastic drug therapy.

• The single-photon emission computed tomography (SPECT) scan uses a more readily available radioisotope than the PET scan. The SPECT scan can detect perfusion defects in CVA patients before there is CT evidence of infarction and during transient ischemic attacks. Like PET scans, the SPECT scan has proved effective in localizing seizure foci.

• Cerebral arteriography, although less precise and more invasive than CT or MRI scans, is still useful in diagnosing atherosclerosis of the extracranial vessels and in evaluating a patient scheduled for vascular surgery, such as endarterectomy.

Disadvantages of arteriography include anaphylactic reaction to the contrast dye, embolization of clots, and dislodgment of arterial plaque. Bleeding and localized spasm at the injection site (usually the femoral artery) can cause occlusion of arterial flow in the affected extremity.

• Doppler imaging, a noninvasive test, can accurately detect atheromatous plaque within the carotid arteries. The Doppler ultrasound probe is placed over the common carotid artery and moved to the bifurcation of the internal and external carotid arteries to determine lumen patency.

• Digital subtraction angiography uses computer imaging to enhance arteriographic images of extracranial blood vessels. Pictures of the vessels are taken before and after injection of contrast dye into the antecubital vein. The images taken without contrast dye are then "subtracted" from the images taken with contrast dye in the vessels.

• In an EEG, electrodes attached to the patient's scalp detect electrical impulses generated by the brain cells. Leadwires transmit these impulses to an EEG machine, which translates them into waveforms. Altered waveforms occur with seizures, hypoxia, hypothermia, hypoglycemia, hypotension, and toxic or metabolic encephalopathy.

• Evoked potential studies record the brain's responses to external visual, auditory, or somatic stimuli. These tests are used to detect brain stem lesions and to evaluate the extent of damage produced by demyelinating spinal cord lesions, as in MS.

Nursing diagnosis

The next step of the nursing process, nursing diagnosis, represents your professional judgment of the patient's clinical status, response to treatment, and nursing care needs. The nursing diagnosis reflects your assessment findings and your interpretation of the patient's ability to meet basic needs.

To formulate a nursing diagnosis, evaluate the essential information de-

rived from your neurologic assessment. Consider such questions as:
• What are the patient's signs and symptoms?
• Which assessment findings are abnormal for this patient?
• How do particular behaviors affect the patient's neurologic health?
• Does the patient understand his illness and its treatment?
• How does his environment affect his health?
• How does he respond to his health problem? Does he want to change his state of health?

Chapters 4 through 10 contain common nursing diagnoses for many neurologic disorders. Keep in mind, however, that diagnostic statements must be tailored to your patient's individual needs. Each patient responds to illness and stress differently, and your nursing diagnoses should never become so standardized that they fail to address individual differences and special needs.

For greater accuracy, you should write an etiology, or "related to" statement, for each nursing diagnosis. The etiology should identify conditions or circumstances that contribute to the development or continuation of that particular nursing diagnosis.

Developing individual nursing diagnoses for each patient can be difficult. You can make this task easier and save time by becoming familiar with the nursing diagnoses most frequently used in neurologic care.

Altered thought processes

This nursing diagnosis describes an inability to process thoughts correctly and accurately. Altered thought processes may be associated with numerous neurologic disorders, such as brain tumors, head trauma, and sensory deprivation from isolation, prolonged bed rest, or septicemia.

High risk for injury

This nursing diagnosis describes an accentuated risk of physical harm. In a neurologic patient, injury may be caused by sensory or motor deficits. Sensory deficits may include decreased or absent vision, hearing, or temperature perception. Motor deficits may include contractures, pain with movement, inflamed joints, muscle spasticity, paralysis, or paresis.

High risk for infection

This nursing diagnosis describes an accentuated risk of introducing pathogenic microorganisms into the body from either internal or external sources. Factors that increase this risk include immobility, the use of an indwelling urinary catheter or an I.V. catheter, the use of invasive monitoring devices, prophylactic antibiotic therapy, chemotherapy, hemodialysis, respiratory treatments, and corticosteroid therapy.

High risk for infection may be associated with numerous neurologic disorders, such as MS and spinal cord injury. It may also be associated with disorders that can have neurologic complications, such as acquired immunodeficiency syndrome.

Pain

This diagnosis describes a subjective sensation of discomfort caused by physical, chemical, biological, or psychological stimuli. The patient with this diagnosis may exhibit altered muscle tone (ranging from flaccid to rigid) and autonomic responses not seen in chronic stable pain, such as diaphoresis, blood pressure and pulse rate changes, dilated pupils, and increased or decreased respiratory rate. He may also moan, cry, or exhibit a pained expression characterized by lackluster eyes, a "beaten" look, or grimacing.

The patient's report of pain is the most important information when formulating this diagnosis. Ask the patient to describe the characteristics of pain, including its location, quality, intensity on a scale of 1 to 10, precipitating factors, and sources of relief.

Sensory or perceptual alterations

This diagnosis refers to a change in the characteristics of sensory stimuli. In your diagnosis, you must specify which of the senses are altered: visual, auditory, gustatory, olfactory, kinesthetic, or tactile.

A patient with this diagnosis may exhibit visual and auditory distortions, anxiety, exaggerated emotional responses, abnormal sensations, altered conceptualization, diminished motor coordination, altered taste sense, altered communication pattern, impaired hearing, and disorientation to time, place, or person.

Sensory or perceptual alterations can be associated with numerous neurologic disorders, such as CVAs, head injury, organic mental syndrome, dementia, Guillain-Barré syndrome, migraine headache, MS, peripheral neuropathy, polyneuropathy, seizure disorders, spinal cord lesions, and transient ischemic attacks.

Impaired physical mobility

This nursing diagnosis describes a limitation of physical movement brought on by neuromuscular impairment. Defining characteristics include:

• decreased muscle strength, control, mass, and endurance
• impaired coordination
• inability to move purposefully, which may affect transfer and ambulation
• limited ROM
• reluctance to attempt movement.

Impaired physical mobility may be associated with amyotrophic lateral sclerosis, cerebral palsy, CVA, MS, muscular dystrophy, myasthenia gravis, Parkinson's disease, and spinal cord injury.

Additional nursing diagnoses

Many additional diagnoses may be used to describe the neurologic patient's response to illness. (See *Identifying common nursing diagnoses in neurologic care.*)

Neurologic injury or disease often has far-reaching effects on the patient's cognitive abilities, affect, and personality. The compounded effects of numerous stresses and losses may strain the coping skills of the patient and family. Changes in a patient's behavior affect interpersonal relationships and family structure. Possible nursing diagnoses to describe the psychosocial effects of neurologic illness include *ineffective individual coping, ineffective family coping (disabling or compromised), anxiety, hopelessness, caregiver role strain, body image disturbance,* and *impaired adjustment.* Although these diagnoses aren't specific to neurologic illness, their importance shouldn't be underestimated.

Patient teaching is vital for the neurologic patient. For example, you may need to teach your patient about tests and procedures or encourage lifestyle changes. *Knowledge deficit* is the diagnosis used most frequently to document learning needs. Because this diagnosis is so broad, you should word the diagnostic statement carefully to ensure that the patient's specific needs are clearly communicated. For example, you might write in your plan of care *Knowledge deficit related to spinal cord injury teaching needs.*

Identifying common nursing diagnoses in neurologic care

Certain nursing diagnoses are used frequently to describe the response patterns of neurologic patients. This list identifies and defines these diagnoses.

Activity intolerance. Fatigue, weakness, or other symptoms brought on by performing a simple activity.
Altered cerebral tissue perfusion. Diminished cellular nutrition and oxygenation related to reduced capillary perfusion.
Altered thought processes. Inability to process thoughts accurately and correctly.
Anxiety. A vague, uneasy feeling arising from an unidentified source.
Body image disturbance. Disruption in self-perception that makes healthful functioning more difficult.
Caregiver role strain. A caregiver's perceived difficulty in providing care of a family member with significant home care needs.
Fear. Feeling of dread related to an identifiable source.
High risk for impaired skin integrity. Accentuated risk of interruption or destruction of skin surface.
High risk for infection. The state in which an individual is at increased risk for being invaded by pathogenic organisms.
High risk for injury. Accentuated risk of physical harm related to sensory or motor deficits.

Hopelessness. A subjective state in which an individual sees few or no available alternatives or personal choices and can't mobilize energy on his own behalf.
Impaired adjustment. Inability to modify lifestyle or behavior consistent with changed health status.
Impaired physical mobility. Limitation of physical movement due to perceptual or cognitive impairment.
Impaired swallowing. Inability to move food, fluid, or saliva from the mouth to the stomach.
Impaired verbal communication. Decreased ability to speak, understand, or use words appropriately.
Ineffective individual coping. Inability to use adaptive behaviors in response to difficult life situations.
Knowledge deficit. An inadequate understanding of information or inability to perform skills needed to practice health-related behaviors.
Pain. Subjective sensation of discomfort generated by physical, chemical, biological, or psychological stimuli.
Sensory or perceptual alterations. Change in the individual's perception of visual, auditory, kinesthetic, tactile, or olfactory stimuli.

Planning

In this next step of the nursing process, you'll create a written plan of care designed to help you deliver quality patient care. The plan of care includes relevant nursing diagnoses, patient outcomes, nursing interventions, and evaluation data and becomes a permanent part of the patient's health record.

When writing your plan, you must assign priorities to nursing diagnoses. Many patients with neurologic disorders have multiple problems requiring multiple nursing diagnoses. High-priority nursing diagnoses involve the patient's most urgent needs (such as emergency, or immediate, physical needs). Intermediate-priority diagnoses involve nonemergency needs, and low-priority diagnoses involve needs that don't directly relate to the patient's illness or prognosis. When establishing priorities, consider how the patient perceives his health problem. (See *Setting priorities among nursing diagnoses*.)

Establishing patient outcomes

Next, you'll need to establish patient outcomes — measurable goals derived from nursing diagnoses that describe behaviors or results to be achieved within a specified time. A patient outcome may specify an improvement in ability to function — for example, an increase in the ability to perform activities of daily living (ADLs) with assistive devices following a spinal injury. Or it may specify an amelioration of a problem — for example, decreased pain for a patient with migraine headache. Each outcome statement should call for a realistic, achievable outcome. For example, suppose the outcome for a newly admitted patient with CVA is: *Patient will ambulate without assistance*. That goal is not realistic until several preliminary outcomes are achieved, such as *Patient maintains active joint range of motion*.

An outcome statement should describe the specific behavior that will show the patient has reached his goal, include criteria for measuring the behavior, state conditions under which the behavior should occur, and include the target date or time by which the behavior should occur. Because patient outcomes are the criteria you'll use to evaluate care, you must express them clearly.

For example, if your patient's nursing diagnosis is *Sensory or perceptual alterations related to sensory overload*, appropriate outcome statements might include:
• Patient becomes oriented to time, place, and person within 2 days (2/20).
• Patient communicates in a lucid manner by 2/22.
• Patient verbalizes when sensory stimuli are excessive by 2/24.
• Patient voices decreased anxiety and irritability by 2/26.
• Patient describes measures to avoid excessive stimuli by 2/27.

Developing interventions

After establishing patient outcomes, you'll develop interventions designed to help the patient achieve these outcomes. Consider such factors as your patient's age, developmental and educational levels, environment, and cultural values. The more you know about the patient, the easier it will be to formulate appropriate interventions. For example, an appropriate intervention for an 80-year-old CVA patient would be to assist him in performing ADLs in a safe, supervised environment by:

Setting priorities among nursing diagnoses

For many patients, your assessment will reveal multiple problems that must be addressed. When planning care for these patients, you'll need to identify all of the problems, establish appropriate nursing diagnoses, and rank them from highest to lowest priority. To understand how to set these priorities, consider the case history of Ruben Collins, a 73-year-old retired carpenter.

Subjective data

Mr. Collins was admitted to the hospital with the complaint that his right arm felt "heavy and clumsy." He tells you that, unlike previous episodes, this sensation hasn't gone away.

Mr. Collins says, "I have spells when I can hardly move my right hand or arm. It feels numb and tingling, like it's asleep. When I try to tell my wife what's happening, I can't seem to find the right words, or else they get jumbled and won't come out right."

He reports that the spells started about 8 months ago. They begin suddenly, last 10 to 20 minutes, and resolve spontaneously. According to Mr. Collins, the spells initially occurred about once a month. During the last 2 weeks, though, he's had at least one every other day.

Mr. Collins continues, telling you that he's had high blood pressure for 40 years. He had been taking an antihypertensive drug but stopped taking it last year because he was "feeling good and not having any headaches." He adds that his father died of a stroke at age 82.

Objective data

Your examination of Mr. Collins reveals the following:
• temperature, 98.8° F (37.1° C); pulse rate, 78 beats/minute and regular; respiratory rate, 22 breaths/minute, even, and unlabored; blood pressure, 182/96 mm Hg
• awake, alert, oriented to person, place, and time; remote and recent memory intact; speech slightly slurred but intelligible; occasionally seems to have trouble finding words
• pupils round, equal, and reactive to light
• right-handed; moves all extremities on command without difficulty; arms and legs strong; right grasp slightly weaker than left; mild paresis indicated by downward drift of right arm when extended with eyes closed; gait slow and steady, unassisted
• light touch, pain, and temperature sensation absent in right hand and forearm, but intact in left arm and both legs.

Identifying problems and establishing priorities

Results of the patient history and physical examination suggest that Mr. Collins has cerebral ischemia. Transient neurologic deficits, caused by transient ischemic attacks (TIAs), are the classic warning signs of an impending cerebrovascular accident. His failure to report his "spells" sooner probably reflects a knowledge deficit but may indicate that he's using denial to cope. His reason for stop-

(continued)

Setting priorities among nursing diagnoses *(continued)*

ping antihypertensive medication suggests a lack of knowledge about hypertension and its treatment.

Thus, your care must first be directed toward educating the patient about the importance of taking his medication and about the warning signs of TIAs. You select *Knowledge deficit related to warning signs of TIAs and importance of adhering to antihypertensive regimen* as the chief nursing diagnosis.

Your next concern is to address Mr. Collins's loss of tactile sensation in his right arm. The change in his sense of touch may cause skin breakdown and lead to accidental injury. You select *Sensory or perceptual alterations (tactile) related to right arm paresthesia* as your second-priority nursing diagnosis.

You're also concerned about Mr. Collins's decreased muscle strength, control, mass, and endurance in his right arm and the possibility that he may not be able to move himself away from danger. You select *Impaired physical mobility related to right arm weakness and clumsiness* as your third-priority nursing diagnosis.

Other suggested nursing diagnoses for Mr. Collins include:
• self-care deficit related to right arm paresis and sensory loss, especially because patient is right-handed
• impaired verbal communication related to difficulty in finding words and slurred speech.

Once you have prioritized your nursing diagnoses, you can proceed to develop appropriate goals, interventions, and evaluation criteria.

• keeping the bed in a low position with side rails up at all times
• assisting the patient with bathing, eating, and other potentially problematic activities.

When documenting interventions, state the necessary action clearly. Many interventions must be continued, and possibly evaluated and modified, by other nurses when you're not present. If family members are participating in your patient's care, they will need to understand the interventions as well. Write your interventions in precise detail. Include how and when to perform the interventions as well as any special instructions.

Implementation

During this fourth step of the nursing process, you put your plan of care into action. Your activities are directed toward resolving the patient's diagnoses and meeting health care needs. You must collaborate with other caregivers, the patient, and the patient's family.

Treatment for the patient with a neurologic disorder is becoming increasingly sophisticated. For example, implanted cerebellar stimulators are used to regulate uncoordinated neuromuscular activity in patients with a seizure disorder and to provide better neuromuscular control in patients with cerebral palsy. Life-threatening disorders may call for emergency surgery, possibly involving a craniotomy. Other complex neurologic treatments include cerebral aneurysm repair, ICP monitoring, and ventricular shunting.

The following is a brief review of nursing interventions you may implement in neurologic care.

Therapeutic interventions

These interventions aim to alleviate the effects of illness or restore optimal function. A common therapy is administration of drugs, such as anticonvulsants (to help control seizures), beta-adrenergic blockers (to prevent migraine headache), or diuretics (to help lower ICP). Other common therapies include maintaining CSF drains, performing comfort measures (such as giving a back massage), checking for the gag reflex before offering small oral feedings of semisolid foods, and performing ROM exercises.

Emergency care

Emergency care may include tending to a patient with increasing ICP who needs surgery (to alleviate the pressure) or a patient with an evolving CVA or thrombus who needs rapid intervention (to decrease the number of residual effects). Patients with head trauma may require rapid resuscitation measures to prevent increased ICP.

Monitoring

Periodic or continuous evaluation of your patient's ICP, neurologic status, and response to therapy is just as important as the initial assessment. ICP can fluctuate, depending on the patient's condition and response to ther-

apy. For further information on ICP monitoring, see Chapter 3, Monitoring neurologic status.

Monitor the patient's vital signs, skin color and temperature, motor and sensory functions, and psychological and emotional status. Also monitor reflexes, intake and output, and laboratory tests, such as serum electrolyte and CSF measurements.

Patient teaching

Teaching may help the neurologic patient live with his disorder and prevent complications resulting from lack of knowledge. Many of your lessons will focus on instructing the patient and family members on how to manage the disorder.

For example, the patient with a seizure disorder may need information on how to manage seizures and how to avoid them, such as diet, medication, stress control, and maintaining a balance between activity and rest. Teaching is particularly important upon the neurologic patient's discharge from the hospital because of the risk of complications and possible complex at-home care requirements.

Timesaving tip: To avoid repeating the same teaching session, plan to teach the patient when family members are present.

Preoperative care

Preoperative nursing measures may include enforcing food and fluid restrictions, washing the patient's hair with an antimicrobial shampoo the night before a craniotomy, administering preoperative corticosteroids to reduce postoperative inflammation, using sequential compression sleeves to improve venous return and reduce the risk of thrombophlebitis, inserting a urinary catheter, establishing an I.V. line, establishing baseline vital signs, and providing sedation. You may also perform and document a complete neurologic assessment to establish a baseline for postoperative evaluation.

Prepare the patient for surgery by teaching him about preoperative and postoperative procedures. For example, arrange a preoperative visit to the intensive care unit (ICU) for the patient and his family to introduce them to staff members and to explain the equipment.

Postoperative care

Postoperative interventions include monitoring the patient's vital signs and neurologic status. Throughout the postoperative period, observe the patient closely for signs of increased ICP and monitor respiratory status, electrolyte and fluid status, intake and output, and weight. Also monitor the patient for declining mental status, pupillary changes, or focal signs, such as increasing weakness in an extremity. Other possible interventions include encouraging deep breathing and coughing, suctioning, changing dressings, checking the patency of postoperative drainage devices (such as Jackson-Pratt drains), administering medications, and monitoring the patient for signs of wound infection.

Counseling and emotional support

You may plan and implement interventions to enhance your patient's emotional well-being. The patient with a neurologic disorder, especially, needs a trusting, open relationship with family members and health care providers. You can be a source of reassurance and calm for the patient and his family, and help relieve their anxiety. For patients with severe emotional problems or adjustment disorders, you may need to provide a referral for psychological counseling.

Preparation for discharge

For many discharged patients with neurologic disorders, dealing with necessary lifestyle changes or limitations on activity is difficult. By preparing the patient for discharge, you can help to make this transition smooth and ensure continued quality of care.

Discharge planning may include:
• instructing the patient to notify the doctor of any signs or symptoms that may signal complications or a deteriorating condition
• reminding him when to return for follow-up appointments
• providing necessary referrals, such as for a home health care agency
• making sure the patient understands the dosage and possible adverse effects of all prescribed drugs
• teaching family members first aid for seizures
• explaining wound care to a patient who has had surgery and instructing him to report to the doctor any redness, warmth, or tenderness at the surgical site.

Evaluation

In this final stage of the nursing process, you'll judge the effectiveness of your plan of care and gauge your patient's progress in meeting expected outcomes. Evaluate the patient by answering the following questions:
• How has he progressed in terms of the plan's projected outcomes?
• Does he have any new needs or problems?
• How did he respond to care, including medications, changes in diet or activity, procedures, and patient teaching?
• Did he achieve the goals outlined in the plan of care?

To ensure a successful evaluation, keep an open mind. Never hesitate to consider new patient data or to revise previous judgments. After all, no plan of care is perfect. In fact, you should anticipate revising the plan of care during the course of treatment.

Reassessment

You'll need to reassess the patient continually while he's under your care. Collect information from all available sources — for example, from the patient, his family, his medical record, and other caregivers. Also include your own observations of the patient and his condition. Next, compare reassessment data with criteria established in the patient outcomes documented in your plan of care. For example, a CVA patient with the nursing diagnosis *High risk for injury related to sensory or motor deficits* might have the following patient outcomes:
• Patient identifies factors that increase potential for injury.
• Patient identifies and implements safety measures to prevent injury.

During your reassessment of this patient, you'd ask him to describe factors that increase his risk of injury and ask him and his family members to describe safety measures to prevent falls. When evaluating your findings, try to determine if the patient's overall condition is improving or deteriorating.

Assess whether the patient has achieved all the expected outcomes by the projected dates. If many problems remain unresolved, determine the factors that are interfering with goal achievement. Consider all possible reasons that a patient may not be able to achieve a desired outcome, such as the following:
• The purpose and goals of the plan of care aren't clear.

• The expected outcomes aren't realistic in light of the patient's condition.
• The plan of care is based on incomplete assessment data.
• Nursing diagnoses are inaccurate.
• The nursing staff experienced conflict with the patient or other members of the health care team.
• Staff members didn't follow the plan of care.
• The patient failed to carry out activities outlined in the plan of care.
• The patient's condition changed.

Reviewing implementation

When trying to determine factors interfering with goal achievement, take a close look at the documented interventions and the manner in which they were implemented.

For example, suppose a patient with the nursing diagnosis *Reflex incontinence related to sensory or neuromuscular impairment* fails to achieve one of his planned outcomes — urinary continence — by the third week of hospitalization. To find out why, consider such questions as:
• Were the patient's elimination patterns accurately monitored?
• Was the patient's reflex arc stimulated to control voiding?
• Was a sufficient fluid volume administered to stimulate the micturition reflex?
• Were the patient's wet clothes changed to prevent him from becoming accustomed to them?

Answering these questions will help you determine why the patient outcome wasn't achieved.

Writing evaluation statements

Evaluation statements provide a method of documenting the patient's response to care. These statements indicate whether expected outcomes were achieved and list the evidence supporting your conclusions. The importance of clearly written evaluation statements cannot be overemphasized: Documentation of patient outcomes is necessary to support the rationales for nursing care and to justify the use of nursing resources. Record your evaluation statements in your progress notes or on the revised plan of care, according to your hospital's documentation policy.

When writing an evaluation statement, describe the patient's progress using active verbs, such as "walk," "demonstrate," or "express." Include criteria used to measure the patient's response to care, and describe the conditions under which the response occurred. Write a separate evaluation for each patient response or behavior that you wish to describe, and date the statement.

Examples of evaluation statements used in neurologic care include:
• Patient clears airway using assisted coughing techniques.
• He states at least two ways to cope with anxiety.
• He takes an active role in planning aspects of care.
• He expresses emotions associated with change in body image.
• He experiences no complications of dysreflexia, as evidenced by an absence of contractures, venous stasis, thrombus formation, skin breakdown, or hypostatic pneumonia.
• His temperature remains within normal limits.
• He experiences no injury to the affected body part.

Modifying the plan of care
During evaluation, you may discover that the plan of care needs to be modified. If patient outcomes have been achieved, be sure to record this information. Revise other patient outcome statements as necessary. Determine which nursing interventions need to be revised or discontinued. Assess whether changes are needed in priorities assigned to nursing diagnoses. You may need to document that a nursing diagnosis has been resolved, or you may find that a nursing diagnosis no longer accurately describes the patient's status.

Like all steps of the nursing process, evaluation is ongoing. Continue to assess, diagnose, plan, implement, and evaluate for as long as you provide care.

CHAPTER 2

Exploring chief complaints

In neurologic disorders, the most common chief complaints include headache, neck pain, back pain, vision loss, sensory disturbances, weakness, dizziness, memory loss, decreased level of consciousness, and confusion. By fully investigating your patient's chief complaint and associated signs and symptoms, you can form a diagnostic impression of his problem to guide your subsequent care.

Headache

The single most common neurologic complaint, headache can stem from many causes. Most headaches are benign and result from muscle contraction (tension headaches), vascular events (migraine headaches), or a combination of the two. (See *Causes of headache.*) Often, performing a thorough history and physical examination can determine the most likely source of the patient's headache.

History of the symptom
To better characterize your patient's headache, consider asking the following questions:
• When did you first experience your headaches?
• What part of your head hurts the most?
• How would you describe the pain? Is it throbbing, dull, stabbing, or squeezing?
• Does any particular activity intensify or relieve your headache?
• Are you taking any prescription or over-the-counter drugs either to relieve headaches or to treat another condition?
• How often do your headaches occur? How long do they last?

• Has the headache pain been worse lately?
• Do any warning symptoms occur before the onset of a headache? (Prodromal symptoms typically consist of visual abnormalities and occasionally transient hemiparesis.)
• Do you experience nausea or vomiting simultaneous to headache? (Migraine headaches commonly cause these problems.)
• Have you recently experienced a head injury?
• Does anyone in your family have a history of headaches?

Associated findings
Note whether the patient has experienced any of the following signs or symptoms:
• confusion
• fever
• head cold, with pain localized in the sinus areas
• nausea (common with migraine headaches)
• neck stiffness (with fever, suggests infection; without fever, suggests muscle contraction)
• numbness or tingling in the extremities or vision changes (can indicate subarachnoid hemorrhage)
• photophobia (common with migraine headaches)
• recent increase in stress (commonly precipitates migraine and tension headaches).

Previous conditions and treatments
Consult with the patient, family members, or members of the health care team to determine the patient's health history.

Timesaving tip: Have family members, the patient's chart, and previous medical records (if possible) present when collecting his-

Causes of headache

Numerous neurologic disorders may cause headache. These include brain abscess or tumor, ruptured cerebral aneurysm, encephalitis, meningitis, postconcussional syndrome, subdural hematoma, and epidural, intracerebral, and subarachnoid hemorrhage.

Brain abscess
Headache is localized to the abscess site. Usually, it intensifies over a few days. Nausea, vomiting, and focal or generalized seizures may accompany the headache. The patient's level of consciousness (LOC) will vary from drowsiness to deep stupor.

Brain tumor
Initially, this disorder causes a localized headache near the tumor site. The headache eventually becomes generalized as the tumor grows. Usually, it's intermittent, deep-seated and dull, and most intense in the morning. It's aggravated by coughing, stooping, Valsalva's maneuver, and changes in head position; it's relieved by sitting and rest. Associated signs and symptoms may include personality changes, altered LOC, motor and sensory dysfunction, and eventual signs of increased intracranial pressure (ICP), such as vomiting, increased systolic blood pressure, and widened pulse pressure.

Ruptured cerebral aneurysm
Sudden, excruciating headache characterizes this life-threatening disorder. The headache may be unilateral and usually peaks within minutes of aneurysmal rupture. The patient may lose consciousness immediately or display an altered LOC. Depending on the severity and location of the bleeding, he may also have nausea and vomiting, signs of meningeal irritation, and hemiparesis.

Encephalitis
A severe, generalized headache is characteristic of this disorder. Typically, the patient's LOC deteriorates within 48 hours from lethargy to coma. Associated signs and symptoms include fever, nuchal rigidity, irritability, seizures, nausea, vomiting, photophobia, hemiparesis, and cranial nerve palsies (such as ptosis).

Meningitis
Sudden onset of a severe, constant, generalized headache that worsens with movement is common in this disorder. Associated signs include nuchal rigidity, positive Kernig's and Brudzinski's signs, hyperreflexia, photophobia, and possibly opisthotonos. Fever occurs early in meningitis and may be accompanied by chills. As ICP increases, vomiting and, occasionally, papilledema develop. Other features may include altered LOC, seizures, ocular palsies, facial weakness, and hearing loss.

Postconcussional syndrome
One to thirty days after concussion, a generalized or localized headache may develop and last for 2 to 3 weeks. The patient may report an aching, pounding, pressing, stabbing,

(continued)

Causes of headache *(continued)*

or throbbing pain. The patient's neurologic examination will be normal, but he may have giddiness or dizziness, blurred vision, fatigue, insomnia, inability to concentrate, and noise and alcohol intolerance.

Subdural hematoma
Both acute and chronic subdural hematomas may cause headache and decreased LOC. In acute subdural hematoma, the patient may experience headache, drowsiness, confusion, agitation and, eventually, coma. In chronic hematoma, he may experience a dull pounding headache over the hematoma, fluctuating in severity.

Acute epidural hemorrhage
Usually preceded by head trauma, acute epidural hemorrhage causes a progressively severe headache accompanied by nausea, vomiting, bladder distention, confusion, and a rapid decrease in LOC. Because loss of consciousness is so fast, the patient may not have time to complain of the headache.

Intracerebral hemorrhage
This disorder may cause a severe generalized headache. Clinical features vary with the hemorrhage's size and location. A large hemorrhage may produce a rapid, steady decrease in LOC, possibly resulting in coma. Other common findings may include hemiparesis, abnormal pupil size and response, aphasia, dizziness, nausea, vomiting, seizures, decreased sensations, irregular respirations, positive Babinski's reflex, decorticate or decerebrate posture, and increased blood pressure.

Subarachnoid hemorrhage
Commonly, this type of hemorrhage produces a sudden, violent headache. Related signs and symptoms include nuchal rigidity, altered LOC that may rapidly progress to coma, nausea, vomiting, seizures, dizziness, and ipsilateral pupil dilation. The patient will also have positive Kernig's and Brudzinski's signs, photophobia, blurred vision, and possibly fever. Hemiparesis, hemiplegia, sensory or vision disturbances, and aphasia may also occur. Signs of elevated ICP, such as bradycardia and increased blood pressure, may also occur.

Nonneurologic causes
Headache may occur secondary to a variety of nonneurologic causes, such as glaucoma, hypertension, influenza, infection, temporal arteritis, typhoid fever. Headache may also occur following use of vasodilators, such as caffeine, ergotamine, or sympathomimetic drugs.

tory information from the patient. You can confirm facts and fill in gaps without having to conduct multiple interviews and record searches.

Ask if the patient has a history of any of the following risk factors:
• acquired immunodeficiency syndrome (can cause central nervous system [CNS] infection)

- bruxism (grinding teeth during sleep)
- cancer
- depression
- ear or upper respiratory infections or sinus problems
- hypertension
- muscle weakness of the arms or legs (suggests cerebrovascular accident)
- personality changes (with increasing headaches, may suggest CNS tumor)
- recent change in medications
- recent dental work
- seizure disorder or head trauma
- substance abuse.

Drug therapy
Note any past or current use of the following drugs:
- alcohol
- caffeine (recent stoppage commonly causes a headache that lasts 3 to 4 days)
- calcium channel blockers, such as nifedipine
- indomethacin
- nitrates
- oral contraceptives (may cause migraine headaches)
- theophylline.

Physical examination
Examine the patient according to the steps described below.

Vital signs
- Note if the patient has a fever, a common cause of headache.
- Observe the character of the patient's respirations.
- Assess the patient's blood pressure. Severe hypertension can cause early morning occipital headaches.

Inspection
- If the patient has a history of head trauma, examine his head for evidence of bruising, bleeding, swelling, or obvious bone abnormalities. Check for neck stiffness, otorrhea, rhinorrhea, raccoon eyes, or Battle's sign.
- Assess the patient's level of consciousness, and check his pupils for equality, size, and reaction to light. Note photophobia, if present. If possible, use an ophthalmoscope to check for retinal abnormalities or swelling of the optic nerve (papilledema).
- Observe for symmetrical muscle movement.
- If the patient is alert, check for cranial nerve involvement by having him raise his eyebrows and smile (tests cranial nerve VII) and clench his teeth (tests cranial nerve V).
- If the patient complains of acute, severe headache, it may indicate a serious problem, such as meningitis. If you suspect meningeal irritation, test for *Kernig's sign*. With the patient on his back, flex one leg at the hip and knee. Then attempt to straighten the leg (with the hip still flexed). If meningeal irritation is present, the patient will feel pain in his spine or head.

You can also test for *Brudzinski's sign*. With the patient on his back, attempt to flex his head so that his chin touches his chest. If meningeal irritation is present, the patient will respond by flexing his hip and knee (to counteract the increased traction on the meninges caused by this maneuver).

Palpation
- Palpate the posterior skull at the base for tenderness (common in tension headaches) and over the temples and jaw hinges (tenderness here may indicate temporomandibular joint disorder).

• Palpate over the maxillary and frontal sinuses for the discomfort associated with sinus headaches.

Neck pain

This symptom can result from numerous conditions affecting the meninges, the cervical vertebrae, and the neck's blood vessels, muscles, and lymphatic tissues. The pain's location, onset, and pattern help determine its origin and underlying causes. (See *Causes of neck pain.*)

If your patient reports neck pain, take a health history and perform a physical examination according to the guidelines below.

History of the symptom
To better characterize your patient's neck pain, consider asking the following questions:
• Did the neck pain occur suddenly or gradually? If it occurred suddenly, find out if the patient suffered a traumatic injury, and consider immobilizing the neck to prevent spinal cord injury. Also, try to get an accurate description of the trauma from the patient or witnesses.
• If trauma occurred, has there been limb paralysis, numbness, tingling, or bladder or bowel incontinence?
• If the neck pain developed gradually, when did it first occur?
• Is the pain constant or intermittent?
• Is it in the front or back of his neck?
• Does the patient have any sensory disturbances in his arms?
• Does he have any weakness in his arms or hands?
• Is his neck stiff?
• Does he have a fever?
• Has he recently started an activity that keeps his head in a fixed position, such as typing?

• What aggravates the pain and what alleviates it?

Associated findings
Note whether or not the patient has experienced any of the following signs or symptoms:
• ear pain (a common complaint with disorders of the temporomandibular joint, which also can cause neck pain)
• enlarged lymph nodes in the neck
• headache
• increased stress
• meningeal signs (such as neck stiffness with fever or headache)
• sensory or motor deficits of the upper extremities.

Previous conditions
Consult with the patient, family members, or members of the health care team to determine if the patient has a history of any of the following risk factors:
• cancer
• degenerative or rheumatoid arthritis
• history of alcohol abuse
• history of cervical injury or infection
• motor vehicle accident (may cause whiplash)
• osteoporosis.

Drug therapy
Neck pain may occur as an adverse effect of certain drugs. Note any past or current use of nonsteroidal anti-inflammatory drugs or prednisone (which may cause osteoporosis).

Physical examination
After obtaining vital signs, examine the patient according to the steps described below. Remember that acute trauma may require immobilization of the neck, making it impossible to perform a complete examination.

Causes of neck pain

Neurologic disorders linked to neck pain include cervical extension injury; cervical spine fracture, infection, or tumor; herniated cervical disk; meningitis; spinous process fracture; and subarachnoid hemorrhage.

Cervical extension injury
Anterior or posterior neck pain may develop within hours or days of whiplash. Anterior pain usually diminishes within several days, but posterior pain persists and may intensify. Associated findings include tenderness, swelling and nuchal rigidity, occipital headache, muscle spasms, visual blurring, and unilateral miosis.

Cervical spine fracture, infection, or tumor
Fracture at the C-1 to C-4 levels often results in sudden death. Survivors may experience severe neck pain that restricts all movement, intense occipital headache, quadriplegia, and respiratory paralysis.

Infection can cause fever, muscle spasms, local tenderness, dysphagia, paresthesia, muscle weakness, and moderate neck pain that restricts movement.

Metastatic tumors typically produce persistent neck pain that increases with movement and isn't relieved by rest. Primary tumors cause mild to severe pain along a specific nerve root. Other findings depend on the site of the lesions and may include paresthesia, arm and leg weakness that progresses to atrophy and paralysis, and bladder and bowel incontinence.

Herniated cervical disk
This disorder may cause variable neck pain that restricts and is aggravated by movement. It also causes referred pain, paresthesia and other sensory disturbances, and arm weakness.

Meningitis
Neck pain may accompany characteristic nuchal rigidity. Related findings include fever, headache, photophobia, positive Brudzinski's and Kernig's signs, and decreased level of consciousness (LOC).

Spinous process fracture
Fracture near the cervicothoracic junction produces acute pain radiating to the shoulders. Associated findings include swelling, extreme tenderness, restricted range of motion, muscle spasms, and deformity.

Subarachnoid hemorrhage
This life-threatening condition may cause moderate to severe neck pain and rigidity, headache, and a decreased LOC. Kernig's and Brudzinski's signs may be present.

Nonneurologic causes
Other causes of neck pain include ankylosing spondylitis, cervical fibrositis, cervical spondylosis, cervical stenosis, esophageal trauma, Hodgkin's lymphoma, laryngeal cancer, lymphadenitis, neck sprain, osteoporosis, Paget's disease, rheumatoid arthritis, and thyroid and tracheal trauma.

Inspection
• Check for obvious evidence of trauma, such as lacerations, swelling, or bruising.
• Observe the patient's head movement to assess for range of motion (ROM). If acute neck trauma has been ruled out, have the patient rotate his head from side to side. Next, have him flex his neck so that he touches his chin to his chest and then have him extend his neck by looking directly up at the ceiling. (Elderly patients may have limited neck flexion and extension.) Finally, have the patient bend his head toward each shoulder. From this, determine if neck ROM is normal or restricted.
• Assess for torticollis (deviation of the head toward one shoulder).
• Observe for evidence of limb paralysis.
• Assess for bladder or bowel incontinence, which may suggest spinal cord trauma.
• Assess for any sensory changes — for example, loss of certain types of sensation or increased sensitivity.

Palpation
• Palpate the neck muscles, particularly the posterior ones, where muscle discomfort frequently occurs. Assess for enlarged lymph nodes.
• Check hand and arm strength if paresthesia is present.

Percussion
• If the patient complains of paresthesia of the upper extremities along with neck pain, check the tendon reflexes at the biceps, triceps, and brachioradialis muscles. If paresthesia affects only one arm, compare the findings in both arms.

Back pain

Back pain affects an estimated 80% of the population; in fact, next to the common cold, it's the most frequent cause of time lost from work. While back pain can reflect disorders unrelated to the spine and its associated structures, its most common cause is strain of the paravertebral muscles and ligaments. (See *Causes of back pain.*)

History of the symptom
To better characterize your patient's back pain, consider asking the following questions:
• Where does your back hurt? Can you point to the location?
• Did the pain just start, or has it been occurring for a long time? Is the pain constant or intermittent?
• When did the pain first begin?
• Is the pain made worse by activity or other factors? Is it relieved by rest? (Muscle strain is usually aggravated by activity and relieved by rest.)
• Do you have any pain in your legs? If so, is it a dull ache, or does it tingle or burn? Does it seem to shoot down the legs? This symptom often indicates sciatica.

Timesaving tip: Ask the patient to describe his pain rather than asking him numerous yes-or-no questions. Only if the pain description is incomplete will further (and probably fewer) questions be necessary.
• Can you find a position that relieves the pain?
• How severe is the pain? (Use a scale of 1 to 10.)
• Have you taken medication to relieve the pain? If so, what was it, and did it help?

Causes of back pain

Neurologic causes of back pain include chordoma, herniated intervertebral disk, lumbosacral sprain, metastatic tumors, myeloma, sacroiliac strain, spinal neoplasm, spinal stenosis, spondylolisthesis, transverse process fracture, vertebral compression fracture, vertebral osteomyelitis, and vertebral osteoporosis.

Chordoma
A slow-developing malignant tumor, chordoma causes persistent pain in the lower back, sacrum, and coccyx. As the tumor expands, pain may be accompanied by constipation and bowel and bladder incontinence.

Herniated intervertebral disk
This disorder produces gradual or sudden lower back pain with or without leg pain (sciatica). Rarely, it produces leg pain alone. More often, pain begins in the back and radiates to the buttocks and leg. The pain is exacerbated by activity, coughing, and sneezing and is eased by rest. It's accompanied by paresthesia (most commonly, numbness or tingling in the lower leg and foot), muscle spasm, and decreased reflexes on the affected side.

This disorder also affects posture and gait. The patient's spine is slightly flexed and he leans toward the painful side. He walks slowly and rises from a sitting to standing position with extreme difficulty.

Lumbosacral sprain
This disorder causes aching, localized pain and tenderness associated with muscle spasm on lateral motion. The recumbent patient will typically flex his knees and hips to help ease pain. Flexion of the spine intensifies pain, whereas rest helps relieve it.

Metastatic tumors
These tumors commonly spread to the spine, causing lower back pain in at least 25% of patients. Typically, the pain begins abruptly, is accompanied by cramping muscular pain, and isn't relieved by rest.

Myeloma
Back pain caused by this primary malignant tumor frequently begins abruptly and worsens with physical activity. It may be accompanied by arthritic symptoms, such as achiness, joint swelling, and tenderness. Other clinical effects include fever, malaise, peripheral paresthesia, and weight loss.

Sacroiliac strain
This disorder causes sacroiliac pain that may radiate to the buttock, hip, and lateral aspect of the thigh. The pain is aggravated by weight bearing on the affected extremity and by abduction with resistance of the leg. Associated signs and symptoms include tenderness of the symphysis pubis and a limp.

(continued)

Causes of back pain *(continued)*

Spinal neoplasm (benign)
Typically, this disorder causes severe, localized back pain and scoliosis.

...bral

...n. ...pain may progress to numbness or weakness unless the patient rests for relief.

Spondylolisthesis
A major structural disorder characterized by forward slippage of one vertebra onto another, spondylolisthesis may cause no symptoms or cause lower back pain with or without nerve root involvement. Associated symptoms of nerve root involvement include paresthesia, buttock pain, and pain radiating down the leg. Flexion of the spine may be limited.

Transverse process fracture
This fracture causes severe localized back pain with muscle spasm and hematoma.

Vertebral compression fracture
Initially, this fracture may be painless. Several weeks later, it causes back pain aggravated by weight bearing and local tenderness. Fracture of a thoracic vertebra may cause referred pain in the lumbar area.

Vertebral osteomyelitis
Initially, this disorder causes intermittent back pain. As it progresses, the pain may become constant, more pronounced at night, and aggravated by spinal movement. Accompanying signs and symptoms include vertebral and hamstring spasms, tenderness of the spinous processes, fever, and malaise.

Vertebral osteoporosis
This disorder causes chronic, aching back pain that is aggravated by activity and somewhat relieved by rest. Tenderness may also occur.

Nonneurologic causes
Back pain may also be caused by abdominal aortic aneurysm (dissecting), ankylosing spondylitis, appendicitis, cholecystitis, endometriosis, pancreatitis (acute), perforated ulcer, prostatic carcinoma, pyelonephritis (acute), Reiter's syndrome, renal calculi, and neurologic tests, such as lumbar puncture and myelography.

• Have you experienced any trauma to your back?
• Have you had a fever?
• Have you had uncomfortable or frequent urination?

• Have you had problems with constipation?
• Have you had abdominal, pelvic, or back surgery?

- Do your legs feel weak? Do they ever "give out" on you?
- Also, ask the female patient if she has back pain related to her menstrual cycle.

Associated findings

Note whether the patient has experienced any of the following signs or symptoms:
- abdominal pain (can cause referred pain to the lower back)
- bladder or bowel incontinence (suggests a cauda equina syndrome, caused by pressure on the nerves at the base of the spinal cord)
- gait disturbance (could reflect sciatica)
- leg weakness (could indicate worsening sciatica or spinal cord compression)
- sensory disturbances in the legs (also reflects sciatica or other types of nerve compression).

Previous conditions and treatments

Consult with the patient, family members, or members of the health care team to determine if the patient has a history of any of the following risk factors:
- arthritis (can cause compression of spinal cord or nerve roots)
- back trauma (can frequently cause muscle spasm, ligament tears, or disk prolapse)
- chiropractic treatment for back pain
- endometriosis (can cause back pain that varies with the menstrual cycle)
- history of cancer (especially colon or pelvic)
- obesity (can pull the lumbar spine forward, straining muscles and ligaments)
- osteoporosis (can weaken vertebrae)

- Paget's disease (can weaken vertebrae)
- pancreatitis (can refer pain to the middle of the back)
- peptic ulcer disease (can cause referred back pain)
- previous back, abdominal, or pelvic surgery
- prostatitis (can cause referred back pain).

Drug therapy

Note any past or current use of the following drugs:
- corticosteroids (can cause osteoporosis)
- etidronate (used in osteoporosis and Paget's disease)
- muscle relaxants
- narcotic analgesics
- nonsteroidal anti-inflammatory drugs.

Physical examination

After obtaining the patient's vital signs, observe the patient's gait (if he is ambulatory). Watch how he sits — sitting is uncomfortable for most patients with back pain. Next, examine the patient according to the steps described below.

Inspection

Inspect the spine for obvious abnormalities such as *kyphosis,* which is an anteroposterior spinal curve that causes the back to bow; *scoliosis,* which is a lateral deviation of the spine; and *lordosis,* which is an exaggerated dorsal concavity of the lumbar spine.

Have the patient perform range of motion of the spine. Note which areas of the back the patient identifies as painful during these maneuvers. Make sure he flexes the spine by bending as far forward as possible; then have him extend the spine by arching backward as far as possible.

Straight-leg-raising test

The straight-leg-raising test helps to determine if back pain is related to sciatica. It is conducted with the patient lying supine on the examination table or in bed, as shown. The examiner asks the patient to keep the leg straight while the examiner lifts it. If back pain is related to sciatica, the patient will report burning, pain, or pins and needles in the buttocks or leg.

Pain in the back caused by this maneuver is not considered indicative of sciatica. Pain caused by the hamstring muscle being stretched behind the knee is a commonly found, normal occurrence.

In the illustration at right, symptoms of sciatica in the buttocks or leg are precipitated on the left side with the straight left leg raised to 45 degrees.

In crossed straight-leg-raising, pain on the left side is precipitated by straight-leg-raising on the right side.

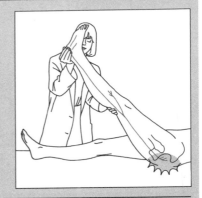

Dorsiflexion of the foot sometimes exaggerates sciatica.

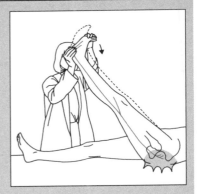

Next, have him bend laterally to one side, then to the other. Finally, have him twist from side to side to test rotation of the spine; make sure his feet don't move during this procedure.

Palpation
Palpation of the spinal column isn't helpful because much of it is inaccessible. However, sore back muscles can often be palpated and often have a characteristic hardness caused by spasm. Ask the patient to guide your fingers to the area of greatest pain. This may enable you to locate the most tender area quickly.

If the history indicates a possible abdominal or pelvic problem, such as peptic ulcer disease, appendicitis, or pelvic inflammatory disease, palpate the abdomen and pelvis.

Percussion
Test the reflexes at the knees, thereby evaluating spinal nerves that exit at L-2 to L-4. Also test reflexes at the ankles, thereby evaluating spinal nerves that exit at L-5 to S-2.

If the patient complains of sciatica in one leg, compare his reflexes on one side with the other side. The affected leg will often demonstrate a diminished reflex.

Special tests
You also may need to perform the straight-leg-raising test during your assessment if the patient complains of sciatica. (See *Straight-leg-raising test*.) This test assesses flexion and muscle strength of the lower extremities.

Timesaving tip: You can quickly test leg muscle strength by having the patient walk on his toes, then on his heels. Observe to see if the patient exhibits any signs of leg weakness. (He may start to fall, so be prepared to give support if the patient loses his balance.)

Vision loss

Loss of vision can be gradual or sudden, partial or complete, painful or painless. The affected eye may appear normal or abnormal. An abnormal appearance may suggest trauma, infections, or burns.

Loss of vision can also be temporary or permanent. Episodes of temporary loss of vision, *amaurosis partialis fugax,* may precede permanent loss of vision. (See *Causes of vision loss,* page 54.)

History of the symptom
To better characterize your patient's vision loss, consider asking the following questions:
• Is vision lost in one eye or both?
• Was the loss sudden or gradual?
• Has all vision been lost or just some of it?
• When did the vision loss occur?
• Did any activities precipitate the loss of vision?
• Are you having any eye pain? If so, when did the pain begin? Is it constant or intermittent? How would you describe it?
• Was there any trauma to the eye or head?
• Do you wear contact lenses? (These can cause infection and subsequent loss of vision.)

Associated findings
Note whether the patient has experienced any of the following signs and symptoms:
• halos around electric lights at night (found in glaucoma)
• increasingly poor night vision, beginning in childhood (a frequent complaint in retinitis pigmentosa and a possible sign of vitamin A deficiency)

Causes of vision loss

Neurologic disorders that cause vision loss include concussion, optic atrophy, and optic neuritis.

Concussion
Immediately or shortly after blunt head trauma, vision may be blurred, double, or lost. Vision loss is usually temporary. Other findings may include headache, anterograde and retrograde amnesia, transient loss of consciousness, nausea, vomiting, dizziness, irritability, confusion, lethargy, and aphasia.

Optic atrophy
Degeneration of the optic nerve may develop spontaneously or follow inflammation or edema of the nerve head, causing irreversible loss of the visual field with changes in color vision. Pupillary reactions are sluggish, and optic disk pallor is evident.

Optic neuritis
An umbrella term for inflammation, degeneration, or demyelinization of the optic nerve, optic neuritis usually produces temporary but severe unilateral vision loss. Pain around the eye occurs, especially with movement of the globe. This may be accompanied by visual field defects and a sluggish pupillary response to light. Ophthalmoscopic examination commonly reveals hyperemia of the optic disk, blurred disk margins, and filling of the physiologic cup.

Nonneurologic causes
Other causes of vision loss include cataracts, diabetic retinopathy, endophthalmitis, glaucoma, hereditary corneal dystrophies, herpes zoster, keratitis, Paget's disease, pituitary tumor, retinal artery occlusion (central), retinal detachment, retinal vein occlusion (central), senile macular degeneration, Stevens-Johnson syndrome, temporal arteritis, trachoma, uveitis, and vitreous hemorrhage.

Vision loss may also be caused by methanol toxicity and drugs such as chloroquine, digitalis glycosides, ethambutol, indomethacin, phenylbutazone, and quinine sulfate.

• loss of central vision, with preservation of peripheral vision (a common finding in macular degeneration)
• photophobia, a common complaint in migraine headaches, which can occasionally cause transient, usually monocular loss of vision (commonly occurs in disorders of the cornea and iris)
• significant weakness or paralysis of one side of the body (hemiplegia) occurring at the same time as vision loss (suggests cerebrovascular accident or transient ischemic attack)
• tenderness of the temporal artery in the scalp on the same side as the affected eye or a history of jaw claudication (local weakness and pain when eating, which may indicate temporal arteritis).

Previous conditions and treatments

Consult with the patient, family members, or members of the health care team to determine if the patient has a history of any of the following risk factors:

- acquired immunodeficiency syndrome (can lead to both eye and central nervous system infections)
- atrial fibrillation (can cause emboli, which form in the atria and travel to the retinal artery)
- autoimmune disorders, such as juvenile rheumatoid arthritis, ankylosing spondylitis, and Reiter's syndrome (can lead to uveitis, which can cause severe eye pain and diminished or hazy vision)
- cancer
- cataracts (causes a gradual loss of vision)
- concussion (can cause transient vision loss)
- corneal burns, trauma, or infections (can result in scarring of the cornea, leading to blurred, dimmed vision or complete loss of vision)
- diabetes (common cause of retinopathy and subsequent blindness)
- glaucoma (chronic open-angle type that causes gradual vision loss; acute angle-closure type that causes sudden vision loss and severe eye pain)
- hypercholesterolemia or tobacco use (can lead to atherosclerosis and blockage of the retinal artery)
- hypertension (if untreated, can increase risk of retinal artery occlusion or hemorrhage)
- I.V. drug abuse (can cause endophthalmitis, an infection in the vitreous humor of the eye leading to a loss of vision)
- macular degeneration
- multiple sclerosis (common cause of optic neuritis with subsequent loss of vision)
- Paget's disease (increasing bone growth that can impinge on cranial nerves, causing blurred or lost vision)
- pituitary tumors (can exert pressure on the optic nerve, leading to blurred or lost vision)
- retinal detachment (can recur)
- sickle cell anemia (can occlude retinal artery)
- temporal arteritis (an inflammatory process of the extracranial arteries that can cause occlusion of the lumen of the retinal artery).

Drug therapy

Note any past or current use of the following drugs:

- chloroquine (an antimalarial that can cause retinopathy if used for an extended duration)
- corticosteroid eyedrops (can precipitate glaucoma)
- hydroxychloroquine (used in rheumatoid arthritis; can cause retinopathy if used for an extended duration)
- lithium carbonate (may be associated with pseudotumor cerebri, which can cause pressure on the optic nerve)
- oral prednisone (associated with the development of cataracts when use is long-term).

Physical examination

Assess the patient's vital signs, including temperature, blood pressure, respiratory rate and depth, and pulse rate and rhythm. Then examine him according to the steps described below.

Inspection

- Observe both eyes, noting edema around the orbit or involving the eyelids.
- Check for ptosis (drooping of the upper eyelid, found in cranial nerve III disorders and Horner's syndrome).

• Observe for redness of the sclera, and note any discharge from the eye.

• Check for obvious signs of trauma to the eye or surrounding tissue.

• Note any bulging of the eyes, which is sometimes found in hyperthyroidism.

• Using a penlight, examine the cornea and iris for scars, cloudiness, irregularities, and foreign bodies.

• Observe pupillary size and shape, and look for discoloration of the pupil (a cloudy cornea, in conjunction with severe eye pain, scleral redness, and loss of vision, often indicates acute glaucoma). A whitish cornea commonly results from corneal scarring, which can stem from trauma or corneal burns.

• Test the patient's direct and consensual light reflexes and accommodation.

• Test visual acuity.

• Evaluate extraocular muscle function by having the patient hold his head still while his eyes follow your finger as it moves through the cardinal fields of vision.

Palpation

• Gently palpate the patient's closed eye, feeling for firmness. Firmness may indicate acute glaucoma.

• Palpate the eye orbit and skull to detect obvious fractures or puncture wounds.

Auscultation

• Listen over the patient's carotid and temporal arteries for bruits when you suspect embolism as the cause of vision loss.

Sensory disturbances

Because they're almost entirely subjective, sensory disturbances may prove especially difficult to assess. Common sensory disturbances include:

• *paresthesia,* which refers to abnormal sensations, such as tingling (pins and needles)

• *dysesthesia,* which refers to unpleasant sensations, such as burning

• *numbness,* which is more accurately described as anesthesia, but is often considered a paresthesia. (See *Causes of sensory disturbances.*)

The distribution of the patient's sensory complaints can help determine a lesion's presence and location. (See *Location of lesions in sensory disturbances,* page 58.)

History of the symptom

To better characterize your patient's sensory disturbance, consider asking the following questions:

• How long have you had the sensation?

• Can you describe the sensation?

• Where is the sensation occurring?

• Do any of your muscles feel weak?

• Is the sensation more noticeable now than before?

• Is it constant or intermittent?

• How severe is it? (Use a scale of 1 to 10, with 1 equaling the slightest sensation and 10 equaling maximum severity.)

• What activities increase or decrease the abnormal sensation?

Associated findings

Note whether the patient has experienced any of the following signs or symptoms:

• circulatory deficits (coldness of the extremities, skin pallor)

• head, neck, or back pain (especially if it is related temporally to the paresthesia)

• trauma of head, spine, or limbs

• weakness or muscle wasting.

Causes of sensory disturbances

Neurologic causes of sensory disturbances include herniated intervertebral disk, head trauma or cerebral tumors, spine trauma or spinal tumors, migraine headache, or transient ischemic attacks (TIAs).

Herniated intervertebral disk
When a herniated intervertebral disk presses on the spinal cord, sensation may be disturbed in the corresponding dermatome. Abnormal sensations may include paresthesia, dyesthesia, or anesthesia. Herniated intervertebral disk may occur at any location in the spine, but is most common in the cervical and lumbar regions.

Head trauma or cerebral tumors
Damage to the parietal lobe or sensory cortex can cause loss of stereognosis. Damage to the sensory cortex may also cause loss of touch discrimination on the opposite side of the body from the lesion. Damage to the thalamus can cause diminished sensation on the opposite side of the body.

Spine trauma or spinal tumors
A spinal tumor, depending on its location, may cause local pain and loss of sensation in corresponding dermatomes. Complete transection of the spinal cord can cause loss of all sensation below the level of injury. In a partial transection of the spinal cord, some sensory function is usually preserved.

Migraine headache
Many types of sensory disturbances can occur with a migraine. The most common are visual abnormalities, unilateral paresthesia or numbness, unilateral weakness, and aphasia or other speech disorders.

Transient ischemic attacks
Paresthesia, numbness, and weakness occur on the opposite side of the body from the ischemic area. If recovery of sensation (and motor function) from a TIA isn't complete — a cerebrovascular accident (CVA) has occurred. TIAs are often precursors to more serious neurologic problems.

Nonneurologic causes
Other causes of sensory disturbance include acute arterial occlusion, such as Buerger's disease, embolism, and arteriosclerosis obliterans; diabetes; alcohol abuse; malnutrition; vitamin deficiencies; hyperventilation; hypocalcemia; and pernicious anemia.
   Certain drugs may cause sensory disturbances, including chloroquine, isoniazid, nitrofurantoin, parenteral gold, and phenytoin. Chemotherapeutic agents, such as procarbazine, vinblastine, and vincristine, have been known to cause paresthesia and dyesthesia of the hands and feet.

Location of lesions in sensory disturbances

The distribution of the patient's sensory complaints can be helpful in determining the presence and anatomic level of a lesion. The table below correlates patient symptoms with the location of a lesion.

Location	Symptoms
Central nervous system	Graphesthesia and stereognosis are lost, while primary modes of sensation such as touch, pain, and vibration are preserved.
Spinal cord	Disease of posterior column leaves pain and temperature sensations intact, while altering ipsilateral sense of touch and vibration. Anterolateral spinothalamic disorders cause contralateral loss of pain and temperature sensations, leaving sense of touch and vibration intact.
Nerve root	Sensory abnormalities, such as tingling and pain, develop.
Peripheral nerve	Sensory symptoms, such as tingling, a crawling sensation, or pain, develop.

Previous conditions

Consult with the patient, family members, or members of the health care team to determine if the patient has a history of any of the following risk factors:
• acquired immunodeficiency syndrome (can cause central nervous system [CNS] infection)
• alcohol or narcotic abuse
• arthritis
• atherosclerosis or clotting disorders
• cardiovascular accident
• diabetes
• herniated intervertebral disk
• hyperventilation
• migraine
• multiple sclerosis (can cause widespread paresthesia)
• past history of head, neck, or back trauma
• poor nutrition
• seizure disorders.

Drug therapy

Note any past or current use of the following drugs:
• chemotherapeutic drugs, such as vincristine, vinblastine, and procarbazine
• chloroquine
• isoniazid
• nitrofurantoin
• parenteral gold
• phenytoin.

Physical examination

Assess the patient's vital signs, including temperature, blood pressure, respiratory rate and depth, and pulse rate and rhythm. Then examine the patient according to the steps described below.

Inspection
• Observe the affected area for muscle atrophy.

• Observe skin color. Autonomic nervous system disorders (such as multiple sclerosis, spinal cord lesions, and reflex sympathetic dystrophy) and circulatory disturbances can cause pallor or redness.

Timesaving tip: Perform two tasks at once by inspecting affected area and skin color while performing palpation.

Palpation
• Check for muscle strength and tone.
• Check capillary refill (slow capillary filling indicates arterial occlusion).

Percussion
• Check tendon reflexes in affected area.

Special tests
During your assessment, you may also need to test for the following:
• pain sensation. To test for this, use a sharp instrument, such as a pin, and prick various areas of the patient's skin. Ask him to indicate whether he feels a sharp or dull sensation.
• temperature sensation. To test for this, fill two test tubes, one with hot water and one with cold. Briefly place each test tube separately on the patient's skin and ask him to identify which one is touching the skin.

Timesaving tip: If pain sensation is intact, you can omit testing temperature sensation because both sensations are transmitted by the same spinal cord tract.
• light-touch sensation. To test for this, touch the major dermatomes with a wisp of cotton. Ask the patient to identify when and where he feels something.

Timesaving tip: The longest nerves are affected first in peripheral neuropathy, so first

check for pain and light-touch sensations at the toes. If sensation in the toes is intact, you don't need to test further.
• vibration. To test for this, apply the base of a vibrating fork to the interphalangeal joint of the patient's big toe. Ask the patient what he feels. Typically, he should report a vibration or buzzing.
• stereognosis, graphesthesia, and proprioception. To test for *stereognosis,* place different-sized objects, such as coins, in the patient's hand while his eyes are closed and ask him to correctly identify them. To test for *graphesthesia,* have the patient close his eyes while you trace letters or numbers in his palm; he should be able to identify them by feel. To test for *proprioception,* have the patient close his eyes while you move one of his fingers rapidly up and down. Then pause with the fingertip pointing either up or down, and ask the patient to describe the position of his finger.

Abnormal stereognosis, graphesthesia, and proprioception may indicate a CNS lesion or a peripheral nerve disorder.

Weakness

A classic sign of motor disturbance, weakness may be either partial or complete. It may also be temporary, such as occurs with a pinched nerve, or permanent, such as after a severe cerebrovascular accident (CVA). (See *Causes of weakness,* page 60.)

History of the sign
To better characterize your patient's weakness, consider asking the following questions:
• Do you feel weak throughout your whole body or in one particular area?

Causes of weakness

Various neurologic disorders may cause weakness. These include cerebrovascular accident (CVA), central nervous system (CNS) trauma, CNS neoplasms, herniated disk, Parkinson's disease, peripheral nerve compression, and peripheral polyneuropathy.

Cerebrovascular accident
In a CVA, weakness often affects an entire side of the patient's body (hemiparesis). Deep tendon reflexes, absent immediately after the CVA on the side opposite of the lesion, become hyperreflexive after a few weeks and remain that way. Muscles on the affected side become atrophic and tone is increased, leading to the characteristic flexion contractures.

CNS trauma and neoplasms
A similar pattern of muscle weakness and increased tone such as that found in CVA will occur. The motor abnormalities will occur on the side of the body opposite the lesion.

Herniated disk
A herniated disk will eventually cause weakness in the muscles served by the nerves in the affected dermatome. Unlike CNS lesions, however, muscle tone is diminished, and reflexes in the affected dermatome become hyporeflexive.

Parkinson's disease
Parkinson's disease typically causes bradykinesia (slowness of movement), which can progress to akinesia (inability to initiate a desired movement). A resting tremor is typically present, which often improves when the patient moves the affected limb. Muscle tone increases dramatically, leading to rigidity. Reflexes can be normal, but can become impaired as muscle rigidity worsens.

Peripheral nerve compression
Compression of a peripheral nerve (carpal tunnel syndrome, for example) causes paresthesia and pain below the level of compression and eventual weakness of muscles served by the compressed nerve. Along with weakness, muscle atrophy and fasciculations eventually appear.

Peripheral polyneuropathy
Symptoms here present a picture very similar to peripheral nerve compression, except that they are not limited to only one extremity. The weakness and sensory abnormalities typically appear first in the feet, then in the hands (the so-called stocking-and-glove distribution). In contrast to the local nature of the peripheral nerve compression, peripheral polyneuropathy may reflect an underlying metabolic or nutritional disorder such as diabetes mellitus or vitamin B deficiency. It can also appear as a consequence of alcoholism.

Nonneurologic causes
Weakness may also result from diabetes, nutritional deficiencies, and infection.

- How would you describe the weakness?
- When did you first feel weak? Did it begin abruptly? (An abrupt onset suggests a CVA.)
- Is the weakness constant or intermittent?
- Do you have any pain? If so, how would you describe it?
- Was there any precipitating trauma?
- What seems to aggravate your weakness?
- What seems to make it better?
- Is the weakness getting worse?

Associated findings

Note whether the patient has experienced any of the following signs or symptoms:
- bowel or bladder dysfunction
- fever (may indicate central nervous system [CNS] infection)
- gait abnormalities
- mental status changes (if present and gradual, may suggest a tumor or dementia; if present and sudden, may suggest trauma, cerebral aneurysm, or CVA)
- tingling or numbness
- tremor (suggests extrapyramidal problem).

Previous conditions and treatments

Consult with the patient, family members, or members of the health care team to determine if the patient has a history of any of the following risk factors:
- acquired immunodeficiency syndrome (can cause CNS infection)
- amyotrophic lateral sclerosis
- anxiety
- arthritis (especially rheumatoid)
- cancer (both cancer itself and chemotherapy can cause neuropathic lesions)

- CNS infection (brain abscess, encephalitis, meningitis)
- CVA, or past history of clotting disorder
- depression (causes a generalized fatigue, which some patients may describe as weakness)
- diabetes, alcohol abuse, or malnutrition (can cause distal weakness, secondary to polyneuropathy)
- history of exposure to toxins, such as lead, mercury, or poisons
- hypertension or hypercholesterolemia (suggests CVA in patients with acute hemiplegia)
- migraine (can cause transient hemiparesis)
- multiple sclerosis
- muscular dystrophy
- myasthenia gravis
- Parkinson's disease
- polio (can lead to post-polio syndrome)
- polymyalgia rheumatica (causes shoulder and hip weakness)
- thyroid disorders
- trauma to the head, spinal cord, or extremities.

Drug therapy

Note any past or current use of the following drugs:
- alcohol, nicotine, or cocaine
- antidepressants
- antihypertensive agents
- carbidopa-levodopa (used in Parkinson's disease)
- insulin or oral antidiabetic medications
- thyroid medications
- tranquilizers.

Physical examination

Assess the patient's vital signs, including temperature, blood pressure, respiratory rate and depth, and pulse rate and rhythm. Then examine the patient according to the steps described below.

Inspection
• With the patient seated, observe the muscles of his hands, arms, shoulders and legs for their bulk. Atrophied muscles demonstrate loss of bulk. Compare one side to the other. If you suspect muscle atrophy, consider using a tape measure to determine muscle circumference.

• Observe the patient's face for unilateral drooping and expression.

Palpation
• Feel for muscle tone by passively extending and flexing the patient's elbows and knees.

• Assess muscle strength, comparing both sides of the body.

Timesaving tip: You can quickly assess motor strength from the waist down by having the patient stand, do a deep knee bend, and then return to the standing position. This tests all the major muscle groups in the hips and legs at once. (You may have to hold an older patient's hands to provide balance when he does this.)

Percussion
• Assess the patient's reflexes. Upper motor neuron lesions cause hyperactive, forceful reflexes because of the loss of inhibition of the reflex arc normally provided by the brain. Lower motor neuron lesions, such as those from nerve compression in the spinal cord caused by a herniated intervertebral disk, cause diminished or absent reflexes. Metabolic disorders, such as hyperthyroidism, and anxiety can cause exaggeration of all types of reflexes.

Dizziness

A common neurologic symptom, dizziness refers to the sensation of illusory movement. It may be felt, for example, when stepping off a merry-go-round or spinning around a fixed point and suddenly stopping. Dizziness may be categorized as vertigo, presyncope, disequilibrium, or lightheadedness. (See *Four types of dizziness,* opposite, and *Causes of dizziness,* page 64.)

History of the symptom
To better characterize your patient's dizziness, consider asking him these questions:
• Can you describe your symptoms without using the word "dizzy?" Although difficult for some patients to answer, the question can help pinpoint the patient's type of dizziness.
• When did you first feel dizzy?
• Are you dizzy all of the time or only sometimes?
• Can you continue to function with your symptoms, or are they disabling?
• Can you describe what activities precipitate your dizziness?
• Does anything aggravate or alleviate the dizziness?

Determine which type of dizziness most closely fits the patient's description, keeping in mind that the types can overlap, and then focus history questions on that type. However, if you cannot establish a pattern leading to only one type, you will need to ask the history questions specific for each type.

Vertigo
• Have you experienced hearing loss and tinnitus? (Vertigo, hearing loss,

Assessment TimeSaver

Four types of dizziness

Dizziness can be categorized as vertigo, presyncope, disequilibrium, and light-headedness.

Vertigo

Vertigo involves a definite sense of motion, often rotational (although it can be described as a tilting or up and down motion, such as a boat might make). Usually the patient complains of the external environment moving — less commonly, that he is spinning.

Presyncope

Presyncope describes the sensation that occurs just before loss of consciousness. Often, the patient will abort the sensation by sitting down abruptly or lying flat. Most people experience periodic presyncope when they stand up quickly after squatting. The sensation commonly results from the gravitational pooling of blood in the lower extremities caused by rapid assumption of the upright position.

Disequilibrium

Disequilibrium is the sensation of poor balance, most typically during ambulation, but without the sense that fainting is about to occur. Patients are also free of any vertigo symptoms.

Light-headedness

Light-headedness is a vague symptom of wooziness or spaciness. It usually can be distinguished from vertigo and presyncope by the patient. It can be constant and can occur at rest and with activity, thus distinguishing it from disequilibrium.

and tinnitus are found in Ménière's disease.)
• Does your symptom only occur with changes in the position of your head, such as when you turn over in bed? (This classic symptom of benign positional vertigo typically occurs in middle-aged to elderly patients. The vertigo usually lasts less than 30 seconds and is relieved by remaining still.)
• Have you experienced nausea or vomiting? (Both are almost always present with vertigo, except when the episodes are extremely brief.)

• Do you have ear or sinus pain? (Middle ear and sinus infections can cause vertigo.)
• Have you experienced any recent head trauma? (Postconcussional syndrome can include vertigo.)

Presyncope
• Do you feel faint when you stand up? (Orthostatic hypotension is the most common cause of presyncope.)
• Can you describe exactly what you were doing just before you felt faint?
• Have you ever passed out? If so, were there any witnesses? (Seizures usually require an observer for a description; syncope can be distin-

Causes of dizziness

Neurologic causes of dizziness include postconcussional syndrome, transient ischemic attack, and benign positional vertigo.

Postconcussional syndrome

Occurring 1 to 3 weeks after head injury, this syndrome is marked by dizziness, headache (throbbing, aching, band-like, or stabbing), emotional lability, alcohol intolerance, fatigue, anxiety, and possibly vertigo. Dizziness and other symptoms are intensified by mental or physical stress. The syndrome may persist for years, but symptoms eventually abate.

Transient ischemic attack

Lasting from a few seconds to 24 hours, a transient ischemic attack frequently signals impending cerebrovascular accident. Dizziness of varying severity may occur during an attack. Dizziness is accompanied by unilateral or bilateral diplopia, blindness or visual field deficits, ptosis, tinnitus, hearing loss, paresis, and numbness. Other findings include dysarthria, dysphagia, vomiting, hiccups, confusion, decreased level of consciousness, and pallor.

Benign positional vertigo

Episodes of violent vertigo, lasting more than 30 seconds, can occur in older patients. These events are al-ways triggered by sudden movements of the head, such as turning over in bed. Nystagmus occurs, but there is no associated hearing loss or tinnitus, such as in Ménière's disease. Attacks usually subside within several weeks or months, but may recur after months or years.

Nonneurologic causes

Dizziness may occur secondary to anemia, cardiac arrhythmias, vestibular disease, Ménière's disease, hypertension, hyperventilation syndrome, orthostatic hypotension, anemia, hypothyroidism, carotid sinus hypersensitivity, emphysema, cataract excision, chronic diplopia, micturition syncope, generalized anxiety disorder, and panic disorder.

Drugs

Drugs that may cause dizziness include:
- antianxiety drugs
- central nervous system depressants
- decongestants
- narcotics
- vasodilators.

guished from seizures by the presence of brief hypoxic twitches and cyanosis and the lack of incontinence and postictal confusion.)
- Have you had problems recently with vomiting or diarrhea?
- Have you had black stools? (This sign can indicate GI bleeding, causing anemia and diminished blood volume and precipitating presyncope.)

- Have you had a fever? (Fever can lead to dehydration and syncope.)
- Have you had frequent urination? (Frequent urination can cause dehydration and syncope.)

Disequilibrium
- Does walking make your dizziness worse? (Impaired ambulation is the most common finding in disequilibrium.)
- How is your vision? Hearing? Sensation in your feet? (Multiple sensory deficits are the most common cause of disequilibrium.)
- Does using a cane or walker or holding on to another person's arm improve the dizziness? (Patients with disequilibrium will frequently respond positively to this question.)

Light-headedness
- Do you become short of breath frequently? (Hyperventilation is probably the most common cause of dizziness.)
- Do you ever feel that you can't get a satisfying breath?
- Do you also have symptoms such as chest pain, rapid heart rate, and weakness and tingling in the extremities? (These are classic symptoms of hyperventilation.)
- Have you been under more stress recently? (Hyperventilation is usually related to anxiety.)

Associated findings
Note whether the patient has experienced any of the following signs or symptoms:
- tachycardia, peripheral paresthesia (common in light-headedness)
- nausea and vomiting (frequently present with persistent vertigo)
- orthostatic blood pressure changes (found in presyncope)
- visual impairment, peripheral neuropathy (found in disequilibrium).

Previous conditions
Consult with the patient, family members, or members of the health care team to determine if the patient has a history of any of the following risk factors:
- acquired immunodeficiency syndrome (can cause central nervous system infections or neoplasms)
- alcoholism (causes disequilibrium)
- Alzheimer's disease or other type of dementia (may cause disequilibrium)
- anemia (causes presyncope)
- arrhythmias (can cause presyncope or syncope)
- arthritis (painful joints in back, hip, knees, ankles, and toes can cause painful ambulation and disequilibrium)
- bleeding disorders (may cause presyncope)
- cancer
- cerebrovascular accident (causes disequilibrium)
- congestive heart failure, cardiac valvular disorders (can lead to impaired cardiac output, causing presyncope)
- diabetes (can cause multiple sensory deficits, leading to disequilibrium)
- history of anxiety (causes light-headedness)
- Ménière's disease (commonly causes vertigo)
- multiple sclerosis (causes disequilibrium)
- parkinsonism (causes disequilibrium)
- vision problems (contributes to disequilibrium).

Drug therapy
Note any past or current use of the following drugs. In particular, pay close attention to any *new* medications:
- antiarrhythmics and antihypertensives
- anticonvulsants

- antidepressants
- antihistamines
- digoxin
- diuretics
- histamine$_2$-receptor antagonists
- insulin and oral antidiabetic drugs
- tranquilizers
- warfarin.

Physical examination
Assess the patient's vital signs, including temperature, blood pressure, respiratory rate and depth, and pulse rate and rhythm. Then examine the patient according to the steps described below.

Inspection
• Observe the patient's gait. Patients with acute vertigo usually walk with great difficulty, if at all. Patients with disequilibrium usually have obviously abnormal gaits.
• Observe the patient with presyncope for signs of transient light-headedness when he arises from a sitting position.
• Check the patient's blood pressure while he stands, sits, and lies down. Avoid standing and sitting readings if the patient has acute vertigo. Normally, systolic pressure drops no more than 10 mm Hg when the patient stands. However, in some healthy elderly patients, systolic pressure may drop as much as 20 to 30 mm Hg. Diastolic pressure usually rises slightly (2 to 5 mm Hg) on standing. If the patient's systolic or diastolic pressure drops 20 mm Hg or more *and* he complains of light-headedness as he stands, suspect orthostatic hypotension.
• Observe for nystagmus (may indicate acute vertigo).

Percussion
• Test the patient's reflexes if hemiplegia or a cranial nerve abnormality is present.

Special tests
Special tests, such as the Romberg test, may also be performed during your assessment. The Romberg test evaluates the patient's ability to maintain his balance with his eyes open and closed.

If you suspect that dizziness results from hyperventilation, have the patient lie on his back, and ask him to breathe deeply and rapidly for 3 minutes. You may need to demonstrate deep breathing for the patient. The goal is for the patient to take approximately 30 breaths/minute. Most people will experience light-headedness when performing this maneuver. Ask the patient if the sensations he experiences resemble his dizziness. If they do, suspect hyperventilation as the probable cause of the dizziness.

Memory loss

Also known as amnesia, memory loss can develop gradually (as in dementia), suddenly (such as after head trauma), or as a result of hypoxia, cerebrovascular accident (CVA), or prolonged hypoglycemia. Sudden memory loss is a dramatic symptom that usually causes the patient to seek professional help.

Retrograde memory loss refers to the loss of memory of events that took place *before* the causative episode. For example, retrograde loss can occur after head trauma, a condition referred to as Korsakoff's psychosis. In this condition, memory for events immediately before the trauma, and occasionally for events extending back months to years in the past, is lost.

Anterograde memory loss refers to memory loss that occurs *after* the causative episode. Anterograde loss is associated with high doses of benzodiazepines, such as triazolam and diazepam. For example, diazepam administered to patients before diagnostic procedures may cause anterograde memory loss.

Memory can be divided into three major components: *immediate,* covering the past few seconds; *intermediate,* or *short-term,* covering the interval from a few seconds past to a few days past; and *remote,* or *long-term,* extending further back in time. (See *Causes of memory loss,* page 68.)

History of the symptom
Besides interviewing the patient, you may need to ask family members, friends, or witnesses (if trauma was involved) questions about the patient's memory loss. To better characterize the patient's memory loss, consider asking the following questions:
• When did loss of memory first become a problem?
• What things are you having trouble remembering?
• Is your memory problem getting worse?
• Have you had a head injury recently?
• Do you consume alcohol? If so, how often and how much?
• Do you know what the date is today? Can you tell me where you are?
• Do you take any prescription or nonprescription medications?

Associated findings
Note whether the patient has experienced any of the following signs and symptoms:

• altered level of consciousness (LOC) (commonly associated with disorders that cause loss of memory)
• dyspnea (may cause hypoxia)
• headache
• sensory or motor disturbance (suggests a CVA, head trauma, or dementia)
• urinary incontinence or gait disturbance
• weakness, diaphoresis, or tremor.

Previous conditions
Consult with the patient, family members, or members of the health care team to determine if the patient has a history of any of the following risk factors:
• acquired immunodeficiency syndrome (may predispose to central nervous system [CNS] infection and dementia)
• alcoholism (causes thiamine deficiency and destruction of CNS neurons)
• Alzheimer's disease (the most common cause of memory loss)
• anxiety disorder (may lead to hysterical loss of memory, a psychiatric problem)
• carbon monoxide poisoning (related hypoxia may cause CNS damage)
• depression (especially in elderly people; can cause pseudodementia with memory loss)
• diabetes
• head trauma
• herpes simplex encephalitis (commonly associated with loss of memory in recovered patients)
• history of clotting disorders or atherosclerosis (may cause vertebrobasilar thrombus or insufficiency, with frequent loss of memory)
• hypertension (may cause CVA)
• insomnia
• malnutrition (may cause thiamine deficiency)
• respiratory disease

Causes of memory loss

Neurologic disorders that may cause memory loss include Alzheimer's disease, head trauma, seizure disorders, vertebrobasilar circulatory disorders, and Wernicke-Korsakoff syndrome.

Alzheimer's disease
In this disorder, retrograde amnesia progresses slowly, eventually producing severe and permanent memory loss. Associated findings include agitation, inability to concentrate, disregard for personal hygiene, confusion, irritability, and emotional lability.

Head trauma
Head trauma may produce retrograde or anterograde amnesia varying in severity. Usually, amnesia of the event persists, as well as brief retrograde and longer anterograde amnesia. Severe head trauma can cause permanent amnesia or difficulty in retaining recent memories. Related findings include altered respirations and level of consciousness (LOC); headache, dizziness, confusion; and visual, motor, and sensory disturbances (such as hemiparesis and paresthesia on the side opposite the injury).

Seizure disorders
In temporal lobe seizures, amnesia occurs suddenly and lasts for several seconds to minutes. The patient may recall an aura or nothing at all. An irritable focus on the left side of the brain primarily causes amnesia for verbal memories; an irritable focus on the right side of the brain, graphic and verbal amnesia. Associated signs include decreased LOC during the seizure, confusion, motor and sensory disturbances, and blurred vision.

Vertebrobasilar circulatory disorders
Vertebrobasilar ischemia, infarction, embolus, or hemorrhage typically cause complete, abrupt, short-term amnesia. Associated findings include dizziness, decreased LOC, ataxia, blurred or double vision, vertigo, nausea, and vomiting.

Wernicke-Korsakoff syndrome
This neuropsychiatric disorder results from thiamine deficiency, most commonly due to chronic alcohol abuse. The patient may experience severe anterograde and retrograde amnesia. Associated clinical findings include confusion, ataxia of gait, nystagmus, and ophthalmoplegia.

Nonneurologic causes
Memory loss may occur secondary to hysteria, cerebral hypoxia, herpes simplex virus, alcoholic blackouts, electroconvulsive therapy, temporal lobe surgery, or frontal lobe tumor.

Drugs
Anterograde amnesia can be precipitated by the use of barbiturates, benzodiazepines and general anesthetics.

• seizure disorder (usually causes loss of memory just before and after a seizure).

Drug therapy
Note any past or current use of the following drugs:
• anticonvulsants
• barbiturates
• benzodiazepines, particularly triazolam and diazepam
• general anesthetics, especially fentanyl, halothane, and isoflurane
• insulin (prolonged insulin shock can damage CNS).

Physical examination
Assess the patient's vital signs, including temperature, blood pressure, respiratory rate and depth, and pulse rate and rhythm. Then examine the patient according to the steps listed below:
• Determine the patient's LOC.
• Assess short-term memory, which is usually affected before other types of memory. Test short-term memory by asking the patient to repeat three items, such as cat, dog, and bridge, immediately after you. Then ask him to repeat those three items 3 to 5 minutes later. An inability to repeat them may indicate short-term memory impairment.
• Test long-term memory by asking the patient for his age and place of birth.
• If the patient is also complaining of motor or sensory disturbance, conduct a neurologic examination of the motor and sensory system.

Decreased level of consciousness

Level of consciousness (LOC) is the most immediate and obvious indica-

tion of neurologic function. Assessing arousal and awareness is the key to determining LOC. Arousal refers to the patient's ability to react to environmental stimuli. Awareness refers to his ability to properly interpret the meaning of the stimuli.

Suddenly decreased LOC often signals catastrophic central nervous system (CNS) disorders, such as cerebrovascular accident (CVA), trauma, and increased intracranial pressure (ICP), and requires emergency measures. (See *Emergency interventions for decreased LOC*, page 70.) Assessment scales, such as the Glasgow Coma Scale, are useful tools in determining the patient's LOC. These scales are used during the initial assessment and throughout the patient's care to monitor his progress and determine his prognosis.

Decreased LOC may result from many factors (See *Causes of decreased LOC,* pages 71 to 74). The patient may be unable to provide an adequate history, so determining the nature of his problem may be difficult. However, proceeding in the systematic manner described below will often reveal important clues.

History of the sign
To better characterize the patient's level of consciousness, consider asking the following questions:
• Was the change in consciousness sudden or gradual?
• Was there any trauma, particularly to the head?
• If the patient was found unconscious, ask about the environment he was found in. Was there evidence of trauma, exposure to heat or cold, ingestion of poisons or drugs, or exposure to smoke or carbon monoxide?
• How did the patient act before his LOC declined? Was there vomiting, headache, pain, or bleeding?

Emergency interventions for decreased LOC

Use the Glasgow Coma Scale to quickly determine the severity of decreased level of consciousness (LOC) and to obtain baseline data. If the patient's score is 13 or less, and the patient's overall hemodynamic status is deteriorating, emergency interventions may be necessary. Perform the following:

• Insert an artificial airway.
• Elevate the head of the bed 30 degrees.
• If spinal cord injury has been ruled out, turn the patient's head to the side.
• Prepare to suction the patient, if necessary.
• Remember to hyperventilate him first to reduce carbon dioxide levels. Then determine the rate, rhythm, and depth of spontaneous respirations. Support breathing with mechanical ventilation, if necessary.
• Examine the patient's circulation by checking carotid pulse, heart rate and rhythm, and blood pressure.
• Continue to monitor his vital signs, being alert for signs of increasing intracranial pressure, such as bradycardia and widening pulse pressure.
• When you're confident his airway, breathing, and circulation are stabilized, perform a neurologic examination.

If the patient's Glasgow Coma Scale score is 7 or less, intubation and resuscitation may be necessary.

• Was he depressed?
• Was there evidence of seizures?
• Has there been any recent respiratory problem or complaints of chest pain?

Associated findings

Note whether the patient has experienced any of the following signs or symptoms:
• chest pain or dyspnea (can indicate heart or lung dysfunction, leading to impaired CNS oxygenation)
• fever
• headache (if sudden and severe, can indicate subarachnoid hemorrhage)
• hemorrhage (suggests hypovolemic shock)
• neck rigidity (in the absence of trauma, suggests meningitis)
• personality changes (can indicate depression or possibly a CNS tumor or hemorrhage)
• polyuria and polydipsia (suggests uncompensated diabetes)
• visual disturbances (found in a wide range of CNS disorders)
• vomiting and diarrhea (causes dehydration; if only vomiting, may indicate increasing CNS pressure).

Previous conditions

Consult with the patient, family members, or members of the health care team to determine if the patient has a history of any of the following risk factors:
• acquired immunodeficiency syndrome (may cause CNS malignancy, infection, or dementia)
• angina
• atrial fibrillation (may cause embolic CVA)
• cancer (may cause CNS metastasis)
• clotting disorder
• diabetes
• history of alcohol or drug abuse

(Text continues on page 74.)

Causes of decreased LOC

Neurologic disorders that may cause decreased level of consciousness (LOC) include brain tumor, cerebral aneurysm, cerebral contusion, cerebrovascular accident, encephalitis, encephalomyelitis, encephalopathy, epidural hemorrhage, intracerebral hemorrhage, meningitis, pontine hemorrhage, seizure disorders, subdural hematoma, subdural hemorrhage, and transient ischemic attack.

Brain tumor
LOC decreases slowly, from lethargy to coma. The patient may also experience apathy, behavior changes, memory loss, and decreased attention span; he may complain of morning headache, dizziness, vision loss, ataxia, or sensorimotor disturbances. Aphasia and seizures are possible, along with signs of hormonal imbalance, such as fluid retention or amenorrhea. In later stages, papilledema, vomiting, bradycardia, and widening pulse pressure also appear. The patient may exhibit a decorticate or decerebrate posture.

Cerebral aneurysm
Somnolence, confusion and, at times, stupor characterize an episode of moderate bleeding; deep coma occurs with severe bleeding. Usually, onset is abrupt, with sudden, severe headache, nausea, and vomiting. Nuchal rigidity, back and leg pain, fever, restlessness, irritability, occasional seizures, and blurred vision may occur, reflecting meningeal irritation. The type and severity of other findings depend on the site and severity of the hemorrhage and may include hemiparesis, hemisensory defects, dysphagia, and visual defects.

Cerebral contusion
In this disorder, the patient is usually unconscious for a prolonged period. He may develop dilated, nonreactive pupils and decorticate or decerebrate posture. If he's conscious or recovers consciousness, he may be drowsy, confused, disoriented, agitated, or even violent.

Cerebrovascular accident
In this disorder, LOC changes vary in degree and onset. Thrombotic cerebrovascular accident (CVA) is typically preceded by multiple transient ischemic attacks and may occur abruptly or evolve over several minutes, hours, or days. Embolic CVA occurs without warning, and deficits reach their peak almost at once. Hemorrhagic CVA deficits usually develop progressively over minutes or hours.

Encephalitis
Within 24 to 48 hours after onset, the patient may experience changes in LOC ranging from lethargy to coma. He may also have abrupt onset of fever, headache, nuchal rigidity, vomiting, irritability, seizures, aphasia, ataxia, hemiparesis, nystagmus, photophobia, myoclonus, and cranial nerve palsies.

(continued)

Causes of decreased LOC *(continued)*

Encephalomyelitis (postvaccinal)

This life-threatening disorder produces rapid LOC deterioration from drowsiness to coma. The patient also experiences rapid onset of nuchal rigidity, vomiting, and seizures.

Encephalopathy

Decreased level of consciousness is an important finding in hepatic, hypertensive, hypoglycemic, and uremic encephalopathy.

Hepatic encephalopathy

Signs and symptoms develop in four stages. In the prodromal stage, the patient exhibits slight personality changes (disorientation, forgetfulness, slurred speech) and slight tremor. In the impending stage, he develops tremor progressing to asterixis (the hallmark of hepatic encephalopathy), lethargy, aberrant behavior, and apraxia. In the stuporous stage, stupor is accompanied by hyperventilation and the patient is noisy and abusive when aroused. In the comatose stage, coma is accompanied by decerebrate posture, hyperactive reflexes, positive Babinski's reflex, and fetor hepaticus.

Hypertensive encephalopathy

In this life-threatening condition, LOC progressively decreases from lethargy to stupor to coma. In addition to markedly elevated blood pressure, the patient may experience severe headache, vomiting, seizures, visual disturbances, transient paralysis, and eventually Cheyne-Stokes respirations.

Hypoglycemic encephalopathy

Early signs and symptoms include nervousness, hunger, alternate flushing and cold sweats, headache, trembling, and palpitations. The patient also appears confused and restless, with cyanosis and increased heart and respiratory rates and blood pressure. Blurred vision progresses to motor weakness, hemiplegia, dilated pupils, pallor, decreased pulse rate, shallow respirations, and seizures.

Hypoxic encephalopathy

LOC rapidly deteriorates from lethargy to coma. Later, the patient's respiratory pattern becomes abnormal, and assessment reveals decreased pulse rate, blood pressure, and deep tendon reflexes; Babinski's reflex; absent doll's eye reflex; and fixed pupils. Flaccidity and decerebrate posture appear late. Depending on its severity, hypoxic encephalopathy can cause brain death.

Uremic encephalopathy

LOC decreases gradually from lethargy to coma. In the early stage, the patient may appear apathetic, inattentive, confused, and irritable and may complain of headache, nausea, fatigue, and anorexia. Other findings may include vomiting, tremors, edema, papilledema, hypertension, cardiac arrhythmias, dyspnea, rales, Kussmaul's and Cheyne-Stokes respirations, and oliguria.

Causes of decreased LOC *(continued)*

Epidural hemorrhage (acute)
This life-threatening posttraumatic disorder produces momentary loss of consciousness followed by a lucid interval. While lucid, the patient has severe headache, nausea, vomiting, and bladder distention. Rapid deterioration in consciousness follows, possibly leading to coma.

Intracerebral hemorrhage
This life-threatening disorder produces rapid, steady loss of consciousness within hours, often accompanied by severe headache, dizziness, nausea, and vomiting.

Meningitis
The patient usually exhibits confusion and irritability. Stupor, coma, and seizures may occur in severe meningitis. Fever develops early, possibly accompanied by chills.

Pontine hemorrhage
This disorder causes a sudden, rapid decrease in LOC resulting in coma within minutes and death within hours. The patient may also exhibit total paralysis, decerebrate posture, Babinski's reflex, absent doll's eye reflex, and bilateral miosis although pupils remain reactive to light.

Seizure disorders
Decreased LOC is an important finding in complex partial seizure, absence seizure, generalized tonic-clonic seizure, and atonic seizure.

Complex partial seizure
In this type of seizure, decreased LOC is evidenced by a blank stare, purposeless behavior (picking at clothing, wandering, lip-smacking, or chewing motions), and unintelligible speech. The seizure may be heralded by an aura and followed by several minutes of mental confusion.

Absence seizure
This seizure usually involves a brief change in LOC, indicated by blinking or eye rolling, blank stare, and slight mouth movements.

Generalized tonic-clonic seizure
This type of seizure typically begins with a loud cry and sudden loss of consciousness. Muscle spasm alternates with relaxation. Tongue biting, incontinence, labored breathing, apnea, and cyanosis may also occur. Consciousness returns after the seizure, but the patient remains confused. He may complain of drowsiness, fatigue, headache, muscle aching, and weakness and may fall into a deep sleep.

Atonic seizure
This type of seizure produces sudden unconsciousness for a few seconds.

Subdural hematoma (chronic)
LOC deteriorates slowly. Signs and symptoms include confusion, decreased ability to concentrate, and

(continued)

Causes of decreased LOC *(continued)*

personality changes accompanied by headache, giddiness, seizures, and a dilated ipsilateral pupil with ptosis.

Subdural hemorrhage (acute)
In this potentially life-threatening disorder, consciousness progressively decreases from somnolence to coma, preceded by agitation and confusion. The patient may also experience headache, fever, unilateral pupil dilation, decreased pulse and respirations, widening pulse pressure, seizures, hemiparesis, and Babinski's reflex.

Transient ischemic attack
The patient may experience an abrupt decrease in LOC, which varies in severity and disappears gradually within 24 hours. Site-specific findings may include vision loss, nystagmus, aphasia, dizziness, dysarthria, unilateral hemiparesis or hemiplegia, tinnitus, paresthesia, dysphagia, or staggering or incoordinated gait.

Nonneurologic causes
Decreased LOC may also occur secondary to adrenal crisis, diabetic ketoacidosis, heatstroke, hypercapnia with pulmonary disease, hyperglycemia, hyperosmolar nonketotic coma, hypernatremia, hyperventilation syndrome, hypokalemia, hyponatremia, hypothermia, myxedema crisis, poisoning, shock, thyroid storm, and alcohol use.

Drugs
Sedation and other degrees of decreased LOC can result from an overdose of barbiturates, other central nervous system depressants, and aspirin.

• hypercalcemia (may result from cancer, bone disease, or parathyroidism; causes lethargy and coma)
• hypertension and hypercholesterolemia (may suggest CVA)
• hypokalemia (may cause lethargy)
• kidney disease (may cause uremic encephalopathy)
• liver disease (may cause hepatic encephalopathy)
• pulmonary disease (may cause decreased LOC secondary to hypoxia or hypercapnia)
• recent head trauma
• recent exposure to extremes of heat or cold
• transient ischemic attacks.

Drug therapy
Note any past or current use of the following drugs:
• alcohol, cocaine, or opiates
• anticonvulsants
• antihypertensives
• aspirin or acetaminophen (overdose may lead to lethargy and coma)
• insulin or oral antidiabetic drugs
• tranquilizers or barbiturates

• warfarin (may indicate previous clotting disorder).

Physical examination
Examine the patient according to the steps listed below.

Vital signs
• Observe the rate, quality, and depth of the patient's respirations.
• Check for a widened pulse pressure, which may indicate increasing ICP.
• Check apical pulse rate and rhythm.
• Check his temperature.

Inspection
• Determine the patient's orientation using the Glasgow Coma Scale.
• Note the quality of his speech.
• Observe his behavior for any unusual patterns.
• Examine the skin for pallor, cyanosis, icterus (jaundice), the cherry-red color of carbon monoxide poisoning, and diaphoresis. Look for evidence of hypodermic injections.
• Observe his pupils for equality and reaction to light and accommodation. Pinpoint pupils suggest either opiate overdose or a pontine CVA. Fixed and dilated pupils, an ominous sign, suggest severe CNS trauma. Lift the eyelids and let them close. Lagging of one lid suggests hemiplegia. In suspected hemiplegia, look for conjugate deviation of the eyes.
• Check for nystagmus by performing extraocular muscle testing.
• If the patient is unconscious, test his eyes for the doll's eye reflex (oculocephalic response) by briskly rotating the head from side to side or by briskly flexing and extending the neck. When the head is rotated, the eyes should move in the direction opposite to the head movement. When the neck is flexed, the eyes should ap-

pear to look upward. When the neck is extended, the eyes should look downward. When the doll's eye reflex is absent, the eyes do not move in the sockets, but follow the direction of passive rotation. Loss of the doll's eye reflex in the comatose patient indicates a severe lesion at the pontine-midbrain level of the brain stem. Do not test for doll's eye reflex in a trauma patient who may have a cervical vertebral fracture.
• Inspect his scalp and skull for contusions, lacerations, gunshot wounds, and clear CNS fluid or blood draining from his nose or ears.
• Check for evidence of incontinence, which may result from seizure activity.
• Observe for facial symmetry. Asymmetry of the face suggests hemiplegia. If the patient is comatose, pressure on the supraorbital bone will often cause a lopsided grimace, revealing the asymmetry.
• Examine the oral cavity. Look for evidence of tongue biting, pharyngitis, or evidence of discoloration that might suggest poisoning.
• Smell the breath for alcohol or the sweet fruity scent of diabetic ketoacidosis.
• Observe for seizure activity, abnormal posturing, or muscle spasm.

Palpation
• Palpate the skull for depressions, which may indicate a skull fracture.
• Palpate the facial bones for obvious deformities.
• If the patient can follow commands, have him bite down. Doing this without pain suggests an absence of facial bone fractures.
• If spinal cord injury has been ruled out, assess the neck for mobility.
• If the patient is comatose, lift each arm and let it drop, checking for muscle tone. In hemiplegia, the more

flaccid arm indicates the affected side.
• Test motor function and check for abnormal sensations.
• For comatose or stuporous patients, test for pain response by applying firm pressure to the nail beds (fingernails and toenails) and observing the motor response. Pinching the trapezius muscle or grasping the gastrocnemius muscle are other methods of providing a painful stimulus.
• If the patient can cooperate, test the cranial nerves.
• Palpate the abdomen for liver or spleen enlargement.

Percussion
• Test the patient's reflexes. Reflexes on the affected side are absent during the acute phase of a CVA. A patient in a deep coma will have no reflexes.
• Test the patient for Babinski's sign. With hemiplegia, the affected side demonstrates a positive Babinski's sign, but in a deep coma, there will be a bilateral Babinski's sign.

Auscultation
• Auscultate all lung fields, noting whether airflow is present bilaterally. Listen for adventitious breath sounds such as crackles, rhonchi, and wheezing.
• Auscultate heart sounds, noting rate, rhythm, and the presence of murmurs.

Confusion

This general term describes disordered thought processes. The patient may complain that he can no longer think quickly and coherently. Depending on its cause, confusion may arise suddenly or gradually and may

be temporary or irreversible. (See *Causes of confusion.*)

When severe confusion arises suddenly and the patient also has hallucinations and psychomotor hyperactivity, his condition is classified as *delirium*. Long-term, progressive confusion with deterioration of all cognitive functions is classified as *dementia*.

Delirium often results from alcohol or drug withdrawal, systemic illnesses (particularly when accompanied by fever), or head trauma. It's characterized by fluctuations in alertness and attention, disruption of the sleep cycle, disorganized thinking, incoherent speech, hallucinations, and disorientation. In elderly debilitated patients, delirium can signal the onset of a potentially fatal systemic illness. Delirium and acute psychosis produce similar clinical signs.

In contrast, dementia typically has a slowly progressive course. However, nonprogressive, static dementia can occur after head trauma or a cerebrovascular accident (CVA). Memory loss is usually the earliest symptom and eventually the patient's ability to carry out the activities of daily living is impaired. Pseudodementia refers to depression in elderly people that is mistaken for dementia. The distinction is important because depression is often treatable, while true dementia generally is not. (See *Distinguishing between delirium and dementia*, page 78.)

History of the symptom
In patients with delirium or dementia, an accurate history can only be obtained from family members, friends, or colleagues. In early dementia, the patient may be able to supply the history. To better characterize your patient's confusion, consider asking the following questions:

Causes of confusion

Neurologic disorders that may cause confusion include brain tumor, head injury, dementia, and seizure disorders.

Brain tumor
In the early stages of brain tumor, confusion is usually mild and difficult to detect. As the tumor impinges on cerebral structures, however, the patient's confusion worsens, and he may display personality changes, bizarre behavior, or sensory and motor deficits. He may also have visual field deficits and aphasia.

Head injury
Concussion, contusion, and brain hemorrhage may produce confusion at the time of injury, shortly afterward, or months or even years later. The patient may be delirious, with periodic loss of consciousness. Vomiting, severe headache, pupillary changes, and sensory and motor deficits are also common.

Dementia
This group of progressive brain diseases, such as Alzheimer's disease, eventually produces severe and irreversible confusion along with memory loss and intellectual deterioration. Disorientation, tremors, and gait disturbances may also occur.

Seizure disorders
Mild to moderate confusion may immediately follow any seizure and disappears within several hours.

Nonneurologic causes
Confusion may also occur secondary to acute psychosis, infections, heatstroke, high fever, hypothermia, systemic diseases, and severely impaired cardiac output.

Confusion may also result from metabolic disorders such as uremia, hepatic encephalopathy, severe hypoxemia or hypercarbia, hypoglycemia, hyperosmolarity, hyponatremia, hypercalcemia, Cushing's disease, thyroid hormone disorders, and thiamine, niacin, or vitamin B_{12} deficiency.

Drugs
Confusion may also be caused by intoxication or adverse effects secondary to the use of the following agents:
• alcohol
• analgesics
• antiarrhythmics, such as lidocaine and amiodarone
• antihistamines
• corticosteroids
• decongestants
• digitalis glycosides
• diuretics
• indomethacin
• psychotropics.

Acute confusion, possibly with delirium, may be caused by withdrawal from central nervous system depressants.

Distinguishing between delirium and dementia

Characteristics	Delirium	Dementia
Onset	Acute or slow	Insidious
Duration	Days to weeks; almost always worse at night	Permanent; commonly worse at night
Associated conditions	Drug abuse or withdrawal or systemic illness always present	No systemic conditions necessary
Attention span	Poor	Usually unaffected
Appearance	Slovenly	Often neat
Arousal level	Fluctuates from lethargy to agitation	Normal
Orientation to person, place, and time	Variably impaired for person and place, almost always for time	Impaired if disease results in social isolation
Cognition	Disorganized thoughts; hallucinations and illusions common	Delusions common
Speech and language	Dysarthric, slow, often not coherent and inappropriate	Aphasia possible
Memory	Impaired	Loss of recent memory with impaired remote memory

• Have you noticed any changes in your memory, speech, mood, behavior, or judgment? If so, how would you describe these changes?
• Have you had problems remaining alert? (typical in delirium)
• Have you had problems with vision, hearing, or walking?
• Have these changes been gradual, or did they occur suddenly?
• Are the changes becoming more noticeable? If yes, to whom?
• Have you had a similar problem in the past?
• Has there been a recent change in your medications?
• What other medical problems do you have, if any?

• Has there been any history of head trauma?

Associated findings

Note whether the patient has experienced any of the following signs or symptoms:
• altered respirations (hypoxia can cause confusion)
• arrhythmias or murmurs (may cause emboli and decreased central nervous system [CNS] perfusion)
• difficulty ambulating
• fever (may precipitate delirium)
• hypertension (a common cause of multi-infarct dementia)
• incontinence (incontinence and gait disturbance in dementia suggest normal pressure hydrocephalus)

- motor weakness or paralysis (suggests a CVA)
- muscle wasting (malnutrition can cause confusion)
- myoclonus (may indicate seizure disorder, severe liver or kidney disease, or advanced Alzheimer's disease)
- polyuria or polydipsia (can lead to dehydration, precipitating delirium)
- skin pallor and diaphoresis (suggest shock or hypoglycemia); cyanosis (suggests hypoxia); cherry-red color (suggests carbon monoxide poisoning).

Previous conditions

Consult with the patient, family members, or members of the health care team to determine if the patient has a history of any of the following risk factors:

- acquired immunodeficiency syndrome (dementia occurs in 50% of these patients and is related to CNS lesions and infection)
- atrial fibrillation (may cause a CVA from embolization)
- cancer (may cause CNS metastasis)
- diabetes (may lead to hypoglycemic or hyperglycemic coma)
- depression (pseudodementia)
- drug abuse, particularly of alcohol, barbiturates, and cocaine (abrupt withdrawal from these agents may precipitate delirium and seizures)
- head trauma
- Huntington's disease (causes eventual severe dementia)
- hypertension, smoking, or hypercholesterolemia (known risk factors for a CVA)
- hypothyroidism (may cause dementia if untreated)
- liver or kidney disease (may cause hepatic or uremic encephalopathy)
- Lyme disease (causes CNS symptoms in 8% of patients)
- malnutrition (may cause vitamin B deficiencies and anemia, both of which can cause dementia)
- Parkinson's disease
- severe heart failure
- severe lung disease
- syphilis (may cause neurosyphilitic dementia).

Drug therapy

Note any past or current use of the following drugs:

- alcohol
- antibiotics (particularly isoniazid and aminoglycosides)
- anticholinergic agents
- anticonvulsants
- antidepressants
- antihypertensives and other cardiovascular drugs
- antiparkinsonian agents
- chemotherapeutic drugs
- cocaine, amphetamines, or opiates
- GI drugs, such as cimetidine and metoclopramide
- high-dose vitamin therapy
- narcotics
- sedatives
- tranquilizers.

Physical examination

Conducting a physical examination of a delirious patient may require the help of other staff members or the judicious use of restraints. Physical examination findings may indicate significant, immediate health problems.

Demented patients, unless suffering from severe dementia, are usually cooperative. Physical examination findings are usually normal, apart from the cognitive impairment. Consider having a family member or friend present during the examination to reassure the patient.

Examine the patient according to the steps described below.

Vital signs

• Check the patient's temperature. Fever may indicate infection or dehydration, a possible cause of the delirium.

• Check his pulse. A weak or absent pulse suggests severely impaired peripheral perfusion from low cardiac output.

• Check his blood pressure. With diminished cardiac output, it will be low. A widened pulse pressure can indicate increasing intracranial pressure. High systolic and diastolic readings may be related to a CVA.

• Observe the rate, quality, and depth of the patient's respirations. Respiratory difficulty can lead to hypoxia or, in hyperventilation, to hypocarbia. High levels of oxygen in patients with long-standing respiratory disease can cause respiratory depression, with secondary hypoxia.

Inspection

• Perform a mental status test if the patient appears to be suffering from dementia.

• Complete a full neurologic evaluation of the patient.

CHAPTER 3

Monitoring neurologic status

Because signs and symptoms do not always provide a reliable indicator of neurologic deterioration, you may need to implement neurologic monitoring. The most commonly used techniques include intracranial pressure and cerebral blood flow monitoring. Two newer techniques are jugular venous oxygen saturation and regional cerebral oxygen saturation monitoring. (See *New techniques for monitoring neurologic status.*)

Intracranial pressure monitoring

Intracranial pressure (ICP) monitoring allows you to detect increases in ICP before signs and symptoms become evident. Prolonged increases in ICP can diminish cerebral blood flow and cause permanent brain damage or death. With ICP monitoring, interventions can be initiated before cerebral function is threatened. Prompt intervention can help avert or diminish neurologic damage caused by cerebral hypoxia and shifts of brain mass. (See *Understanding normal and elevated ICP,* pages 84 and 85, and *Detecting increased ICP promptly,* page 86.)

ICP monitoring is most often used for trauma patients, who are susceptible to cerebral edema. It's also used for patients with subarachnoid hemorrhage, tumors that obstruct the ventricular system, cerebral aneurysm, intracranial hemorrhage, or Reye's syndrome.

Types of monitoring devices

Although continuous ICP monitoring systems vary, all systems share three basic components: a sensor, a pressure transducer, and a recording de-

vice. The intracranial sensor, once implanted, signals changes in ICP to a transducer. The transducer then converts mechanical or light impulses into electrical impulses. A recording device converts the signals to visible tracings, which appear on an oscilloscope or are transferred to graph paper. Some systems also provide a digital readout of pressures. (See *Components of an ICP monitoring system,* page 87.)

Depending on the patient's condition and the doctor's preference, the intracranial sensor may be surgically implanted within the ventricle; subarachnoid, epidural, or subdural space; or brain parenchyma.

Implementation

A neurosurgeon inserts the ICP monitoring device into the patient in the operating room or emergency department, or at the bedside in the intensive care unit (ICU). You'll need to provide reassurance for the patient and his family members and assist the neurosurgeon in placing the device, as ordered.

Preparation

• Make sure that the patient is fully informed about the procedures involved in ICP monitoring and obtain a signed consent form. If the patient is unconscious, ask a family member to sign the consent form after you've explained the procedure.

• If the patient is awake, inform him that the surgeon will place a device inside his head to allow ICP monitoring. Mention that his head will be shaved beforehand and that a dressing will be placed over the site after the device is in place. Tell him that the monitoring system will restrict his movement. Reassure him that you'll check him frequently and that he'll receive analgesics as needed during the procedure.

• Whenever possible, the doctor will insert the monitoring device in the operating room. If he must insert it in the emergency department or ICU, be sure to use aseptic technique when preparing the area to prevent infection. Shave the insertion site; then clean it with a povidone-iodine solution.

• Also use aseptic technique when setting up and maintaining the external components that will be attached to the implanted device.

Timesaving tip: Talk to the patient while checking his ICP monitoring equipment and parameters. This conversation will allow you to assess his level of consciousness (LOC) and help you detect signs of deterioration more quickly.

• If you're using the fluid-filled catheter system, you'll probably have to prime the system before connecting it to the patient. Prime the pressure tubing — a one-piece unit consisting of a short length of tubing, a stopcock, and another length of tubing — with preservative-free 0.9% sodium chloride solution. Priming eliminates air in the tubing, which can cause inaccurate pressure readings. Prime the equipment completely from the point at which the pressure tubing attaches to the implanted device past both stopcocks to the drip chamber. You may attach the transducer at either stopcock. Then attach the tubing to the device to be implanted.

Timesaving tip: To save time, the transducer, stopcock, and pressure tubing may be primed in advance and placed inside a sterile towel or container until the time of insertion.

• If the patient will have a subarachnoid bolt inserted, gather a short length of pressure tubing and a stop-

New techniques for monitoring neurologic status

Jugular venous oxygen saturation monitoring

Continuous jugular venous oxygen saturation ($SjvO_2$) monitoring can detect cerebral ischemia after traumatic brain injury. In this technique, a fiber-optic oxygen saturation catheter is implanted percutaneously into the internal jugular vein with the tip of the catheter in the jugular bulb. When connected to a co-oximeter, oxygen saturation can be measured. Improvement in cerebral oxygen delivery is assessed by monitoring the arteriovenous difference of oxygen and $SjvO_2$.

Regional cerebral oxygen saturation monitoring

Regional cerebral oxygen saturation (rSO_2) monitoring, or cerebral oximetry, provides data about brain perfusion, ischemia, and hypoxia. This noninvasive technique focuses on the microvasculature of the brain, using infrared light sensors to monitor rSO_2. These sensors penetrate scalp, bone, and brain to a depth of several centimeters.

When an infrared sensor (adhesive pad) is affixed to the forehead, light-absorbing molecules in cerebral hemoglobin weaken the light and return a nonpulsating signal. This signaling provides brain oximetry values.

cock, or just a stopcock that fits directly onto the hollow bolt. Prime it completely with 0.9% sodium chloride solution, using aseptic technique.

Understanding normal and elevated ICP

Intracranial pressure (ICP) is the pressure exerted by the brain tissue, cerebrospinal fluid (CSF), and blood within the skull. ICP continuously fluctuates. Healthy individuals experience transient elevations with such movement as coughing, sneezing, and straining during bowel movements (Valsalva's maneuver). However, in patients with cranial insults or injuries, prolonged increases in ICP can diminish cerebral blood flow and cause irreversible brain damage or death.

Because the cranium is rigid and can't expand, maintaining normal ICP requires that intracranial volume remain nearly constant. Intracranial volume consists of brain volume (about 1,400 ml), blood volume (150 ml), and CSF volume (150 ml). An increase in the volume of any one of these components without a compensatory drop in another will cause ICP to rise above normal.

Compensatory mechanisms
Normally, several compensatory mechanisms maintain ICP within normal limits. These mechanisms are activated whenever intracranial volume

How decreasing compliance affects ICP

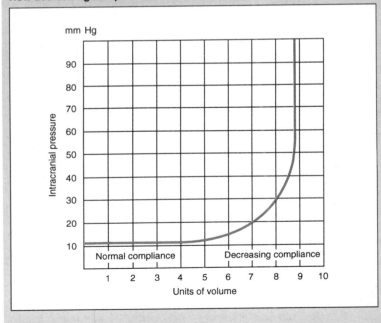

begins to increase. The most important compensatory mechanisms are:

• CSF displacement from the ventricles into the spinal subarachnoid space

• reduction of cerebral blood volume through shunting of venous blood out of the skull or reduced cerebral blood flow

• increased absorption of CSF into the arachnoid villi.

Cerebral compliance

Small increases in intracranial volume cause only minimal rises in ICP because compensatory mechanisms are able to handle the increased volume. *Cerebral compliance* is the ability of the brain to tolerate an increase in intracranial volume without a corresponding increase in pressure. However, large increases in volume can exhaust compensatory mechanisms, causing sharp elevations in ICP. As compensatory mechanisms fail and compliance decreases, ICP rises rapidly, leading to life-threatening complications.

As the graph at left shows, ICP remains within normal limits because of cerebral compliance when small volume increases occur. However, as intracranial volume continues to increase, compensatory mechanisms begin to fail. When compliance decreases, even small volume additions can cause dangerously sharp rises in ICP.

• If you're using the fiber-optic transducer–tipped catheter, preparation of the equipment usually involves only zeroing the system immediately before catheter insertion. Follow the manufacturer's directions closely. (See *Understanding ICP monitoring systems,* pages 88 to 90.)

Procedure

If the monitor will be inserted in the ICU or the emergency department, assist the surgeon as needed. Begin by preparing all required equipment.

• Using aseptic technique, prepare an insertion tray with a twist drill and various needles, syringes, hemostats, and sutures.

• Position the patient as ordered. Usually, the patient is placed in a supine position, with his head slightly elevated. The monitoring device is commonly placed on the right side anteriorly. However, if the device will be inserted during a craniotomy for hematoma or tumor removal, the surgical site determines monitor placement.

Attempt to determine from the patient or a family member if the patient is right-handed (left hemisphere dominant) or left-handed (right hemisphere dominant). Whenever possible, the ICP monitoring device is inserted on the side of the nondominant hemisphere.

Timesaving tip: To prevent unnecessary delay before the monitoring device's insertion, include the patient's right- or left-handedness in his initial history.

• If a fiber-optic transducer–tipped catheter or an epidural sensor will be inserted, help the surgeon balance the system. As he holds the cable at the patient end, attach the monitor end to the cable and turn the monitor on.

• If mean pressure on the monitor doesn't read zero, adjust the system

Assessment TimeSaver

Detecting increased ICP promptly

The earlier you recognize signs of increased intracranial pressure (ICP), the quicker you can intervene and the better the patient's chances of recovery. By the time late signs appear, intervention may not be able to avert irreversible brain damage. This chart shows you both early and late signs of increased ICP.

	Early signs	Late signs
Level of consciousness	• Subtle orientation loss • Restlessness • Sudden quietness	• Nonreactive pupils
Pupils	• Pupil changes on side of lesion • Unilateral pupil constriction, then dilation (unilateral hippus) • Sluggish bilateral pupil reaction • Unequal pupil size	• Fixed, dilated bilateral pupils ("blown pupils")
Motor response	• Sudden weakness • Motor changes on side opposite the lesion • Positive pronator drift (with palms up, one hand pronates)	• Profound weakness • Decerebration • Decortication
Vital signs	• Intermittent increases in blood pressure	• Increased systolic pressure • Profound bradycardia • Abnormal respirations (Cushing's response)

according to the manufacturer's guidelines until a zero appears.

• Monitor the patient's vital signs and neurologic response (unless he has received a paralytic agent).

• After the surgeon has inserted the device and sutured it in place, help him connect the transducer component.

• Document the initial ICP reading, waveform, and neurologic findings at the time of the monitoring device's insertion.

Timesaving tip: To save time, be sure to make a hard copy of the initial ICP waveform to help you troubleshoot the system later, if needed. Keep the hard copy readily available.

• After the procedure, clean the insertion site with a povidone-iodine solution and apply a dry, sterile occlusive dressing over the site.

Nursing considerations

After the monitoring system is in place, continue to assess the patient's

Components of an ICP monitoring system

Intracranial pressure (ICP) monitoring systems vary in the type of sensors they use and the location of sensor placement. The system illustrated here shows a fiber-optic transducer–tipped ventricular catheter in which the transducer and the sensor are combined in the tip. Other systems used to monitor ICP may have an external transducer.

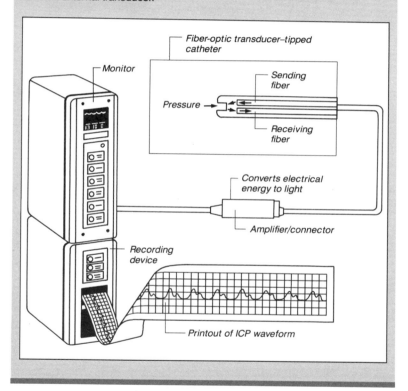

vital signs and neurologic status and check for signs of infection.
• Be sure to obtain ICP readings at the same time every day. Make sure the patient's head is in the same position for each reading. Keep the patient calm and relaxed before obtaining a reading.
• Check for trends, not isolated values, when measuring ICP. (See *Managing increased ICP,* page 91, and *Evaluating ICP measurements,* page 92.)

(Text continues on page 91.)

Understanding ICP monitoring systems

Intracranial pressure (ICP) monitoring systems use a variety of sensors, including the intraventricular catheter, subarachnoid bolt, epidural sensor, subdural sensor, and fiber-optic transducer–tipped catheter (for intraparenchymal monitoring). Besides monitoring ICP, some of these systems can also be used to drain cerebrospinal fluid (CSF) and relieve pressure.

How ICP monitoring systems work

Although ICP monitoring system designs vary, most work similarly. A fluid-filled line connects the catheter or bolt to a disposable transducer. This fluid-filled catheter system communicates the patient's ICP to the external transducer. The transducer then transmits pressure readings to a monitor for display.

When a fiber-optic transducer–tipped catheter is used, a fluid-filled transducer isn't required. The fiber-optic transducer–tipped catheter uses optical fibers and a specialized diaphragm to transmit light impulses produced by pressure changes inside the cranium. A miniature transducer at the tip of the catheter has a mirrored diaphragm, which reflects pressure changes and produces changes in light intensity. The light is transmitted by fiber optics to an amplifier, which converts the light impulses to electrical signals. These signals, in turn, produce oscilloscopic images.

Intraventricular catheter monitoring

This monitoring system measures ICP directly, allows evaluation of cerebral compliance, and permits CSF drainage. First, the surgeon drills a burr hole in the skull and inserts a small polyethylene or silicone rubber catheter into the lateral ventricle. Then he connects the catheter to a fluid-filled line that has an external transducer. (Alternatively, he may use a fiber-optic transducer–tipped catheter.)

Disadvantages

Because the monitoring catheter penetrates the cerebrum, the insertion procedure carries a risk of infection and brain damage. Contraindications typically include stenotic cerebral ventricles, a cerebral aneurysm in the path of catheter placement, or suspected vascular lesions.

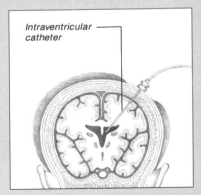

Intraventricular catheter

Subarachnoid bolt monitoring

In this monitoring system, a special bolt is inserted into the subarachnoid space through a twist-drill burr hole in the front of the skull. The bolt connects to a fluid-filled line that has an external transducer. Because the bolt doesn't penetrate the cerebrum, there is less risk of infection and parenchymal damage than with the intraventricular catheter. This system allows collection of small amounts of CSF for culture.

Disadvantages

Because this system doesn't penetrate the cerebrum, it doesn't allow drainage of large amounts of CSF. It also tends to become occluded more readily than the intraventricular catheter. This system can be used only in patients with an intact skull.

Epidural sensor monitoring

This monitoring system is the least invasive and carries the lowest infection risk. It uses a tiny fiber-optic sensor inserted into the epidural space through a burr hole. A cable connects the sensor to a monitor. Unlike an intraventricular catheter or a subarachnoid bolt, the sensor can't become occluded by blood or brain tissue. It can, however, become wedged against the bone of the skull (wedge effect).

Disadvantages

Because the epidural sensor doesn't measure ICP directly from a CSF-filled space, measurements may be less accurate. This method is contraindicated in patients who don't have an intact skull.

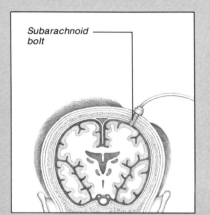

Subarachnoid bolt

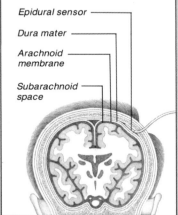

Epidural sensor

Dura mater

Arachnoid membrane

Subarachnoid space

(continued)

Understanding ICP monitoring systems *(continued)*

Subdural sensor monitoring

In this monitoring system, a tiny fiber-optic sensor is inserted into the subdural space through a burr hole. A cable connects the sensor to a monitor. Unlike an intraventricular catheter or a subarachnoid bolt, a subdural sensor can't become occluded by blood or brain tissue. It can, however, become wedged against the bone of the skull.

Disadvantages

This system cannot be used for CSF drainage.

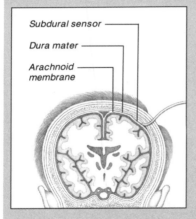

Subdural sensor

Dura mater

Arachnoid membrane

Intraparenchymal monitoring

In this monitoring system, the surgeon inserts a fiber-optic transducer–tipped catheter through a small subarachnoid bolt. After puncturing the dura mater, the surgeon advances the catheter a few centimeters into the brain's white matter. There's no need to balance or calibrate the equipment after insertion.

Although this method doesn't provide direct access to CSF, measurements of ICP are accurate because brain tissue pressures correlate well with ventricular pressures. This system may be used to obtain ICP measurements in patients with compressed or dislocated ventricles.

Disadvantages

This system cannot be used for CSF drainage.

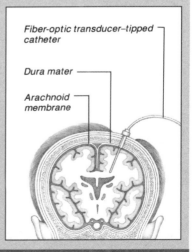

Fiber-optic transducer–tipped catheter

Dura mater

Arachnoid membrane

Managing increased ICP

By performing interventions carefully, you can avoid further increases in intracranial pressure (ICP) and even reduce it significantly. Here are steps you can take to manage increased ICP.

• Plan your care to include rest periods between activities. This planning allows the patient's ICP to return to baseline, thus avoiding lengthy and cumulative pressure elevations.

• Try to speak to the patient before attempting any procedures, even if he appears comatose. Touch him on an arm or leg first before touching him in a more personal area, such as the face or chest. This is especially important if the patient doesn't know you or if he's confused or sedated.

• Suction the patient only when needed to remove secretions and maintain airway patency; suctioning may increase ICP. Avoid depriving him of oxygen for long periods and monitor his heart rate while suctioning; always hyperventilate the patient with oxygen before, during, and after the procedure.

• Promote venous drainage. Keep the patient's head in the midline position, even when he's lying on his side. Avoid neck or hip flexion greater than 90 degrees, and keep the head of the bed elevated 30 to 45 degrees.

• To avoid increasing intrathoracic pressure, which raises ICP, discourage Valsalva's maneuver and isometric muscle contractions. To avoid isometric contractions, distract the patient when giving him painful injections (by asking him to wiggle his toes and by massaging the area before injection to relax the muscle). Have him concentrate on breathing during difficult procedures such as bed-to-stretcher transfers. Tell the patient to relax as much as possible during position changes so that he doesn't hold his breath when moving around in bed. If necessary, administer a stool softener to help prevent constipation and unnecessary straining during bowel movements.

• If the patient is heavily sedated, monitor respiratory rate and arterial blood gas levels. Depressed respirations will compromise ventilations and oxygen exchange. Maintaining adequate respiratory rate and volume helps reduce ICP.

• If you're in a specialty unit, you may be able to routinely hyperventilate the patient to counter sustained ICP elevations. This procedure is one of the best ways to reduce high ICP at bedside for short periods. Follow your hospital's policy.

• If the patient will have a fluid-filled monitoring system in place, ensure that all connections are tight and that the system is air-free. Air in the system can cause damped waveforms and alter ICP values. Zero the system at least every 8 hours, and maintain the transducer at the level of the foramen of Monro.

Assessment TimeSaver

Evaluating ICP measurements

When you assess your patient's intracranial pressure (ICP), keep in mind that clinical trends are far more important than isolated values. Whenever possible, correlate ICP trends with clinical findings. Use the chart below as a quick reference to help you identify values that are within normal limits or moderately or severely elevated.

	ICP measurement	
Description	mm Hg	mm H_2O
Normal	4 to 15	50 to 200
Moderately elevated	15 to 40	200 to 540
Severely elevated	40 or greater	540 or greater

• If the patient has an implanted catheter attached to a drainage system, maintain the height of the drip chamber at the ordered level so that the system drains at the desired pressure. When draining, observe the fluid flowing into the drip chamber; drainage of more than 3 ml of fluid at a time may cause ventricular collapse. Assess the system's patency by observing drainage for color, clarity, blood, and sediment. Also document the amount of drainage.

• Observe the monitor insertion site every 8 hours, if accessible, for redness and drainage. If you see drainage, determine whether it's cerebrospinal fluid (CSF) by checking for a blood-tinged spot surrounded by a lighter ring of CSF (halo sign) on the patient's pillow or by testing drainage for glucose. Notify the doctor if you suspect CSF leakage because it increases the risk of infection.

• To help prevent infection, change the sterile dressing daily. After removing the old dressing, clean the site with a povidone-iodine solution.

Then apply a new sterile occlusive dressing.

• If the surgeon orders prophylactic antibiotics given through an intraventricular catheter, monitor the patient's cerebral compliance. Instilling antibiotics into this type of catheter may compromise a patient with low cerebral compliance. Carefully observe how much ICP increases after antibiotic therapy; an increase of 5 mm Hg may suggest low cerebral compliance.

• Make sure all caregivers know that an ICP monitoring system is in place, especially if the patient has an intraventricular catheter (which may cause CSF loss).

• If the doctor has ordered CSF drainage, unplug the bed to prevent accidentally changing the level of the patient's head relative to the drainage bag. Minimize activities around the patient to avoid causing a rise in ICP. Turn alarm volumes low, keep bright lights to a minimum, and schedule diagnostic tests and procedures so the patient gets adequate rest and ICP can return to baseline between periods of stimulation. Alert all caregivers to use sterile gloves when manipulating the dressing.

• Use aseptic technique and follow hospital policy when obtaining CSF specimens for culture and analysis. Ideally, you should obtain specimens from the port closest to the ventricle. Most systems have a stopcock or a Y-port just distal to the patient connection point.

• To prevent infection, use a sterile drape under the stopcock when you are withdrawing CSF from invasive devices, such as intraventricular catheters and subarachnoid bolts.

• Document all ICP trends, the condition of the monitoring site, and vital signs. If you see CSF leakage, document the amount and color.

Complications

Each ICP monitoring system carries certain inherent risks, but infection is always the most serious threat. The risk of infection rises when an intraventricular catheter is used, monitoring lasts more than 5 days, the system is flushed, and an open system is used. To prevent infection, always use strict aseptic technique when setting up and maintaining the system. Also monitor the patient for signs of infection (such as chills, fever, elevated white blood cell count) or signs of redness or swelling around the catheter insertion site. Be alert for other complications of ICP monitoring, such as excessive drainage of CSF, clots in the catheter or pressure tubing, and increased ICP.

Interpretation of findings

Continuous ICP monitoring usually provides two types of data: a digital readout of the patient's actual ICP and a dynamic recording of ICP waveforms.

Digital readout

Begin by noting the digital readout of actual ICP. Compare this reading to normal ICP values, which range from 4 to 15 mm Hg (50 to 200 mm H_2O).

ICP waveforms

Examine the ICP waveform. Abnormal waveforms are classified as A, B, and C waves. These waveforms provide important clues about your patient's condition. (See *Interpreting ICP waveforms,* pages 94 and 95.)

A waves are an ominous sign of intracranial decompensation and poor cerebral compliance. They may be sudden and transient, spiking from temporary rises in thoracic pressure or from any other condition that increases ICP beyond cerebral compliance limits. Typically, A waves denote cerebral ischemia and further brain injury. In pressure readings above 20 mm Hg, they presumably reflect permanent cell damage from hypoxia. A waves may be accompanied by changes in neurologic status, such as deterioration in LOC, altered respiratory pattern, headache, nausea, vomiting, abnormal pupil reaction, and altered motor function.

B waves correlate with changes in respiration and may occur more frequently with decreasing compensation. Because B waves sometimes precede A waves, you should notify the doctor if your patient has frequent B waves.

C waves, which are considered clinically insignificant, reflect normal changes in systemic arterial pressure. They may fluctuate with respirations.

Be aware that unusual waveforms also may be signs that equipment isn't working properly. For example,

(Text continues on page 96.)

Interpretation

Interpreting ICP waveforms

You may see various types of intracranial pressure (ICP) waveforms on your patient's bedside monitor.

Normal waveform
A normal waveform shows a steep upward systolic slope, followed by a downward diastolic slope with a dicrotic notch.

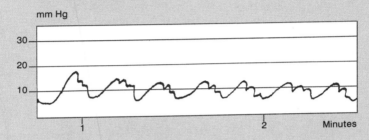

A waves
A waves, which usually occur when ICP is elevated, are commonly called plateau waves because of their shape. A waves may reach an amplitude of 50 to 100 mm Hg, last for 5 to 20 minutes, then drop sharply — signaling exhaustion of cerebral compliance mechanisms. A waves are the most clinically significant ICP waveforms, typically denoting cerebral ischemia and brain injury.

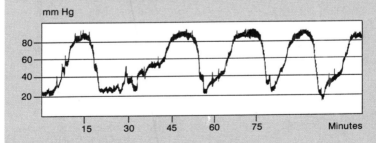

Interpretation

Interpreting ICP waveforms *(continued)*

B waves

Sharp and rhythmic, with a sawtooth pattern, B waves may occur as frequently as every 1½ to 2 minutes and may reach an amplitude of 50 mm Hg. B waves correlate with changes in respiration and may occur more frequently with decreased compensation. They may precede A waves.

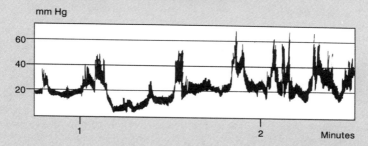

C waves

C waves are rapid and rhythmic, but not as sharp as B waves. They usually occur every 4 to 8 minutes and have an amplitude of about 20 mm Hg. Clinically insignificant, C waves may fluctuate with respirations. They reflect normal changes in systemic arterial pressure.

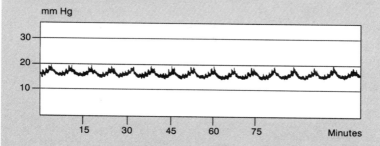

if the waveform is a flat line, suspect that tissue herniation has occluded the catheter tip. Notify the doctor immediately.

Monitoring device removal

The surgeon may discontinue ICP monitoring if the patient's ICP has been stable for 2 to 3 days or if CSF drainage is not required. To assist in removal of the monitoring device, follow these steps:

• Obtain sterile gloves, a dry dressing, suture material, sterile scissors, and forceps for the surgeon. The surgeon removes the anchoring suture and the monitoring device. Then he closes the insertion site with a suture and places a dry dressing over it.

• For the first 24 hours, observe the site frequently for CSF leakage. Also observe carefully for any sign of infection, including meningitis.

• For 2 to 3 days after monitor removal, maintain the site with sterile dressings.

Cerebral blood flow monitoring

This type of monitoring provides information about the adequacy of blood flow to the brain. For the brain to function normally, about 20% of the resting body's cardiac output is needed to supply adequate amounts of oxygen and nutrients. In an average adult, normal resting cerebral blood flow (CBF) is 50 ml/100 g/ minute. Normally, CBF remains relatively constant, despite changes in systemic arterial pressure. (See *How CBF is maintained.*)

If CBF exceeds the amount of blood required for metabolism, hyperemia — an excess of blood — oc-

curs, causing intracranial hypertension. If CBF falls too low, cerebral ischemia occurs, depriving the brain of adequate oxygen and placing the patient at risk for permanent neurologic damage or death.

Monitoring techniques

Traditionally, CBF in neurologically compromised patients has been estimated by calculating cerebral perfusion pressure (CPP), which is the pressure required to perfuse brain cells. (See *Estimating CPP,* page 98.) However, this method provides only an estimate of CBF and may not be reliable in patients with severely injured cerebral tissue.

Continuous regional blood flow monitoring, a newer and more accurate method, permits monitoring at the bedside. A sensor placed on the cerebral cortex continuously measures cortical blood flow, then calculates CBF in the capillary bed by thermal diffusion. Thermistors within the sensor detect the temperature differential between two metallic plates — one heated and one neutral. The temperature differential is inversely related to CBF: The smaller the differential, the higher the CBF — and vice versa. The sensor is attached to a computer data system, or a small, battery-powered, easily transported analog monitor.

CBF monitoring is indicated whenever alterations in the patient's CBF are anticipated. It yields continuous real-time values, which are essential in conditions such as ischemia and infarction, where compromised blood flow may put the patient at risk. It also provides important information about the effects of interventions on CBF. It's used most commonly in patients with subarachnoid hemorrhage (in which a vasospasm may restrict blood flow), trauma as-

How CBF is maintained

In healthy people, autoregulation maintains cerebral blood flow (CBF) at near-normal levels despite a wide variation in mean arterial pressure (MAP). This mechanism allows cerebral vessels to dilate or constrict to maintain a constant blood flow to cerebral tissues. Both metabolic and pressure-related factors contribute to autoregulation.

Metabolic factors
When by-products of cellular metabolism accumulate, the result is excess carbon dioxide and hydrogen ions, which are potent vasodilators. They increase blood flow to the brain.

Pressure-related factors
When MAP drops, the cerebral arteries dilate. This response ensures adequate blood flow to the brain despite low arterial pressures. Conversely, the cerebral arteries constrict with high distending pressures, thereby preventing the delivery of high systemic arterial pressure to brain tissue. After brain injury, autoregulation may fail. When this occurs, vasomotor tone diminishes and CBF becomes passively dependent on changes in systemic blood pressure.

Maintaining cerebral autoregulation
For the brain to maintain cerebral autoregulation:
• intracranial pressure must be lower than 35 mm Hg
• the MAP must range from 60 to 160 mm Hg
• cerebral perfusion pressure must range from 50 to 150 mm Hg.

sociated with high intracranial pressure (ICP), or vascular tumors.

Implementation
Typically, the surgeon inserts the sensor in the operating room, during or at completion of a craniotomy, far from major blood vessels. (See *Placing a CBF sensor,* page 99.) You'll need to reassure the patient and family members, assist the surgeon as needed, and monitor the patient afterward.

Preparation
• Make sure that the patient or a family member is fully informed about the procedures involved in CBF monitoring, and obtain a consent form.
• If the patient will need CBF monitoring after surgery, inform him that a sensor will be in place for about 3 days postoperatively to measure CBF. Tell him that the insertion site will be covered with a dry, sterile dressing. Mention that the sensor may be removed at the bedside.
• Depending on the type of system you're using, you may need to verify that a battery has been inserted in the monitor to allow CBF monitoring during patient transport to the ICU. Otherwise, no special equipment setup is needed.

Assessment TimeSaver

Estimating CPP

Although continuous monitoring is the optimal method to evaluate cerebral blood flow (CBF), you can get a quick estimate by calculating cerebral perfusion pressure (CPP), which serves as a rough index of the adequacy of CBF.

To determine CPP, simply subtract the patient's intracranial pressure (ICP) from his mean arterial pressure (MAP). Be aware of the following:

• In adults, CPP normally ranges from 50 to 150 mm Hg. Inadequate CPP results in ischemia, which progresses to neuronal hypoxia and cell death.

• When CPP falls below 60 mm Hg, the patient is in danger of irreversible ischemia.

• When ICP and MAP are equal, CPP is 0 mm Hg and CBF ceases.

Procedure
• Be prepared to assist the surgeon in setting up the monitoring system.

• If ordered, attach the distal end of the sensor to the monitor. After the sensor is in place, turn the monitor on. To calibrate the system, turn the RUN/CAL switch to CAL, and adjust the ZERO ADJUST knob until the digital readout is 0.00. Then adjust the knob to the lock position, and turn the RUN/CAL switch to RUN.

• Document the baseline CBF value.

Nursing considerations
• Document CBF values hourly. Be sure to check for trends and correlate values with the patient's clinical sta-

tus. Lack of correlation may indicate monitoring system malfunction. Record CPP readings on a regular basis to permit assessment of trends.

• Be aware that stimulation or activity may cause a 10% increase or decrease in CBF. If you note a 20% change, suspect poor contact between the sensor and the cerebral cortex. To correct this, turn the patient toward the side of the sensor or gently wiggle the catheter back and forth (using a sterile gloved hand). Determine if these maneuvers have improved contact between the sensor and the cortex by observing the CBF value on the monitor as you perform them.

• If your patient has low CBF but no neurologic symptoms that indicate ischemia, suspect a fluid layer (a small hematoma) between the sensor and the cortex. Notify the doctor.

• Change the dressing at the insertion site, as ordered, to reduce the risk of infection. After cleaning the site with a povidone-iodine solution (if ordered), apply a new dry, aseptic dressing. Be sure to use sterile technique during dressing changes. Administer prophylactic antibiotics if prescribed.

• Observe the site for cerebrospinal fluid (CSF) leakage, which increases the risk of infection.

Complications
As with ICP monitoring, CBF monitoring may lead to infection. To reduce the risk of this complication, administer prophylactic antibiotics, as prescribed, and maintain a sterile dressing around the insertion site. CSF leakage, another potential complication, may occur at the sensor insertion site. To prevent leakage, the surgeon may place an additional suture at the site.

Placing a CBF sensor

Typically, the surgeon inserts a cerebral blood flow (CBF) sensor during a craniotomy. He tunnels the sensor toward the craniotomy site and then carefully inserts the neutral and heated metallic plates of the thermistor to make sure that they are always in contact with the surface of the cerebral cortex. After closing the dura and replacing the bone flap, he closes the scalp. The CBF sensor, once connected to a monitor, continuously measures cortical CBF.

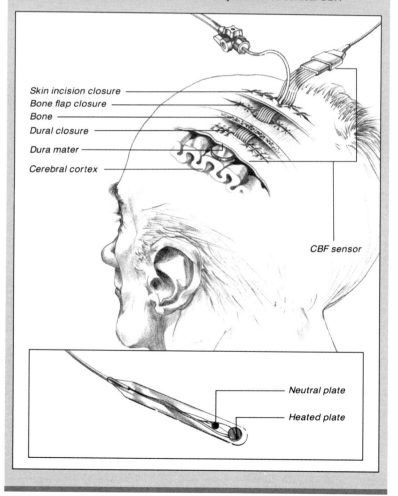

Skin incision closure
Bone flap closure
Bone
Dural closure
Dura mater
Cerebral cortex

CBF sensor

Neutral plate
Heated plate

Interpretation of findings
CBF fluctuates with the brain's metabolic demands, normally ranging from 60 to 90 ml/100 g/minute. However, the patient's neurologic condition dictates the acceptable range. For instance, in a comatose patient, CBF may be half the normal value; in a patient in a barbiturate-induced coma with burst suppression on the EEG, CBF may be as low as 10 ml/100 g/minute. Vasospasm secondary to subarachnoid hemorrhage may result in a CBF that is below 40 ml/100g/minute. In a patient who is awake, CBF above 90 ml/100 g/minute may indicate hyperemia.

Sensor removal
When the surgeon decides to discontinue monitoring (usually after 72 hours), gather a suture removal set and sterile gloves. The surgeon removes the anchoring suture and then gently removes the sensor from the insertion site. He closes the wound with a stitch.
• Carefully observe and document the condition of the site, and document leakage, if any.
• For the first 24 hours, observe carefully for any sign of infection, including meningitis.
• For 2 to 3 days after sensor removal, maintain the site with sterile dressings.

CHAPTER 4

Caring for patients with head, neck, or spinal injuries

Concussion

The most common closed head injury, concussion occurs when the brain is mildly jostled inside the skull. It causes a transient loss of cerebral function but no structural damage. A mild concussion doesn't usually cause loss of consciousness or memory loss; it merely dazes the patient. A severe concussion may cause temporary neurologic dysfunction, unconsciousness, and memory loss. Recovery usually occurs swiftly, within minutes to hours.

Causes
Any blow to the head can cause a concussion. Most often, it results from a fall, a motor vehicle accident, or a punch to the head.

ASSESSMENT

Your assessment should include careful consideration of the patient's history (including probable cause of the concussion), physical examination findings, and diagnostic test results.

Health history
The patient may report headache, nausea, transient vomiting, and dizziness. He may also experience confusion, irritability, giddiness, impaired memory, and fatigue.

Find out as many details as you can. Did the patient receive a blow to the head? If he did, he may report a period of unconsciousness or visual disturbances, such as "seeing stars." If he was knocked unconscious, does he know for how long? Does he recall the injury and the events leading up to it? Can he remember what happened after the injury?

If the patient has postconcussional syndrome, he may report symptoms that have persisted for several weeks or months. (See *Recognizing postconcussional syndrome.*)

Physical examination
The physical examination may not reveal any neurologic deficits. However, you may observe transient gait disturbances or abnormal pupil responses. In some instances, the patient may have an area of scalp tenderness as a result of the injury.

Diagnostic test results
The following tests can help evaluate the extent of injury:
• Computed tomography scan may reveal a focal lesion.
• Skull X-rays will help to rule out fractures and more serious injuries.
• Magnetic resonance imaging may reveal focal lesions, fractures, or tissue damage.

NURSING DIAGNOSIS

Common nursing diagnoses for a patient with concussion include:
• Pain (headache) related to a blow to the head or postconcussional syndrome
• High risk for injury related to impaired judgment
• Sleep pattern disturbance related to headache, nausea or vomiting, and the need for frequent neurologic evaluations.

PLANNING

Based on the nursing diagnosis *pain,* develop appropriate patient outcomes. For example, your patient will:
• rate his headache on a scale of 1 to 10

• report relief from headache within 45 minutes of drug administration
• describe pain-relief strategies to be used after discharge.

Based on the nursing diagnosis *high risk for injury,* develop appropriate patient outcomes. For example, your patient will:
• remain free from injury while post-concussional symptoms are present
• describe which activities to avoid to prevent injury.

Based on the nursing diagnosis *sleep pattern disturbance,* develop appropriate patient outcomes. For example, your patient will:
• sleep a minimum of 2 hours without interruption
• identify strategies to return to sleep quickly after arousal
• report that he feels rested.

IMPLEMENTATION

Treatment for concussion includes maintaining stable vital signs and monitoring for seizures, especially in children. Most patients require only bed rest, observation, and acetaminophen for headache.

Nursing interventions
• Initially, monitor vital signs continuously and check for additional injuries.
• Continue to check vital signs, level of consciousness (LOC), and pupil size every 15 minutes. If the patient's condition worsens or fluctuates, he should be admitted for further neurologic evaluation. If he remains stable after a few hours of observation, he can be discharged (with a head injury instruction sheet) in the care of a responsible adult.
• Observe the patient for signs of headache, dizziness, irritability, and anxiety. If his condition worsens, per-

Assessment TimeSaver

Recognizing post-concussional syndrome

Signs and symptoms of postconcussional syndrome may persist for several weeks or months. So, when assessing the patient with lingering complaints after a concussion, be alert for:
• headache (most common complaint)
• fatigue
• dizziness and loss of balance
• occasional double vision
• increased sensitivity to light and noise
• loss of memory and an inability to concentrate
• emotional lability (easily upset, irritable)
• desire to avoid crowds
• difficulty relating to others
• loss of inhibitions
• loss of libido
• change in alcohol tolerance.

form a complete neurologic evaluation and notify the doctor.
• Observe seizure precautions if the patient has a history of seizures.
• Administer prescribed analgesics and promote rest to help relieve the patient's headache.

Patient teaching
Focus on teaching the patient and his family how to manage the aftereffects of concussion.
• Explain to the patient that headache is common and should be relieved with acetaminophen and rest. Tell him to avoid activities that may cause fatigue. Occasionally, a cool compress applied to the frontal region also helps.

Discharge TimeSaver

Ensuring continued care for the patient with concussion

Review the following teaching topics, referrals, and follow-up appointments to make sure that your patient is adequately prepared for discharge.

Teaching topics
Make sure that the following topics have been covered and that your patient's learning has been evaluated:
☐ explanation of the disorder, its risk factors, and its complications
☐ signs of a worsening condition (increased drowsiness or difficulty awakening, confusion, worsened headache, and persistent vomiting)
☐ who to call if symptoms worsen during the first 48 hours
☐ an understanding of postconcussional syndrome and amnesia.

Referrals
Make sure that the patient has been provided with necessary referrals to:
☐ home health care agency
☐ rehabilitation facility for physical, occupational, or speech therapy
☐ head injury support group, if necessary.

Follow-up appointments
Make sure that the necessary follow-up appointments have been scheduled and that the patient has been notified:
☐ doctor or clinic
☐ neurologist if necessary.

• Instruct the caregiver to observe the patient closely for the first 24 hours after injury. Tell him to wake the patient every 2 hours during the night to assess how easily he's aroused and to evaluate his degree of alertness once awake. Emphasize the importance of bringing the patient to the hospital if he's difficult to arouse or disoriented or if his headache worsens.

• If the patient becomes nauseated or vomits more than once, tell him or the caregiver to call the doctor or return to the hospital. This may be a sign of a more serious injury.

• Instruct the caregiver to be alert for seizures (most common with children). If they occur, he should bring the patient to the hospital promptly.

• Give the patient and his family written information about necessary follow-up care and postconcussional syndrome. (See *Ensuring continued care for the patient with concussion*.)

EVALUATION

When evaluating the patient's response to your care, gather reassessment data and compare this information to the patient outcomes specified in your plan of care. Consider asking the following questions:

• Does the patient report that headache pain has diminished after receiving prescribed medications?

• Can he describe pain-relief strategies to be used after discharge?

• Can he list which activities to avoid to prevent injury?

• Can he sleep at least 2 hours without interruption, and can he describe strategies to return to sleep quickly?

• Does he report feeling rested?

Cerebral contusion

Cerebral contusion is an ecchymosis of brain tissue that results from acceleration-deceleration or coup-contrecoup injuries. Contusions can occur at any place on the cortical surface. Most commonly, they affect the cerebral hemispheres, especially the undersurface of the temporal and frontal lobes and the anterior segments of the temporal lobes.

Seizures may occur immediately after the trauma or months later. Other complications may include hemorrhage of surface vessels, increased intracranial pressure (ICP), herniation, hydrocephalus, coagulopathy, residual headache, and vertigo. Complications associated with immobility may include pneumonia, urinary tract infection, and pressure ulcers.

Causes and types

A contusion occurs when the head strikes or is struck by an object. A *coup* injury indicates a contusion directly beneath the site of impact. A *contrecoup* injury indicates a contusion directly opposite the site of impact. A combination of these injuries, called a *coup-contrecoup* injury, may also occur. Common coup-contrecoup sites include bilateral temporal regions and frontal-occipital lobes. A blow to the vertex of the head may cause cerebellar or brain stem contusions.

ASSESSMENT

Signs and symptoms reflect the area of injury. Large, bilateral lesions cause a frontal lobe syndrome characterized by inappropriate behavior and cognitive deficits. Small, unilateral, frontal lobe lesions may not pro-

Assessment TimeSaver

Signs of increased ICP

Signs of increased intracranial pressure (ICP) depend on its progression.

Early signs
• Deterioration in level of consciousness (LOC)
• Changes in pupillary size, shape, and response to light
• Motor weakness, such as monoparesis or hemiparesis
• Sensory deficits
• Cranial nerve palsy
• Headache
• Seizures

Later signs
• Continued deterioration in LOC, progressing to coma
• Pupillary changes, including bilateral dilation and nonreaction to light, resulting from herniation
• Vomiting
• Headache
• Hemiplegia, decortication, or decerebration
• Altered vital signs, including respiratory irregularities
• Impaired brain stem reflexes, such as corneal and gag reflexes

duce symptoms. If hemorrhage or swelling develops, the patient may exhibit signs of increased ICP. (See *Signs of increased ICP.*)

Health history

The patient's history (usually obtained from family, friends, and emergency personnel) may reveal a severe blow to the head or a hard impact, as occurs in a motor vehicle ac-

Assessment TimeSaver

Signs of common types of contusions

Listed below are signs of the most common types of contusions.

Frontal and parietal lobe contusion
- Depressed level of consciousness
- Dysphasia or aphasia (if the contusion is on the dominant hemisphere)
- Hemiparesis or paralysis
- Flexor posturing
- Focal or generalized seizures
- Pupil alterations (unilateral dilation with slow reaction to light on the same side as the lesion)

Brain stem contusion
- Absent response to verbal or painful stimuli
- Fever above 102.5° F (39.2° C)
- Increased pulse and respiratory rates
- Profuse perspiration
- Pupil changes (constricted, sluggish, or nonresponsive to light)
- Abnormal or absent doll's eye reflex
- Vomiting
- Hiccups
- Otorrhea
- Battle's sign
- Flaccid, bilateral paresis or paralysis
- Cranial nerve palsies

cident or a fall. A period of unconsciousness lasting up to an hour may follow.

Ask any witnesses if the patient has been abusing alcohol or drugs. Substance abuse can affect the patient's neurologic response and may influence the treatment plan.

Physical examination
An unconscious patient may appear pale and lifeless, whereas a conscious patient may appear drowsy or easily disturbed by any form of stimulation, such as noise or light. A conscious patient may even become agitated or violent.

If possible, perform a full neurologic assessment to establish a baseline. Assess for altered level of consciousness (LOC), limb weakness or paralysis, speech difficulty, memory loss, headache, neck stiffness, and vision changes. Observe the patient's pupils — an early indicator of neurologic deterioration — for size, shape, and reaction to light. Be alert for signs of seizure. Check for severe scalp wounds, labored respirations and, possibly, incontinence.

If the patient exhibits signs of shock, look for other injuries. If he's unconscious and in shock, he may have below-normal blood pressure and temperature. His pulse rate may be within normal levels but feeble, and his respirations may be shallow. If he's conscious, his temperature, pulse rate, and respiratory status may vary. (See *Signs of common types of contusions.*)

Diagnostic test results
Computed tomography scans and magnetic resonance imaging can diagnose contusion. Both tests reveal ischemic tissue, cerebral edema, areas of petechial hemorrhage, and subdural, epidural, and intracerebral hematomas. Skull X-rays can rule out fractures.

NURSING DIAGNOSIS

Common nursing diagnoses for a patient with cerebral contusion include:
• Altered cerebral tissue perfusion related to the contusion and resultant edema
• Altered thought processes related to brain injury
• High risk for injury related to altered LOC and seizures.

PLANNING

Based on the nursing diagnosis *altered cerebral tissue perfusion,* develop appropriate patient outcomes. For example, your patient will:
• score between 11 and 15 on the Glasgow Coma Scale
• have an ICP of 15 mm Hg or less
• exhibit pupils that are equal and reactive to light.

Based on the nursing diagnosis *altered thought processes,* develop appropriate patient outcomes. For example, your patient will:
• be oriented to person, place, and time
• be able to make informed decisions.

Based on the nursing diagnosis *high risk for injury,* develop appropriate patient outcomes. For example, your patient will:
• remain free of injury throughout hospitalization
• be able to identify and correct hazards in the home environment.

IMPLEMENTATION

A patient with a small contusion may require only neurologic monitoring. A large contusion may require aggressive treatment. (See *Medical care of the patient with contusion,* page 108.)

Nursing interventions
• Stay alert for signs of increasing ICP, such as changes in LOC, increasing lethargy, restlessness, and altered responses to stimuli, such as flexor or extensor posturing. Also be alert for changes in pupil size or response to light.
• Monitor vital signs and respirations regularly (usually every 15 minutes). Abnormal respirations could indicate damage to the brain's respiratory center and possibly an impending transtentorial herniation — a neurologic emergency.
• Maintain a patent airway and adequate oxygenation.
• If the patient is intubated, hyperventilation may be ordered to control ICP. Keep the partial pressure of arterial carbon dioxide ($PaCO_2$) between 25 and 30 mm Hg. Avoid severe hyperventilation because it can constrict cerebral vessels and lead to infarction of healthy tissue.
• Monitor arterial blood gas values frequently.
• Use an indwelling urinary catheter and closely monitor intake and output. Attempt to keep the patient normovolemic. If ICP rises, osmotic diuretics like mannitol or furosemide can achieve hypovolemia.
• Elevate the head of the bed to 30 degrees, and keep the patient's head in the midline position to promote venous drainage and decrease ICP.
• Protect the patient from injury by raising side rails on the bed.
• If the patient is unconscious, use artificial tears to avoid drying of the eyes and subsequent corneal damage.
• Discuss with the doctor the insertion of a nasogastric (NG) tube if the patient is unconscious and needs enteral feedings. An NG tube should be inserted only if a basilar skull fracture has been ruled out. If tube insertion becomes necessary before the frac-

Treatments

Medical care of the patient with contusion

Treatment of cerebral contusion aims to correct inadequate cerebral oxygenation, control increased intracranial pressure (ICP), and manage complications, such as herniation syndromes.

Providing adequate oxygenation

Adequate oxygen, a patent airway and, possibly, ventilation support, are necessary to correct inadequate cerebral oxygenation. The doctor may insert an endotracheal or tracheostomy tube for secretion removal and oxygen delivery.

Controlling increased ICP

Measures used to treat increased ICP depend on the patient's condition and may include:
- hyperventilating the patient
- administering osmotic diuretics, such as mannitol or furosemide

- giving corticosteroids
- managing blood pressure
- administering skeletal muscle relaxants or neuromuscular blockers, such as pancuronium
- giving sedative-hypnotics, such as benzodiazepines and barbiturates
- controlling body temperature
- limiting fluid intake
- draining cerebrospinal fluid
- controlling seizure activity by administering an anticonvulsant drug such as phenytoin
- inducing barbiturate coma.

Preventing herniation syndromes

If pressure from contused brain tissue threatens to cause herniation, the doctor may perform surgical decompression (probably in the temporal or frontal lobes). In this treatment, necrotic tissue is debrided.

---

ture is ruled out, an orogastric tube is usually recommended. If the patient requires long-term enteral feedings, the doctor may consider the use of a percutaneous endoscopic gastrostomy tube.
- Explain each procedure in a calm, even voice and observe for changes in vital signs. An increase in heart rate or blood pressure in response to a familiar voice may mean a lightening of coma in the unconscious patient.
- Assess frequently for signs of pain and administer analgesics as necessary. Use codeine because it causes less suppression of LOC.

- Observe the patient for agitated behavior. If he's awake and alert, observe for headache, dizziness, increased restlessness, nausea, or vomiting.

Patient teaching

Because of the patient's cognitive difficulties, you may need to include the patient's family or friends in your teaching.
- Forewarn the family that the patient may undergo transient periods of agitation, even aggressive behavior. Also warn them that, in severe instances, he may even undergo a permanent alteration in personality.

Discharge TimeSaver

Ensuring continued care for the patient with contusion

Review the following teaching topics, referrals, and follow-up appointments to make sure that your patient is adequately prepared for discharge.

Teaching topics
Make sure that the following topics have been covered and that your patient's learning has been evaluated:
☐ explanation of the disorder and its complications
☐ potential for seizures
☐ restrictions in activities of daily living
☐ prescribed medications.

Referrals
Make sure that the patient has been provided with necessary referrals to:
☐ rehabilitation facility for occupational therapy, physical therapy, or speech therapy, as needed
☐ head injury support group.

Follow-up appointments
Make sure that the necessary follow-up appointments have been scheduled and that the patient has been notified:
☐ neurosurgeon
☐ doctor or clinic.

• Advise family members to handle the patient in a gentle, positive manner and to correct inappropriate behavior in a matter-of-fact fashion. (See *Ensuring continued care for the patient with contusion.*)
• Caution the family not to assist the patient too much after he resumes activities of daily living.
• Teach the patient and his family techniques to deal with communication and memory deficits. Provide cues to the patient by labeling objects.

EVALUATION

When evaluating the patient's response to your nursing care, gather reassessment data and compare this information with the patient outcomes specified in your plan of care. Ensure that neurologic symptoms, including mental status, have improved following admission.

Teaching and counseling
In evaluating the effectiveness of your patient teaching, consider the following questions:
• Can the patient or his family explain the nature of his brain injury?
• Can they identify and correct hazards in the home environment?
• Are they familiar with the necessary home care measures?

Physical condition
• Is the patient oriented to person, place, and time?
• Can he make informed decisions?
• Is his Glasgow Coma Scale score between 11 and 15?
• Is his ICP 15 mm Hg or less?
• Are his pupils equal in size and shape and reactive to light?
• Was he free of injury throughout hospitalization?

Intracranial hemorrhage and hematoma

Common after head trauma, intracranial hemorrhage occurs when blood accumulates in the ventricles, the brain parenchyma, or the extradural, subdural, or subarachnoid space. Complications include cerebral edema, which may lead to increased intracranial pressure (ICP) and herniation. Hematoma refers to a mass of blood or swelling restricted to a confined space. (See *Understanding intracranial hematomas and subarachnoid hemorrhage.*)

Causes
Intracranial hemorrhage and hematoma most often occur secondary to injury from motor vehicle accidents, falls, assaults, or industrial and sporting accidents. They may also result from hypertension or vascular malformations, such as aneurysms or arteriovenous malformations.

ASSESSMENT

Your assessment should include careful consideration of the patient's history (including the probable cause of trauma), physical examination findings, and diagnostic test results. Many times, you'll find a combination of injuries, such as contusion and hematoma.

Health history
If the patient has no history of trauma, identify any underlying conditions such as hypertension. In nontraumatic subarachnoid hemorrhage, the patient may have a severe headache. Ask about use of alcohol or any medications that might mask or mimic neurologic signs.

Physical examination
Check the patient's level of consciousness (LOC), which may vary from drowsiness to unarousable stupor, depending on the size of the hematoma and the presence of tissue damage.

Check the patient's pupils, which may be large and sluggish or show no reaction to light. Focusing abnormalities may also be present. Pupil dilation is an early sign of increased ICP and occurs ipsilateral to the lesion.

Assess the patient's movement of extremities. If the patient does not follow commands, you'll need to try a painful stimulus. Does he defend or withdraw? Does his response (for example, decorticate or decerebrate posturing) suggest significant cerebral damage?

Observe the patient for signs of ecchymosis, particularly around the eyes (raccoon eyes) and behind the ear (Battle's sign). Look for cerebrospinal fluid (CSF) drainage from the nose or ear.

Check other brain stem reflexes, such as cough and gag reflexes. If no cervical injury is present, assess for the oculocephalic (doll's eye) reflex.

Observe the patient's respiratory pattern for variations that may signal elevated ICP. The following breathing patterns may help you locate the lesion:
• *Cheyne-Stokes respiration* denotes a lesion that usually occurs in both cerebral hemispheres, or in the midbrain or upper pons.
• *Central neurogenic hyperventilation* denotes a lesion in either the lower midbrain or the upper pons.
• *Apneustic breathing* denotes a lesion in the middle or lower pons.
•*Cluster breathing* denotes a lesion in the lower pons or upper medulla.
• *Ataxic breathing* denotes a medullar lesion.

Understanding intracranial hematomas and subarachnoid hemorrhage

Because signs of hematoma or hemorrhage vary greatly, learning about them can speed your assessment and ensure timely interventions. The three types of intracranial hematomas are epidural, subdural, and intracerebral; the most significant type of hemorrhage is subarachnoid.

Epidural hematoma

Bleeding into the epidural space usually occurs as a result of a tear in the middle meningeal artery, resulting from a fracture of the temporoparietal portion of the skull.

Signs and symptoms include headache, ipsilateral pupil change, contralateral motor paralysis, and unconsciousness followed by periods of alertness and lucidity, and then coma.

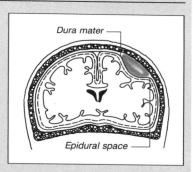

Subdural hematoma

Bleeding into the subdural space may be caused by rupture of the bridging veins, rupture of small branches of cerebral arteries, bleeding from contused or lacerated areas of the brain, or an extension of an intracerebral hematoma. Subdural hematomas are further classified as acute, subacute, or chronic based on the amount of time between the injury and the development of symptoms.

Signs and symptoms include headache, progressive changes in level of consciousness, focal deficits, irritability, confusion, positive Babinski's reflex, and seizures.

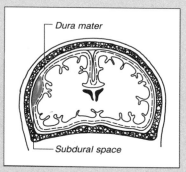

(continued)

Understanding intracranial hematomas and subarachnoid hemorrhage
(continued)

Intracerebral hematoma
Bleeding into the brain tissue itself may follow a severe or, rarely, a mild head injury. It can also result from bleeding secondary to hypertension. Other causes include a ruptured basilar aneurysm, blood dyscrasias, polycythemia, and surgical exploration.

Signs and symptoms include increased intracranial pressure, headache, contralateral hemiplegia, dizziness, vomiting, and seizures.

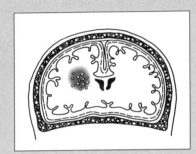

Subarachnoid hemorrhage
In subarachnoid hemorrhage, blood seeps into the subarachnoid space and mixes with the cerebrospinal fluid. Although sometimes the result of trauma, it more commonly stems from a ruptured aneurysm, an arteriovenous malformation, or hypertension.

Signs and symptoms include sudden, violent headache, dizziness and vertigo, nausea and vomiting, drowsiness, sweating, and chills.

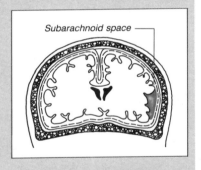

Subarachnoid space

If the history suggests a subarachnoid hemorrhage, assess for signs of meningeal irritation, photophobia, nuchal rigidity, headache, irritability, and restlessness. Check for a positive Kernig's or Brudzinski's sign.

Diagnostic test results
The following tests help to confirm a diagnosis or identify the location of hemorrhage or hematoma:
• Computed tomography scan or magnetic resonance imaging will confirm hemorrhage or hematoma. It will also show any herniation.
• An arteriogram may be performed to identify the source of a subarachnoid hemorrhage.
• A lumbar puncture may confirm the diagnosis of a subarachnoid hemorrhage by revealing blood in the CSF.

NURSING DIAGNOSIS

Common nursing diagnoses for a patient with intracranial hemorrhage or hematoma include:
• Altered cerebral tissue perfusion related to increased ICP
• Ineffective breathing pattern related to increased ICP
• Fluid volume deficit related to treatment for increased ICP.

PLANNING

Based on the nursing diagnosis *altered cerebral tissue perfusion,* develop appropriate patient outcomes. For example, your patient will:
• have a Glasgow Coma Scale score of 11 to 15
• have an ICP of 15 mm Hg or less
• have pupils that are equal in size and reactive to light
• have no or minimal motor deficits.

Based on the nursing diagnosis *ineffective breathing pattern,* develop appropriate patient outcomes. For example, your patient will:
• maintain a respiratory rate of 16 to 24 breaths/minute
• maintain normal arterial blood gas (ABG) levels
• demonstrate a vital capacity of at least 15 ml/kg
• maintain clear breath sounds bilaterally.

Based on the nursing diagnosis *fluid volume deficit,* develop appropriate patient outcomes. For example, your patient will:
• maintain hemodynamic parameters within normal limits for his age
• maintain normal serum electrolyte values
• maintain a urine output greater than 30 ml/hour.

IMPLEMENTATION

Appropriate interventions depend on the location and severity of hemorrhage and hematoma. (See *Medical care of the patient with intracranial hematoma or subarachnoid hemorrhage,* page 114.)

Nursing interventions
• After a craniotomy or any other surgical procedure, perform a quick neurologic assessment every 5 to 15 minutes (frequently enough to establish a trend). Assess LOC, motor response, pupil reaction, brain stem function, and mental status.

Timesaving tip: Between shifts, a health care team member from each shift should complete a neurologic assessment together to allow earlier detection of neurologic changes and to prevent needless duplication of effort.
• Monitor intake and output carefully.
• Monitor electrolyte levels, especially potassium and sodium, because alterations may result from changes in fluid volume.
• Administer an osmotic diuretic, such as mannitol, to help lower ICP.
• Maintain pulmonary function and adequate oxygenation.
• Turn and percuss the patient frequently. Suction him as necessary.
• Hyperventilate the patient as ordered to reduce partial pressure of arterial carbon dioxide ($PaCO_2$), which constricts cerebral arteries and restricts cerebral blood flow, thereby reducing intracranial volume and ICP. Maintain $PaCO_2$ levels of 25 to 30 mm Hg. Monitor $PaCO_2$ carefully; constricting the cerebral blood flow too much can cause infarction.
• Supply enteral feedings as ordered, using a small-bore feeding tube or a percutaneous endoscopic gastrosto-

Treatments

Medical care of the patient with intracranial hematoma or subarachnoid hemorrhage

The type of treatment administered for hematoma depends on whether the hematoma is epidural, subdural, or intracerebral. Subarachnoid hemorrhage is usually treated nonsurgically.

Epidural hematoma

A craniotomy with evacuation is performed to remove the hematoma. Early diagnosis and treatment (long before coma sets in) carry a good prognosis.

Subdural hematoma

A small subdural hematoma may be treated medically because the blood is generally reabsorbed. Serial computed tomography (CT) scans may be ordered so that the size of the lesion can be monitored.

If the hematoma is large or the patient demonstrates significant neurologic compromise, a craniotomy with evacuation will be performed to relieve intracranial pressure. The prognosis in acute and subacute subdural hematoma is poor despite quick surgical intervention because there is usually underlying tissue damage.

Intracerebral hematoma

The condition of the patient, the location of the blood, and the cause and extent of injury determine the type of surgery. If the injury is traumatic, such as a depressed skull fracture, all foreign materials and skull fragments are removed and the hematoma is evacuated by gentle suction. In some cases, postoperative results may show little improvement because of associated complications.

Subarachnoid hemorrhage

The patient is monitored with serial CT scans as subarachnoid blood is reabsorbed. However, if blood is not fully reabsorbed, it blocks subarachnoid villi and interferes with reabsorption of cerebrospinal fluid.

my tube. If enteral feeding is not possible, provide total parenteral nutrition.

• Devise strategies to prevent the complications of immobility. Perform range-of-motion exercises at least four times a day.

• Monitor carefully for signs of seizure activity. Administer anticonvulsants as ordered, and assess for therapeutic levels.

Patient teaching

If the patient's cognitive skills are severely impaired, focus on teaching family members.

• Develop strategies to help the patient and his family adapt to sensory dysfunction and to cope with behavioral changes.

• Emphasize to family members the importance of developing a routine and maintaining a stable environment.

Discharge TimeSaver

Ensuring continued care for the patient with intracranial hematoma or subarachnoid hemorrhage

Review the following teaching topics, referrals, and follow-up appointments to make sure that your patient is adequately prepared for discharge.

Teaching topics
Make sure that the following topics have been covered and that your patient's learning has been evaluated:
☐ explanation of the intracranial hematoma or hemorrhage and how it has affected the brain
☐ causes of intracranial hematoma and hemorrhage, and how to minimize risks
☐ risk factors that could cause rebleeding
☐ modifications in activities of daily living
☐ medications.

Referrals
Make sure that the patient has been provided with necessary referrals to:

☐ rehabilitation facility for physical therapy, occupational therapy, or speech therapy, as needed
☐ home health care agency
☐ social services for assistance with community reentry and financial issues
☐ stroke or head injury support group.

Follow-up appointments
Make sure that the necessary follow-up appointments have been scheduled and that the patient has been notified:
☐ neurologist
☐ neurosurgeon if necessary
☐ internist
☐ neuropsychologist if necessary.

• Teach family members about resources in the community and how to contact them. (See *Ensuring continued care for the patient with intracranial hematoma or subarachnoid hemorrhage.*)

EVALUATION

When evaluating your patient's response to nursing care, gather reassessment data and compare this information with the patient outcomes specified in your plan of care.

Teaching and counseling
• Have the patient and his family developed strategies to help the patient adapt to his sensory dysfunction and cope with his behavioral changes?
• Does the family understand the importance of maintaining a stable environment and developing a routine?
• Do they know about available community resources and how to contact them?

Physical condition
• Is the patient oriented to person, place, and time?
• Is his Glasgow Coma Scale score between 11 and 15?
• Is his ICP 15 mm Hg or less?
• Are his pupils equal in size and reactive to light?

• Has he achieved a respiratory rate of 16 to 24 breaths/minute?
• Are his breathing patterns and ABG levels at baseline?
• Is his vital capacity 15 ml/kg or greater?
• Are his breath sounds clear bilaterally?
• Are his hemodynamic indices within normal limits?
• Are his electrolyte levels within a normal range?
• Is he voiding 30 ml/hour or more?

Skull fracture

This type of head injury results from a blow to the head. Skull fracture can lead to infection, intracranial hemorrhage and hematoma, brain abscess, and increased intracranial pressure (ICP) from edema. Residual effects of the injury, such as seizure disorders, hydrocephalus, and organic mental syndrome, may complicate recovery. (See *Types of skull fractures*.)

Causes
Motor vehicle accidents, falls, and severe beatings are the most common causes of skull fracture.

ASSESSMENT

If the patient is not conscious or alert, find out the injury details from witnesses, family or friends, police, or emergency personnel.

Health history
Find out the velocity and site of the impact. Was the patient hit with a blunt object? If the injury resulted from a car accident, was the patient thrown from the vehicle? Did he ever lose consciousness? How much time has elapsed since the occurrence of the injury and your examination? Does the patient complain of a severe localized headache? Has he experienced any bleeding or other discharge from the nose or ears?

Physical examination
Assume that the patient with a suspected skull fracture has a cervical spine injury until it's been ruled out by the doctor, and take appropriate precautions.

Examine and gently palpate the scalp for lacerations, bleeding, and edema. Check for any areas of swelling. Look for ecchymosis behind the ears (Battle's sign) and around the eyes (raccoon's eyes). Also inspect these areas for cerebrospinal fluid (CSF) and brain tissue leakage. Red-tinged CSF drainage indicates brain injury.

Timesaving tip: For a quick check of CSF drainage in the patient who can sit up, have him bend forward, and watch for drainage from his nose. If you see drainage, test for glucose with glucose reagent strips because CSF tests positive for glucose. (Remember that a positive result will also occur if blood is mixed with another fluid; the test may not be able to differentiate between CSF and the other fluid.) Another CSF indicator is the halo or double-ring sign. When a patient with CSF leakage rests his head on a paper- or cloth-covered pillow, the blood aggregates at the center and a halo of clear CSF surrounds it.

Check for decreased pulse and respiratory rates as well as labored respirations, which may indicate brain stem compression.

Types of skull fractures

Skull fractures may be simple (closed) or compound (open). They are also usually described as linear, comminuted, or depressed. Some fractures, such as basilar fractures, are described in terms of their location.

Linear fracture
A linear, or hairline, fracture is a single, clean break that doesn't displace bone fragments and seldom requires emergency treatment. Of all types of skull fractures, it is the least likely to be fatal.

Comminuted fracture
This type of injury splinters or crushes the bone into fragments.

Depressed fracture
In a depressed fracture, bone fragments are driven toward the dura ma-

ter and brain. It is considered serious only if it compresses underlying structures. A child's thin, elastic skull allows a depression without a fracture.

Basilar fracture
A basilar fracture usually occurs in the anterior or middle fossa at the base of the skull and involves the cribriform plate and the frontal sinuses. Fractures in the middle fossa are most common and typically involve the petrous portion of the temporal bone.

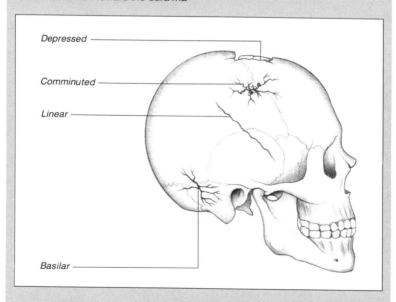

Depressed

Comminuted

Linear

Basilar

Neurologic examination

Be alert for any alteration in the patient's level of consciousness (LOC), agitation and irritability, abnormal deep tendon reflexes, altered pupillary and motor responses, hemiparesis, dizziness, seizures, and projectile vomiting. A patient with a skull fracture could lose consciousness at any time, with little warning.

An altered LOC with signs of increasing ICP suggests contusion or laceration. A patient with residual amnesia, memory loss, and a transient period of unconsciousness may have a concussion.

In a depressed skull fracture, look for focal deficits (such as weakness or paralysis of an arm or leg), and cranial nerve involvement (such as a facial droop, hearing loss, or dysconjugate eye movement).

Diagnostic test results

The following tests may reveal the presence or complications of skull fracture:
• Skull X-rays are the most common way to diagnose a skull fracture, using posteroanterior and lateral views.
• A computed tomography scan identifies basilar fractures, which aren't usually visible on an X-ray, and intracranial hematomas.
• Cerebral angiography locates vascular disruptions from internal pressure or injury.
• A cisternogram may be ordered if CSF leakage is present and the doctor can't locate the fracture area with routine tests.

NURSING DIAGNOSIS

Common nursing diagnoses for a patient with skull fracture include:
• High risk for infection related to CSF leakage

• Altered cerebral tissue perfusion related to edema or increased ICP secondary to fracture
• Altered thought processes related to seizures
• High risk for injury related to agitation, restlessness, or sensory or visual deficits.

PLANNING

Based on the nursing diagnosis *high risk for infection,* develop appropriate patient outcomes. For example, your patient will:
• remain free of central nervous system (CNS) infection throughout hospitalization
• experience a decrease in CSF leakage without surgical intervention.

Based on the nursing diagnosis *altered cerebral tissue perfusion,* develop appropriate patient outcomes. For example, your patient will:
• score between 11 and 15 on the Glasgow Coma Scale
• have an ICP that is less than or equal to 15 mm Hg
• exhibit pupils that are equal in size and reactive to light.

Based on the nursing diagnosis *altered thought processes,* develop appropriate patient outcomes. For example, your patient will:
• appear oriented to person, place, and time
• be able to make decisions following the postictal period.

Based on the nursing diagnosis *high risk for injury,* develop appropriate patient outcomes. For example, your patient will:
• remain free of injury throughout hospitalization
• be able to identify and correct hazards in the home environment.

Treatments

Medical care of the patient with skull fracture

Medical treatment for skull fractures depends on the type of fracture.

Linear fracture
Generally, no special medical intervention is needed. The patient will be maintained on bed rest and observed for underlying cerebral injury for 24 to 48 hours. A mild analgesic may be prescribed for head pain.

Comminuted or depressed fracture
Both of these types of skull fracture commonly require a craniotomy to elevate the depression and debride the tissue of bone fragments. This reduces the risk of infection and further brain damage. If the bone is shattered, the patient may require a cranioplasty to repair the defect. In this operation, the damaged skull section is removed and replaced by mesh or by acrylic plates. Surgery may be postponed for several months if cerebral edema is present.

The patient commonly requires antibiotics and, in profound hemorrhage, blood transfusions.

Basilar fracture
The patient with this type of fracture requires bed rest with frequent assessment of neurologic status. If cerebrospinal fluid (CSF) leakage is present, observe the patient for signs of meningitis. The doctor may prescribe an antibiotic for prophylaxis or a corticosteroid to reduce cerebral edema. If CSF leakage doesn't resolve spontaneously, a lumbar drain or surgical repair may be necessary.

IMPLEMENTATION

Treatment for skull fracture ranges from bed rest to surgical intervention. (See *Medical care of the patient with skull fracture.*)

Nursing interventions
Interventions depend on the type and severity of the fracture and the accompanying complications.

Linear fracture
• Administer a mild analgesic, such as acetaminophen, to control headache.
• Provide wound management as needed, including local injection of procaine, shaving the scalp around the wound, and cleaning and debriding the wound.
• Tell the patient which activities he may resume upon discharge, and advise him to avoid contact sports for 6 weeks.

Depressed or comminuted fracture
The patient with a depressed or comminuted fracture will usually require surgery. Postoperatively, he may require intensive care, including mechanical ventilation and hemodynamic monitoring.
• Monitor neurologic status for signs of increased ICP, especially after surgery. Be especially alert for LOC and pupillary changes.

• As prescribed, provide the patient with an analgesic, such as codeine, for pain.
• Observe the surgical incision for signs of infection, CSF leakage, or bleeding.
• When the patient's condition stabilizes, determine if he has any neurologic deficits. Observe him for short-term memory loss, language difficulties, emotional lability, and poor concentration. Consult with a speech pathologist or a neuropsychologist if necessary.
• Explain all procedures to the patient to help relieve his anxiety.
• Provide emotional support for the patient and his family.
• Help the patient to resume activities of daily living. He may require physical therapy to strengthen muscles and gait training or occupational therapy to regain independence.

Basilar fracture
• Conduct regular neurologic assessments, and watch for signs and symptoms of meningitis. If such signs and symptoms develop, notify the doctor immediately.
• Observe carefully for CSF leakage from the nose or ear. Keep the area clean and allow CSF drainage to flow. Leakage may resolve itself in about 7 to 10 days without surgery.
• If leakage does not resolve itself within 7 to 10 days, intervention may include lumbar drainage. Monitor drainage flow and the catheter insertion site. Since the patient will be kept flat in bed during catheterization, assess him for paresthesia in the lower extremities and for complications of immobility.
• If lumbar drainage does not stop the CSF leakage, surgical repair may be necessary. The surgeon may use temporal muscle for a small repair or

fascia lata from the thigh for a larger repair.
• Postoperatively, observe the patient for signs of infection and CSF leakage. Monitor his vital signs and neurologic status. Report any changes in LOC. Instruct him not to blow his nose or pick his nose or ears since these activities may increase ICP.
• Administer corticosteroids, as prescribed, to reduce the inflammatory response at the sites of pinched peripheral nerves.

Patient teaching
• Instruct the patient to be alert for signs of meningitis, such as headache, stiff neck, photophobia, fever, and malaise, and to report such symptoms immediately to his doctor.
• Teach the patient to identify signs of CSF leakage, including watery drainage from the nose or ear, or a persistent drip in the back of the throat.
• Tell the patient to increase his activity level gradually and to abstain from contact sports until he has been examined by the doctor in a follow-up visit.
• Instruct the patient to take acetaminophen for his headache if a medication has not been prescribed.
• Teach the patient and his family how to care for his scalp wound. Emphasize the need to return for suture removal and follow-up evaluation. (See *Ensuring continued care for the patient with skull fracture.*)

EVALUATION

To evaluate the patient's response to your care, gather your reassessment data and compare this information with the patient outcomes specified in your plan of care.

Discharge TimeSaver
Ensuring continued care for the patient with skull fracture

Review the following teaching topics, referrals, and follow-up appointments to make sure that your patient is adequately prepared for discharge.

Teaching topics
Make sure that the following topics have been covered and that your patient's learning has been evaluated:
□ explanation of the fracture, its risk factors, and its complications
□ prescribed medications, including anticonvulsants and analgesics
□ activity restrictions.

Referrals
Make sure that the patient has been provided with necessary referrals to:

□ rehabilitation facility for occupational therapy, physical therapy, or speech therapy, as needed
□ head injury support group.

Follow-up appointments
Make sure that the necessary follow-up appointments have been scheduled and that the patient has been notified:
□ doctor
□ neurosurgeon
□ plastic surgeon if appropriate.

Teaching and counseling
Determine the effectiveness of your teaching and counseling by considering the following questions:
• Can the patient correct conditions that may have led to the injury?
• Does he understand the need to restrict physical activity?
• Can he identify signs and symptoms of meningitis and CSF leakage?

Physical condition
• Is the patient oriented to person, place, and time?
• Can he cope with the residual effects of his injury?
• Has he received a referral to a head injury support group?
• Has he remained free of injury and CNS infection throughout his hospitalization?
• Is his Glasgow Coma Scale score between 11 and 15?
• Is his ICP 15 mm Hg or less?

• Are his pupils equal in size and reactive to light?
• Does his pain respond to medication within 45 minutes of administration?

Brain laceration

Brain laceration, a traumatic tearing of the cortical surface of the brain, results from the brain striking irregular prominences within the skull.

Brain laceration disrupts cellular activity, resulting in focal deficits. If blood vessels in the injured area tear, hemorrhaging occurs. Contusion and edema may also result. Depending on the injury's location, intracerebral, subdural, or epidural hematomas may develop, causing a dangerous increase in intracranial pressure (ICP). Life-threatening seizures may also occur.

Causes

Brain laceration may occur secondary to a depressed skull fracture, a rotational shearing injury, or penetrating trauma. Many lacerations occur as a result of high-velocity acceleration-deceleration injuries (for instance, car accidents and gunshot wounds). (See *Understanding penetrating wounds.*)

ASSESSMENT

First, check for signs and symptoms of a skull fracture, such as periorbital ecchymosis (raccoon eyes) and leakage of cerebrospinal fluid (CSF) from the nose or ears. Next, assess the patient's level of consciousness (LOC) and his focal neurologic deficits, which will depend on the laceration site. Even if the patient seems minimally impaired, be prepared for emergency intervention. His condition could deteriorate rapidly.

Health history

If the patient can communicate, ask him to describe the incident. Otherwise, obtain information from family members or emergency personnel.

Consider the following questions:
• If the patient was in a motorcycle or bicycle accident, was he wearing a helmet?
• In what position was the patient found?
• How long ago did the injury occur?
• Was the patient unconscious at any time?
• Did he have any episodes of apnea or cyanosis? If so, for how long?
• Was any blood lost? If so, was the loss significant?

Physical examination

Examine the head, inspecting for facial symmetry, skull configuration, and hair color and distribution. Also palpate the entire scalp, and inspect the ears, nose, and mouth. Record your findings on the patient's chart.

Observe the patient for signs and symptoms of increased ICP, such as decreased LOC, extensor or flexor posturing, seizure activity, dilated pupils, elevated systolic blood pressure, widening pulse pressure, bradycardia, and an abnormal respiratory pattern.

In addition, assess the patient's neurologic status by checking his cerebral, cranial, cerebellar, and motor functions and his deep tendon reflexes. Also examine his vital signs. Look for signs of infection, such as a tender and swollen erythematous flap, an elevated white blood cell (WBC) count, and a fever.

Diagnostic test results

The following tests are commonly used to assess the extent and location of injury caused by brain laceration:
• Computed tomography scans and magnetic resonance imaging provide the best diagnostic information about the extent of brain damage and associated injuries, such as contusion, edema, and hematoma.
• X-rays can identify fractures.

NURSING DIAGNOSIS

Common nursing diagnoses for the patient with brain laceration include:
• Altered cerebral tissue perfusion related to severed arterial blood vessels
• High risk for infection related to introduction of microorganisms into the brain
• High risk for injury related to complications such as hematoma formation, seizures, and increased ICP.

Understanding penetrating wounds

A penetrating wound occurs when an object — flying debris, a knife, or a bullet — penetrates the skull. This type of wound may cause many complications, including:
• a sudden rise in intracranial pressure (ICP), which may last for minutes or hours
• contusions
• lacerations
• hemorrhage
• cerebral edema
• tissue necrosis
• a skull fracture
• infection, such as meningitis or brain abscess (may occur when surface debris, such as hair, dirt, or cloth, enters the normally sterile brain).

Examining a penetrating wound
Locate the wound, looking for entry and exit points. An entrance wound appears regular, with even margins or a stellate tear. An exit wound may be larger and less regular.

You may have trouble locating a bullet wound if the bullet penetrated the head through hair or an orifice or if the bullet is small. In such cases, gently palpate the entire scalp, and inspect the ears, nose, and mouth.

Record your findings, including wound configuration, on the patient's chart.

Observe the patient for decreased level of consciousness, extensor or flexor posturing, and dilated pupils. Also check for signs of increased ICP: elevated systolic blood pressure, widening pulse pressure, bradycardia, and an abnormal respiratory pattern.

Treatment
Treatment focuses on preserving body function and preventing associated complications.

The doctor may order prophylactic antibiotics such as nafcillin. However, some doctors believe that prophylactic antibiotics encourage development of resistant organisms. In acute hydrocephalus, the doctor will insert an intraventricular shunt to facilitate cerebrospinal fluid drainage.

If the patient's ICP increases, the doctor may insert an intracranial monitoring device and institute measures to control ICP, such as hyperventilating the patient, administering osmotic diuretics or corticosteroids, inducing barbiturate coma, or performing surgical decompression.

PLANNING

Brain laceration can provoke life-threatening crises. Give these the highest priority. Also, be ready to manage sudden changes in the patient's neurologic status.

Based on the nursing diagnosis *altered cerebral tissue perfusion*, develop appropriate patient outcomes. For example, your patient will:
• show an improved LOC
• maintain a blood pressure high enough to maintain cerebral perfusion pressure but low enough to pre-

vent increased bleeding or cerebral swelling
• experience no hypercarbia
• show a decrease in residual neurologic deficits after the laceration has healed.

Based on the nursing diagnosis *high risk for infection,* develop appropriate patient outcomes. For example, your patient will:
• maintain a normal body temperature and WBC count and differential
• exhibit a head wound that is clean, pink, and free of purulent drainage
• show no evidence of brain abscess or other types of cerebral infections such as meningitis.

Based on the nursing diagnosis *high risk for injury,* develop appropriate patient outcomes. For example, your patient will:
• demonstrate knowledge of signs and symptoms of complications, allowing for prompt treatment
• experience no cerebral injury resulting from complications
• maintain normal cerebral function.

IMPLEMENTATION

Your nursing care will depend on the extent of the patient's neurologic deficits and complications. Monitor the patient's airway, breathing, and circulation closely, and be prepared to intervene immediately if his neurologic status begins to deteriorate. (See *Medical care of the patient with brain laceration.*)

Nursing interventions
• Assess the patient's LOC by checking for pupil size, shape, and reaction to light; corneal and gag reflexes; and motor and respiratory functions.
• Monitor vital signs every 15 minutes. Check for abnormal respirations that might indicate a neurologic emergency, such as a tentorial herniation.
• Maintain a patent airway by endotracheal intubation or a tracheotomy, as necessary.
• Be prepared to intubate and hyperventilate the patient. This will reduce ICP by decreasing the carbon dioxide level.
• Monitor oxygenation by serial arterial blood gas studies.
• Administer medications as ordered.
• Protect the confused or comatose patient from injury by observing him closely and by taking such precautions as raising the side rails of his bed.
• Reassure the patient by explaining your actions, even if he's comatose.
• Insert an indwelling urinary catheter as ordered. Monitor intake and output.
• If the patient is unconscious, insert a nasogastric tube to prevent aspiration. But first make sure that a basilar skull fracture has been ruled out.
• Carefully observe the patient for CSF leakage. Check the bed sheets for a blood-tinged spot surrounded by a lighter ring (halo sign). If CSF leakage develops, raise the head of the bed 30 to 45 degrees (depending on the doctor's recommendation). If you detect CSF leakage from the nose, place a gauze pad under the nostrils. If CSF leaks from the ear, position the patient so that his ear drains naturally; don't pack the ear or nose.
• Monitor the patient for infection by inspecting the head wound regularly for signs of redness, puffiness, or purulent drainage. Maintain strict aseptic technique when changing head dressings. Administer prescribed antibiotics and monitor the patient's WBC count and differential.
• Never clean or suction the ears or nose of a patient with a brain lacera-

Treatments

Medical care of the patient with brain laceration

Medical treatment depends on the laceration's cause and its subsequent complications. Severely injured patients may require intensive care, including hemodynamic monitoring and mechanical ventilation. Treatment may also include anticonvulsant drug therapy, surgery, and interventions to control intracranial pressure (ICP).

Drug therapy
To help prevent seizures, the doctor may order anticonvulsants such as phenytoin and antibiotics such as nafcillin.

Surgery
To elevate a depressed fracture or to remove a hematoma, the doctor may perform surgery. Your postoperative care should include evaluating the patient for complications and promoting recovery of neurologic function.

Monitoring and controlling ICP
If the patient's ICP increases, the doctor may insert an intracranial monitoring device.

The doctor may select a combination of common medical treatments to control increased ICP, depending on the patient's condition. These include:
• hyperventilating the patient
• administering osmotic diuretics, such as mannitol or furosemide
• administering corticosteroids
• managing blood pressure
• administering skeletal muscle relaxants or neuromuscular blockers, such as pancuronium
• administering sedatives such as benzodiazepines
• controlling body temperature
• limiting fluid intake
• draining cerebrospinal fluid
• inducing barbiturate coma
• performing surgical decompression or craniotomy.

---

tion until directed by the doctor. Doing so could introduce microorganisms into the central nervous system.
• Maintain the patient's head and neck in a neutral position. If his head is turned to the side, he may have poor jugular venous return, which can increase ICP.
• Restrict his total fluid intake to 1,500 ml/day to reduce volume and intracerebral swelling, another cause of increased ICP.
• Take precautions against seizures, and administer anticonvulsant medications as prescribed.

• Clean and dress any superficial scalp wounds once the patient is stabilized. If his skin has been broken, consider the possibility of tetanus. Assist with suturing if needed.

Patient teaching
Intensive care is usually required for the patient with brain laceration. In many instances, he may not be mentally alert or stable enough to receive extensive instructions, so keep instructions simple and brief.
• Tell the conscious patient to keep his mouth open when coughing,

Ensuring continued care for the patient with brain laceration

Review the following teaching topics, referrals, and follow-up appointments to make sure that your patient is adequately prepared for discharge.

Teaching topics
Make sure that the following topics have been covered and that your patient's learning has been evaluated:
☐ explanation of neurologic deficits resulting from the brain laceration and possible complications
☐ activity restrictions as needed
☐ proper use of assistive devices, such as a walker or cane
☐ prescribed medications, including dosage and possible adverse effects
☐ dietary recommendations, such as eating high-calorie, protein-rich meals
☐ wound or dressing care if necessary
☐ signs and symptoms of complications, including infection
☐ home safety measures.

Referrals
Make sure that the patient has been provided with necessary referrals to:
☐ home health care agency if needed
☐ rehabilitation program, including physical therapy, occupational therapy, or speech therapy if necessary
☐ medical equipment supplier if needed
☐ social services if financial counseling is needed
☐ support groups if appropriate.

Follow-up appointments
Make sure that the necessary follow-up appointments have been scheduled and that the patient has been notified:
☐ doctor
☐ diagnostic tests for reevaluation
☐ surgeon if necessary
☐ dietitian.

sneezing, or blowing his nose to prevent an increase in ICP.
• Teach the patient and his family the importance of checking for changes in cerebral function and returning to the hospital or calling the doctor if such changes occur.
• Provide an alternative means of communication for the patient with aphasia, such as a note pad and pencil.
• Prepare your patient for rehabilitation therapy if necessary.
• Because infection, hydrocephalus, and seizures can develop after discharge, consult with a community nursing organization to provide follow-up care in the patient's home. (See *Ensuring continued care for the patient with brain laceration.*)

EVALUATION

When evaluating the patient's response to your care, gather reassessment data and compare this information to the patient outcomes specified in your plan of care.

Teaching and counseling
Begin by determining the effectiveness of your teaching. Consider the following questions:
• Does the patient understand the importance of keeping his mouth open when blowing his nose, coughing, or sneezing?
• Has he demonstrated the ability to recognize the signs and symptoms of complications, including infections?
• Do the patient and his family understand diagnostic and treatment measures?
• Can they describe changes in cerebral function?

Physical condition
Evaluate the patient's physical condition by answering the following questions:
• Has the patient regained his normal thought processes?
• Is he oriented to person, place, and time?
• Does he remember recent as well as past events? Does he recognize family members and friends?
• Can he follow simple instructions?
• Has his LOC improved?
• Is his blood pressure high enough to maintain cerebral perfusion pressure, but low enough to prevent increased bleeding or cerebral swelling?
• Has he remained free of residual neurologic deficits?
• Is his carbon dioxide level normal?
• Is he free of infection and other complications?
• Does the patient have a normal body temperature and WBC count and differential?
• Is his head wound clean, pink, and free of purulent drainage?
• Is his neurologic functioning normal?

Herniated disk

Also known as a herniated nucleus pulposus or a slipped disk, a herniated disk occurs when all or part of the nucleus pulposus — an intervertebral disk's gelatinous center — extrudes through the disk's weakened or torn outer ring (annulus fibrosus). (See *How a herniated disk develops,* pages 128 and 129.)

Causes
Herniation of a disk occurs as a result of trauma to or strain on the spine. However, degeneration of vertebral disks occurs as part of the aging process, and in a disk already weakened by the degenerative process, an awkward movement or even a sneeze can result in protrusion of the nucleus pulposus.

ASSESSMENT
The severity of herniated disk symptoms depends on the quantity of protruding disk material, the degree of narrowing of the spinal canal, and the degree of encroachment on the nerve roots. Your assessment should include a thorough health history, a physical examination, and a review of diagnostic test results.

Health history
Pain is the most common characteristic of a herniated disk. Be sure to get a full description of the pain from the patient, including location, extent, intensity, and aggravating factors. Ask the patient if he takes medication for the pain and whether it provides relief.

How a herniated disk develops

A spinal disk has two parts: the soft center called the *nucleus pulposus* and the tough, fibrous surrounding ring called the *annulus fibrosus.* The nucleus pulposus acts as a shock absorber, distributing the mechanical stress applied to the spine when the body moves.

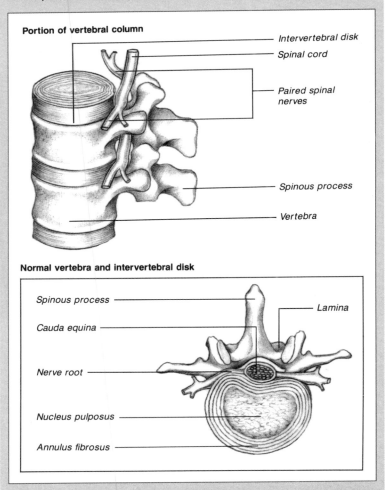

Portion of vertebral column

Intervertebral disk

Spinal cord

Paired spinal nerves

Spinous process

Vertebra

Normal vertebra and intervertebral disk

Spinous process

Cauda equina

Nerve root

Nucleus pulposus

Annulus fibrosus

Lamina

How a herniated disk develops *(continued)*

Protrusion

Physical stress — usually a twisting motion — can cause the annulus fibrosus to tear or rupture, allowing the nucleus pulposus to push through (herniate into) the spinal canal. This process allows the vertebrae to move closer together as the disk compresses. This compression, in turn, causes pressure on the nerve roots as they exit between the vertebrae. Pain and, possibly, sensory and motor loss follow.

Extrusion

A herniated disk can also occur with intervertebral joint degeneration. If the disk has begun to degenerate, minor trauma may cause herniation.

As herniation progresses, the nucleus pulposus begins to protrude against the annulus fibrosus (protrusion), pressing against the nerve root. Eventually, the disk's core bursts through the annulus fibrosus (extrusion), compressing the nerve root.

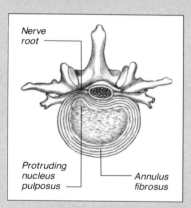

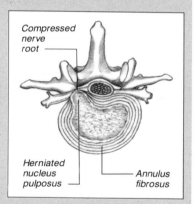

Physical examination

Inspection may reveal a patient with limited ability to bend forward and a posture favoring the affected area. In later stages, you may observe muscle atrophy, and palpation may disclose tenderness over the affected region.

Lumbar region

In the lumbar region, the patient may describe a mild to deep, aching pain radiating from the back into the buttocks and hip and then down the leg. It is intensified by coughing, sneezing, and certain leg positions. You may also detect weak plantar flexion or dorsiflexion of the foot and weakness of the hamstring or quadriceps muscles. Knee or ankle reflexes may be diminished or absent and patches of paresthesia and numbness over the leg and foot may also be evident.

Lumbar and lower thoracic herniations are usually detected by performing the straight-leg-raising test or by testing for Kernig's sign.

Cervical region
In the cervical region, weakness and paresthesias may occur in the neck, shoulder blade, and arm. You may discover a weakness of the arm and hand. Reflexes may be diminished or absent.

Diagnostic test results
The following tests will help identify and locate a herniated disk:
• X-ray studies of the spine are essential to show degenerative changes and rule out other abnormalities.
• Myelography will indicate the presence of herniation, the condition of the spinal canal, and the precise level of herniation.
• Computed tomography scan detects bone and soft-tissue abnormalities. It can show spinal canal compression that results from herniation.
• Magnetic resonance imaging defines tissue in areas usually obscured by bone or other imaging tests, such as X-ray.
• Electromyography confirms nerve involvement by measuring the electrical activity of muscles innervated by the herniated disk.

NURSING DIAGNOSIS

Common nursing diagnoses for patients with a herniated disk include:
• Pain related to the effects of nerve impingement, muscle spasm, or surgery
• Impaired physical mobility related to persistent pain and immobilization devices
• Constipation related to decreased mobility and effects of medications.

PLANNING

Based on the nursing diagnosis *pain,* develop appropriate patient outcomes. For example, your patient will:
• notify his caregiver as soon as pain occurs
• rate pain on a scale of 1 to 10
• express pain relief within 45 minutes after initiation of comfort measure.

Based on the nursing diagnosis *impaired physical mobility,* develop appropriate patient outcomes. For example, your patient will:
• perform activities of daily living (ADLs) as independently as possible and request assistance when needed
• experience no complications related to immobility, such as skin breakdown and venous stasis
• exhibit increased strength and endurance.

Based on the nursing diagnosis *constipation,* develop appropriate patient outcomes. For example, your patient will:
• evacuate soft, formed stools every other day (or according to his normal pattern)
• identify measures to prevent constipation, such as using stool softeners and bulk agents, and ensuring adequate fluid and fiber intake.

IMPLEMENTATION

Focus your nursing care on teaching the patient about herniated disk, enforcing bed rest, alleviating pain, and preventing complications. (See *Medical care of the patient with herniated disk.*)

Nursing interventions
• If the herniated disk is in the lumbar region, keep the patient on his back with his knees slightly flexed.

Medical care of the patient with herniated disk

Management of a herniated disk may consist of conservative or surgical measures.

Initial treatment
Unless neurologic impairment progresses rapidly, initial treatment should be conservative. Options include:
• bed rest or activity restriction
• avoiding unnecessary movements, such as lifting, bending, or twisting
• sleeping on a firm mattress
• applying hot or cold packs
• performing diathermy ultrasound
• employing skin traction
• using supportive devices, such as back braces and hard or soft collars
• drug therapy, including muscle relaxants and anti-inflammatory medications.

Surgical treatment
Surgery is indicated for patients who don't respond to conservative management or for those with progression of marked muscle weakness despite treatment. Surgical treatments include the following:
• *Laminectomy,* the most common surgical procedure, involves excision of a portion of the lamina of the bony vertebra and removal of the protruding disk. A spinal fusion may be performed concurrently to stabilize the spine.
• *Chemonucleolysis* is the injection of the enzyme chymopapain into the herniated disk to dissolve the nucleus pulposus.
• In *microdiskectomy,* a microscope is used to magnify the operative site. Better visualization and illumination decrease the incidence of nerve root trauma. This procedure is performed through a small incision.

Place a pillow under his knees to prevent excessive pressure on the nerve roots.
• If the herniated disk is in the cervical area, placing a small pillow at the nape of the neck may relieve pain.

Timesaving tip: Make sure everything is within easy reach of the bedridden patient before leaving the room to prevent unnecessary and time-consuming visits to the patient's room.
• Avoid complications of prolonged bed rest by applying antiembolism stockings, performing range-of-motion exercises, and ensuring that the

patient performs deep-breathing exercises at least four times a day.
• If the patient is receiving anti-inflammatory or muscle relaxant medications, make sure they are administered on schedule. Be prepared to intervene if adverse effects occur.
• Physical therapy may be instituted to strengthen the cervical muscles, especially if the disk is in the lumbar region. Encourage the patient to actively participate in the exercises and continue them after discharge.
• Make sure the patient's bed has a firm mattress. Elevate the head of the bed slightly. If the herniated disk is in

Teaching TimeSaver

Alleviating back pain

To minimize back pain, instruct the patient to do the following:
• Whenever possible, sit with his knees higher than his hips.
• Avoid reaching, lifting weights above his head, stooping, moving furniture by pulling it in front of him, pushing up windows, or maintaining one position for too long.
• Sleep on a firm mattress.
• Try to sleep on his side with his hips bent.
• When getting up from a sitting position, keep his back straight.
• When lifting, never bend to lift, always use legs to support weight, never hold anything heavier than 10 lb (4.5 kg) more than 2' (60 cm) away from the body, and never lift anything above shoulder level.
• Do back-strengthening exercises regularly.

the cervical area, make sure the patient wears a cervical collar. Assist him with repositioning at least every 2 hours.

Preoperative
• Provide psychological support.
• Apply thigh-high antiembolism stockings to facilitate blood return to the heart and decrease venous stasis. (Venous stasis places the patient at high risk for deep vein thrombosis.)
• Provide patient teaching about the surgical procedure and the recovery period.

Postoperative
• Postoperative care centers on promoting comfort, promoting healing of the operative site, and continually assessing postoperative symptoms.
• After surgery, the patient will still experience some pain, and numbness and weakness will probably continue for some time. Encourage the use of prescribed pain medication, especially in the first 48 hours. Muscle spasms and hematoma are likely to occur at the operative site; reassure the patient that these symptoms are normal and will subside with time and the use of pain and antispasmodic medications.
• The patient may be allowed out of bed on the first postoperative day, but make sure that these periods are short. Caution the patient that even sitting up puts additional strain on the lumbar region. If the operation was in the cervical area, fit the patient with a cervical collar when he is out of bed.
• Observe the patient's dressing for drainage. The dressing is usually removed on the first postoperative day. If the site remains dry, the incision can be left open to the air.
• Leakage of cerebrospinal fluid (CSF) from the incisional area can lead to infection and even meningitis if not treated. Call the doctor immediately if you find evidence of CSF.
• Ask the patient if he's nauseated, and assess his abdomen for bowel sounds and distention. These are both symptoms of paralytic ileus, which can occur following surgery to correct herniation in the lumbar region. If paralytic ileus is present, the patient may require nasogastric intubation.
• Assess the bladder for distention. Urine retention can occur as a result of the anesthesia administered during surgery.
• Check the patient for postoperative voiding. If he is unable to void, he'll require urinary catheterization.

Discharge TimeSaver

Ensuring continued care for the patient with herniated disk

Review the following teaching topics, referrals, and follow-up appointments to make sure that your patient is adequately prepared for discharge.

Teaching topics
Make sure that the following topics have been covered and that your patient's learning has been evaluated:
☐ explanation of disk injury and disease
☐ activity restrictions
☐ medications, including dosage and adverse effects
☐ use of cervical collar if applicable
☐ exercise program.

Referrals
Make sure that the patient has been provided with necessary referrals to:

☐ rehabilitation center for physical or occupational therapy if necessary
☐ home health care facility if necessary.
☐ medical supplier if necessary.

Follow-up appointments
Make sure that the necessary follow-up appointments have been scheduled and that the patient has been notified:
☐ doctor or clinic
☐ neurosurgeon if necessary
☐ diagnostic test center if necessary.

Patient teaching
Patient teaching focuses on alterations in lifestyle that are necessary to avoid exacerbating symptoms. (See *Alleviating back pain*.)
• Work closely with the patient to ensure realistic postoperative expectations about mobility and pain.

Timesaving tip: To save time before patient discharge, begin teaching on the first postoperative day.

• Caution the patient to avoid doing too much even if he feels well. Overexertion will cause additional strain and may result in a setback. (See *Ensuring continued care for the patient with herniated disk*.)

EVALUATION

When evaluating the patient's response to your nursing care, gather

reassessment data and compare this information with the patient outcomes specified in your plan of care.

Teaching and counseling
Begin by determining the effectiveness of your teaching. Note statements by the patient indicating that he understands his condition and intends to make necessary changes in his lifestyle. Consider the following questions:
• Can the patient rate pain intensity on a scale of 1 to 10?
• Does he have realistic expectations with regard to relief of symptoms?
• Can he identify measures to prevent constipation?

Physical condition
When evaluating the patient's physical condition, consider the following questions:

• Is the patient free of complications secondary to immobility?
• Does he perform ADLs independently when possible?
• Does he request assistance when needed?
• Does he demonstrate increased strength and endurance to the greatest extent possible?
• Has his bowel elimination pattern returned to normal?
• Can he demonstrate how to perform prescribed exercises?
• Does he understand instructions for home health care?

Spinal cord injury

Spinal cord injuries usually cause a complete or partial loss of motor, sensory, reflex, and autonomic functions, affecting virtually all body systems below the level of the injury. If the lesion is high enough, the patient may lose pulmonary function and die.

Serious complications associated with spinal cord injury include paralysis, autonomic dysreflexia, and sexual dysfunction.

Classification
Spinal cord injuries may be complete or incomplete and may or may not involve a fracture of the vertebral column.
• *Complete lesions* cause the loss of all voluntary muscle control and all sensations of touch, pain, and temperature on both sides of the body below the level of the lesion. Spinal shock is usually an immediate result of a complete injury.
• *Incomplete lesions* cause some motor loss below the level of injury, accompanied by spotty sensory losses. Incomplete lesions are classified ac-

cording to the area of damage: central, lateral, anterior, or peripheral.

Causes
Injuries to the spinal cord are usually caused by a trauma to the head or neck, often displacing bone from the spinal column, which then encroaches into the spinal canal and compresses, twists, or severs the cord.

Fractures and dislocations can also pinch or tear spinal and vertebral arteries, interrupting blood supply to the spinal cord or causing aneurysms or emboli.

Spinal injuries occur most often in the cervical and lumbar segments of the spine because they are the most mobile parts of the vertebral column.

ASSESSMENT

Keep the patient immobile. Because many spinal cord injuries are associated with head injuries, assess the patient for head injury.

In the unconscious patient, always assume the presence of a spinal cord injury until it is definitively ruled out. Pay careful attention to respirations and other vital signs. Check for signs and symptoms of spinal shock, including:
• decreased blood pressure (systolic pressure below 80 mm Hg)
• peripheral vasodilation due to unopposed parasympathetic stimulation
• a decreased pulse rate (less than 60 beats/minute)
• pink, warm, dry skin
• decreased temperature (less than 98° F [36.7° C])
• immediate areflexia, flaccid paralysis, and loss of skin sensation below the lesion.

Your assessment should include consideration of the patient's health history, physical examination findings, and diagnostic test results.

Health history

When assessing a patient with a spinal cord injury, obtain as much information as possible about how the injury occurred. If the trauma was severe, such as a fall from a height or an automobile accident, determine the patient's position when found, immediate symptoms, and what changes in the patient's status have occurred since the time of the injury. Was extrication from the accident scene difficult, and did rescuers use immobilization equipment?

Find out if the patient has ever had arthritis, a congenital deformity of the spine, degenerative disease of the spine, or underlying pulmonary disease (an important factor if the patient has a high cervical injury).

Physical examination

Depending on the severity and location of the injury, physical findings may vary. Your assessment may reveal the presence of neck or back pain, inadequate respirations, inability to move the extremities, and absent or diminished sensation.

Diagnostic test results

The following tests may be ordered to help identify the type and extent of spinal cord injury:
• X-rays of the spine will identify the fracture type. Initially, a lateral film of the cervical region may be taken. To do this, the X-ray technician (or doctor) puts the patient in a supine position and pulls the patient's arms down while the X-ray is being taken. This allows full visualization of the C7 cervical region. Depending on the results of the lateral X-ray or on the mechanism of injury, complete spinal X-rays may be necessary.
• Computed tomography scan of the region of fracture shows the spinal canal and identifies bone fragments.

• Magnetic resonance imaging (MRI) shows tissue damage, provides information about the spinal canal, and identifies bone fragments. However, MRI is difficult to perform in an unstable, critically ill patient. (See *Functional loss from spinal cord injury,* pages 136 to 138.)

NURSING DIAGNOSIS

Common nursing diagnoses for a patient with spinal cord injury include:
• High risk for injury related to instability of the vertebral column and hazards of immobilization devices
• Ineffective airway clearance related to retained secretions
• Decreased cardiac output related to spinal shock or loss of vasomotor tone
• Dysreflexia related to neurologic injury
• Impaired physical mobility related to neurologic dysfunction
• Ineffective breathing pattern related to paralysis of diaphragm, intercostal, and abdominal muscles.

PLANNING

Based on the nursing diagnosis *high risk for injury,* develop appropriate patient outcomes. For example, your patient will:
• remain free of further sensory or motor impairment throughout hospitalization
• remain free of complications associated with immobilization devices.

Based on the nursing diagnosis *ineffective airway clearance,* develop appropriate patient outcomes. For example, your patient will:
• exhibit clear breath sounds
• maintain baseline arterial blood gas (ABG) levels

(Text continues on page 138.)

Functional loss from spinal cord injury

This illustration of the spinal cord and spinal nerves will help you to visualize the location of nerves that are involved in the specific functional losses (based on complete lesions) that are described on the opposite page.

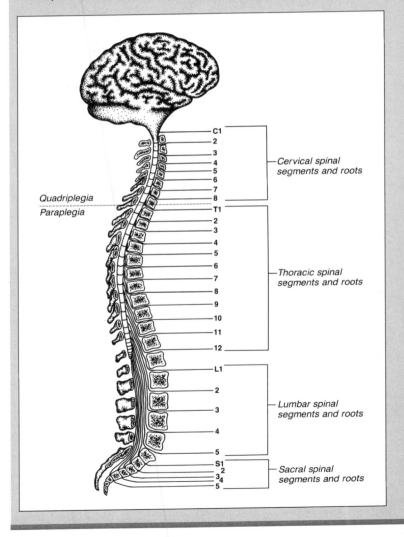

Functional losses from spinal cord injury include variable losses of motor function, deep tendon reflexes, sensory function, respiratory function, and bowel and bladder function, depending on which vertebral level is affected.

Level C1 to C4
- Complete loss of motor function below neck
- No reflex loss
- Loss of all sensory function in neck and below
- Loss of involuntary and voluntary respiratory function
- Loss of bowel and bladder control

Level C5
- Loss of all motor function below upper shoulders
- Loss of deep tendon reflexes in biceps
- Loss of sensation below clavicle and in most of chest, abdomen, and upper and lower extremities
- Phrenic nerve is intact, but not intercostal and abdominal muscles
- Loss of bowel and bladder control

Level C6
- Loss of all function below shoulders; no elbow, forearm, or hand control
- Loss of deep tendon reflexes in biceps
- Loss of sensation below clavicle and in most of chest, abdomen, and upper and lower extremities
- Phrenic nerve is intact, but not intercostal and abdominal muscles
- Loss of bowel and bladder control

Level C7
- Loss of motor control to portions of arms and hands
- Loss of deep tendon reflexes in triceps
- Loss of sensation below clavicle and in portions of arms and hands
- Phrenic nerve is intact, but not intercostal and abdominal muscles
- Loss of bowel and bladder function

Level C8
- Loss of motor control to portions of arms and hands
- Loss of deep tendon reflexes in triceps
- Loss of sensation below chest and in portions of hands
- Phrenic nerve is intact, but not intercostal and abdominal muscles
- Loss of bowel and bladder function

Level T1 to T6
- Loss of all motor function below midchest region, including trunk muscles
- No reflex loss
- Loss of sensation below midchest area
- Phrenic nerve functions independently
- Some impairment of intercostal and abdominal muscles
- Loss of bowel and bladder function

(continued)

Functional loss from spinal cord injury *(continued)*

Level T6 to T12
- Loss of motor control below waist
- No reflex loss
- Loss of all sensation below waist
- No interference with respiratory function
- Impairment of abdominal muscles leading to diminished cough
- Loss of bowel and bladder control

Level L1 to L3
- Loss of most of leg and pelvis control
- Loss of knee jerk reflex (L2, L3)
- Loss of sensation to lower abdomen and legs
- No interference with respiratory function
- Loss of bowel and bladder control

Level L3 to L4
- Loss of control of portions of lower legs, ankles, and feet

- Loss of knee jerk reflex
- Loss of sensation to portions of lower legs, feet, and ankles
- No interference with respiratory function
- Loss of bowel and bladder control

Level L4 to S5
- Varying extent of motor control loss
- Loss of ankle jerk reflex (S1, S2)
- Loss of sensation in upper legs and portions of lower legs (lumbar sensory nerves) and in lower legs, feet, and perineum (sacral sensory nerves)
- No interference with respiratory function
- Possible impairment of bowel and bladder control

- cough and expectorate secretions effectively.

Based on the nursing diagnosis *decreased cardiac output,* develop appropriate patient outcomes. For example, your patient will:
- maintain a systolic blood pressure of 90 mm Hg or above
- maintain a heart rate of at least 50 beats/minute, and a cardiac output and index, pulmonary artery wedge pressure, and systemic vascular resistance within normal limits for the patient's age
- maintain a urine output higher than 50 ml/hour

- maintain a capillary refill time of less than 3 seconds
- exhibit alert, oriented mentation.

Based on the nursing diagnosis *dysreflexia,* develop appropriate patient outcomes. For example, your patient will:
- remain free of episodes of autonomic dysreflexia throughout hospitalization.

The patient or his caregiver also will:
- know the symptoms of dysreflexia
- be familiar with measures to prevent dysreflexia after discharge
- explain measures to manage acute episodes of dysreflexia.

Based on the nursing diagnosis *impaired physical mobility,* develop appropriate patient outcomes. For example, your patient will:

• maintain muscle strength and joint range of motion

• show no evidence of complications such as contractures, venous stasis, or skin breakdown

• achieve the highest level of mobility possible following spinal surgery.

Based on the nursing diagnosis *ineffective breathing pattern,* develop appropriate patient outcomes. For example, your patient will:

• maintain normal respiratory rate and pattern

• demonstrate equal chest expansion

• maintain a vital capacity of 10 to 15 cc/kg and a negative inspiratory force of -25 cm H_2O to avoid the need for mechanical ventilation

• produce clear, odorless sputum and a negative sputum culture while in the hospital.

IMPLEMENTATION

Care of the patient with spinal cord injury requires careful planning and a strong interdisciplinary approach. Nursing interventions will vary with the treatment approach and the type of injury. (See *Medical care of the patient with spinal cord injury,* page 140.)

Nursing interventions
Many patients with spinal cord injuries must be immobilized.

Skeletal traction
• Make sure the proper amount of weight is in place if the patient is maintained in traction to prevent further cervical injury.

• If skull tongs have been ordered, clean the tong site and inspect for infection daily, applying a sterile dress-ing each time. Assess the tongs for tightness and check the patient's alignment. Make sure that the rope doesn't get caught in the mattress and that the weights never rest on the floor. If the patient is being maintained in a hard collar, assess for proper size, position, and tightness.

• If the patient is placed in a halo device, make sure the pins are tight and check the edges of the jacket for fit, which should not be too tight. Perform pin care according to hospital guidelines.

Additional interventions
• After establishing the initial baseline of motor and sensory deficits, assess the patient daily according to hospital guidelines. Also assess him after each transfer, and after weight removal or addition until the fracture is surgically stabilized. The documented assessment should include sensory and motor function, proprioception, and anal reflex.

• Monitor vital signs, report symptomatic bradycardia or hypotension, and maintain crystalloid infusions as needed.

• Consider elevating the patient's legs to increase cardiac volume.

• Discuss the need for a vasopressor if systolic blood pressure is less than 90 mm Hg.

• Maintain fluid intake as directed by the doctor.

• Assess respiratory rate, pattern, and effort and auscultate breath sounds every 2 to 4 hours.

• Assess the use of accessory abdominal and diaphragm muscles.

• Document negative inspiratory force and vital capacity every 8 hours or more often as needed.

• Perform chest percussion, assisted coughing, and suctioning, and change the patient's position every 2 hours, as indicated.

Treatments

Medical care of the patient with spinal cord injury

Medical management of spinal cord injury may include nonsurgical or surgical treatments.

Nonsurgical management
If a fracture is stable, the patient may need skeletal traction using skull tongs or a halo device for immobilization and to reduce the risk of further fracture.

Skull tongs
Tongs can be inserted at the patient's bedside. The procedure involves shaving a small section of the head, injecting a local anesthetic, and placing pins on either side of the skull.

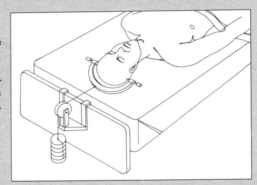

Halo device
This device helps maintain traction and allows for patient mobility.
   Traction must be maintained for 4 to 12 weeks after the injury, depending on the extent of the injury and the prescribed treatment.

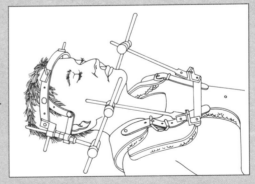

Surgical management
Surgery may be necessary for stabilizing the spine and removing bone fragments from the spinal canal. If the patient has an incomplete lesion, surgery aims to arrest progression of the deficit. Commonly performed procedures include decompression laminectomy with fusion, posterior laminectomy with acrylic mesh and fusion, and insertion of Harrington rods (to stabilize and correct thoracic deformities).

- Use pulse oximetry to monitor oxygenation status if the patient is short of breath.
- Use a touch or call device to enable the patient to call for help.
- Set activity limits when necessary, establish a sense of trust, and involve family and friends in care as much as possible.
- Allow the patient adequate time daily for venting his feelings. Refer him for psychological counseling to assist him in coping.

Patient teaching
- Explain treatment options to the patient, allowing him to participate in decisions related to his care. Let him control as many aspects of his environment as possible.
- Teach the patient and his family how to cope with a completely altered lifestyle. Most patients with spinal cord injury will spend some time in a rehabilitation facility after discharge from the hospital.
- If the patient is discharged in a halo device, teach him and his family how to care for the pin sites and how to assess for tightness of the pins. Advise them to immediately report to the doctor any loosening of the traction device.
- Teach the patient and his family the signs and symptoms of autonomic dysreflexia and interventions necessary to relieve the symptoms.
- Teach them measures to maintain skin integrity.
- Teach the patient to perform range-of-motion exercises as ordered.
- Teach the patient and his family how to maintain bowel and bladder function. Emphasize the importance of adequate fluid intake and implementation of daily routines to avoid incontinence. (See *Ensuring continued care for the patient with spinal cord injury,* page 142.)

EVALUATION

When evaluating your patient's response to nursing care, gather reassessment data and compare this information with the patient outcomes specified in your plan of care.

Teaching and counseling
Talk to the patient and his family to determine the effectiveness of your teaching and counseling. Consider the following questions:
- Has the patient identified ways to manage his environment?
- Does he participate in decisions related to his care?
- Can the patient and his caregiver describe the symptoms of dysreflexia and identify measures to prevent or manage it after discharge?

Physical condition
When evaluating the patient's physical condition, consider the following questions:
- Does the patient remain free of injury related to spinal column instability and immobilization devices?
- Does he exhibit clear breath sounds?
- Does he maintain baseline ABG levels?
- Does he cough and expectorate secretions effectively?
- Does he maintain a systolic blood pressure of at least 90 mm Hg and a heart rate of at least 50 beats/minute?
- Does he maintain a urine output higher than 50 ml/hr?
- Does he maintain a capillary refill time of less than 3 seconds?
- Does the patient appear oriented?
- Does he remain free of episodes of dysreflexia?
- Does he maintain muscle strength and joint range of motion to the greatest extent possible?

Discharge TimeSaver

Ensuring continued care for the patient with spinal cord injury

Review the following teaching topics, referrals, and follow-up appointments to make sure that your patient is adequately prepared for discharge.

Teaching topics
Make sure that the following topics have been covered and that your patient's learning has been evaluated:
☐ understanding of the injury and associated complications
☐ management of halo device if applicable
☐ skin care for the prevention of pressure ulcers
☐ breathing exercises
☐ assisted coughing, if applicable
☐ causes of autonomic dysreflexia and interventions for it
☐ maintenance of body alignment and passive exercises
☐ transfer techniques
☐ proper use of a wheelchair and other adaptive devices designed to aid patient in daily activities.

Referrals
Make sure that the patient has been provided with necessary referrals to:
☐ rehabilitation services
☐ social services
☐ vocational counseling
☐ home health care agency.

Follow-up appointments
Make sure that the necessary follow-up appointments have been scheduled and that the patient has been notified:
☐ psychiatrist
☐ neurosurgeon
☐ orthopedic surgeon
☐ rehabilitative psychologist
☐ physical and occupational therapist
☐ internist if necessary.

• Does he achieve the highest level of mobility possible following surgery?
• Does he maintain a normal respiratory rate and pattern with equal chest expansion?
• Does he maintain appropriate vital capacity and negative inspiratory force measurements?
• Does he produce clear, odorless sputum?

CHAPTER 5

Caring for patients with CNS infections

Meningitis

Meningitis is an inflammation of the membranes surrounding the brain, spinal cord, and cranial and peripheral nerves. It occurs when pathogens invade the central nervous system through the bloodstream. (See *How meningitis affects the brain.*)

Causes

Meningitis usually stems from a bacterial infection but may result from protozoal, fungal, or viral infection. (See *Key points about meningitis,* page 146.) The viral form, known as aseptic viral meningitis, usually has a limited course, with most patients recovering fully. Despite improvements in treatment, bacterial meningitis is a medical emergency that, without prompt care, can cause complications and lead to death within days. (See *Complications of meningitis,* page 147.)

Causative bacterial microorganisms include:
- *Neisseria meningitidis* (also called meningococcus)
- *Haemophilus influenzae*
- *Streptococcus pneumoniae.*

ASSESSMENT

Because of the potential severity of meningitis, you'll need to obtain a timely and thorough history from the patient and family members. Support your findings by reviewing physical examination and diagnostic test results.

Health history

The patient (or his family) may report the following signs and symptoms:
- severe headache
- stiff neck and back
- malaise
- photophobia
- chills
- vomiting
- twitching
- seizures
- altered level of consciousness (LOC).

Vomiting and fever occur more commonly in children than in adults. Affected infants may be fretful, refuse to eat, and suffer from listlessness and bulging fontanels.

Risk factors

In most patients, meningitis results from a preexisting condition, procedure, or infectious disease.

Previous conditions or procedures
The patient may have a predisposing condition or may have undergone a procedure that makes him susceptible to meningitis, such as:
- skull fracture
- penetrating head wound
- human immunodeficiency virus (HIV) infection
- lumbar puncture
- ventricular shunting
- neurosurgery
- ear or sinus surgery.

Previous infections
Many patients with bacterial meningitis have a history of bacterial infection, such as:
- pneumonia
- mastoiditis
- empyema
- osteomyelitis
- endocarditis
- sinusitis
- otitis media.

Patients with viral meningitis may have a history of measles, mumps, or herpes virus.

How meningitis affects the brain

In meningitis, microorganisms invade the central nervous system through the bloodstream, through peripheral nerves, or from adjacent areas. Pathogens in the subarachnoid space then invade the cerebrospinal fluid (CSF) and inflame the pia mater, arachnoidea, and ventricles. Exudate accumulates over the brain and spinal cord and can extend to the cranial and peripheral nerves. Exudate may also block CSF flow and lead to hydrocephalus and increased intracranial pressure (ICP). The meningeal cells may then become edematous, which can further increase ICP, engorge the blood vessels in the meninges, disrupt the blood flow, and possibly cause thrombosis or rupture the vessel walls.

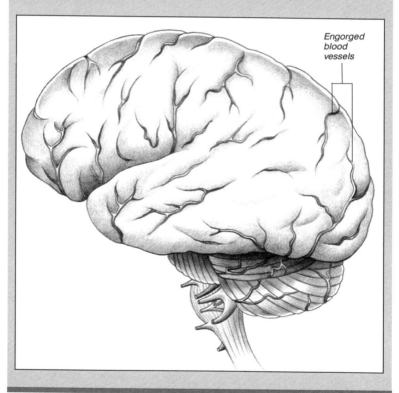

Engorged blood vessels

Additional risk factors
Other risk factors include:
- malnourishment
- radiation therapy
- chemotherapy
- long-term corticosteroid therapy.

Physical examination

Physical findings depend on the infection's severity. Your examination should include assessment of LOC, signs of meningeal irritation, cranial nerves, and other areas.

Level of consciousness
Initially, the patient may have a decreased attention span or memory impairment. However, as meningitis progresses, he may become disoriented and possibly comatose.

Because changes in LOC may indicate rising intracranial pressure (ICP), always establish a baseline using a standard tool such as the Glasgow Coma Scale.

Meningeal signs
Inspection may reveal signs of meningeal irritation, including positive Brudzinski's and Kernig's signs. (See *Two key signs of meningitis,* page 148.) Other signs include exaggerated and symmetrical deep tendon reflexes and opisthotonos (a form of spasm in which the head and heels are bent backward and the body is bowed forward).

Cranial nerves
Testing the cranial nerves may reveal neurologic deficits. Pupils are commonly unequal and sluggish in responding to light. As the patient's condition deteriorates, pupils may become fixed and dilated. Major deficits include:
- ocular palsies if cranial nerves III, IV, and VI are involved
- facial paresis if cranial nerve VII is involved
- hearing loss and vertigo if cranial nerve VIII is affected.

Other deficits may include dizziness, facial weakness, and ptosis.

Additional findings
Early assessment of motor function can reveal muscle hypotonia. Paresis or paralysis may occur later.

In meningococcal meningitis, inspection of the lower body may reveal a petechial, purpuric, or ecchymotic rash. Fever and tachycardia may be present. In bacterial meningitis, fever can remain high throughout the illness and exceed 105° F (40.5° C) in the terminal stages.

Monitor the patient if you suspect increased ICP, which results from purulent exudate and hydrocephalus.

Diagnostic test results

The following tests may reveal predisposing factors and help identify the causes of meningitis:

• A lumbar puncture may reveal changes in cerebrospinal fluid pressure, consistency, protein level, white blood cell (WBC) count, and glucose level.

• A Gram stain and culture can identify the causative bacterium.

• Blood, urine, and respiratory tract cultures can also help identify the source of the infection.

• Chest X-rays reveal pneumonitis, lung abscess, tubercular lesions, cranial osteomyelitis, paranasal sinusitis, skull fracture, or granulomas caused by fungal infection.

• A computed tomography scan may reveal cerebral hematoma, hemorrhage, hydrocephalus, or tumor.

• A complete blood count may reveal an increased WBC count, usually indicating leukocytosis.

• Serum electrolyte studies may indicate hyponatremia and hypochloremia.

Complications of meningitis

Meningitis can cause a range of serious complications, including:
• visual impairment
• optic neuritis
• cranial nerve palsies
• epilepsy
• hearing loss
• personality changes
• headache
• paresis or paralysis
• endocarditis
• pneumonia
• coma
• vasculitis
• cerebral infarction
• encephalitis
• brain abscess
• syndrome of inappropriate secretion of antidiuretic hormone.

Pediatric complications

Other complications seen primarily in children include:
• unilateral or bilateral sensory hearing loss
• mental retardation
• hydrocephalus
• subdural effusions.

NURSING DIAGNOSIS

Common nursing diagnoses for a patient with meningitis include:
• Pain related to meningeal irritation
• Altered cerebral tissue perfusion related to increased ICP
• Hyperthermia related to infection
• High risk for injury related to altered LOC and seizures.

PLANNING

Based on the nursing diagnosis *pain*, develop appropriate patient outcomes. For example, your patient will:
• rate pain on a scale of 1 to 10
• report that pain doesn't interfere with daily activities
• report relief of pain.

Based on the nursing diagnosis *altered cerebral tissue perfusion*, develop

Assessment TimeSaver

Two key signs of meningitis

Brudzinski's sign and Kernig's sign are two diagnostic tests that can help identify meningitis.

Brudzinski's sign
With the patient lying on her back, put your hands behind her neck and bring the head forward to the chest. If she has meningitis, she'll exhibit pain and resistance and flex her hips and knees.

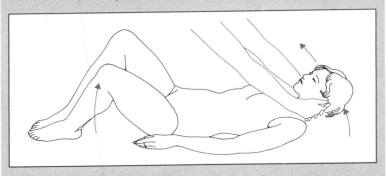

Kernig's sign
With the patient lying on her back, flex her leg at the hip to a 90-degree angle and then straighten the knee. If she has meningitis, she'll resist and experience pain caused by inflammation of the meninges and spinal roots.

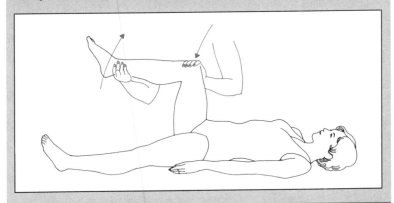

appropriate patient outcomes. For example, your patient will:
• exhibit an ICP less than or equal to 15 mm Hg
• register a score of 11 to 15 on the Glasgow Coma Scale
• exhibit reactive pupils
• demonstrate normal respiration
• exhibit systolic blood pressure within 20 mm Hg of an acceptable baseline level
• have a normal pulse rate
• experience no vomiting or seizures
• demonstrate adequate motor skills.

Based on the nursing diagnosis *hyperthermia,* develop appropriate patient outcomes. For example, your patient will:
• have an oral temperature below 101.6° F (38.7° C)
• be able to detect early signs of hyperthermia, such as fatigue, chills, and general malaise.

Based on the nursing diagnosis *high risk for injury,* develop appropriate patient outcomes. For example, your patient will:
• remain free of injury while hospitalized
• demonstrate compliance with safety measures.

IMPLEMENTATION

Treatment consists of aggressive drug therapy and vigorous supportive care. I.V. antibiotics, commonly prescribed for at least 2 weeks, are followed by oral antibiotics. (See *Medical care of the patient with meningitis,* page 150.)

Nursing interventions
• Follow your hospital's infection control policy. Expect to maintain isolation until the infection's cause is identified and cultures are negative. Consider discharges from the nose and the mouth as infectious.

• Monitor the patient's clinical status continually, including neurologic function and vital signs. (See *Early warning signs in meningitis,* page 151.)
• Assess the cranial nerves and monitor for signs of increasing ICP.
• Obtain arterial blood gas measurements, and maintain partial pressure of arterial oxygen at ordered levels. Mechanical ventilation may be required if the patient can't maintain adequate oxygenation. If necessary, care for his endotracheal or tracheostomy tube.
• Monitor fluid balance to control cerebral edema, but avoid dehydration.
• Administer prescribed medications, and watch for adverse reactions.
• Position the patient carefully to prevent joint stiffness and neck pain. Turn him often, according to a planned positioning schedule. Assist with range-of-motion exercises, but caution against isometric exercises and hip flexion, which may increase ICP. Elevate the head of the bed 30 to 45 degrees to improve venous drainage and decrease ICP.
• Give the patient a mild laxative or stool softener, as ordered, to prevent constipation and minimize the risk of increased ICP.
• Monitor his temperature at least every 2 hours. Administer antipyretics as ordered. Control fever with tepid sponge baths or a hypothermia blanket as needed.
• Ensure the patient's safety by keeping the side rails of his bed up and padded.
• Make certain that suction equipment is on hand.
• Check on the patient frequently, reorienting him when necessary. Keep his call light next to him, and anticipate his needs. Helping the patient go to the bathroom or get a drink may prevent injury.

Treatments

Medical care of the patient with meningitis

Management of meningitis includes appropriate antibiotic therapy and vigorous supportive care.

Drug therapy

Because meningitis usually stems from bacterial infection, I.V. antibiotics are given for at least 2 weeks, followed by oral antibiotics. The regimen usually includes:
- cefotaxime sodium
- ceftriaxone sodium
- ampicillin
- penicillin
- co-trimoxazole (if the patient is allergic to penicillin).

Other drugs appropriate for coexisting conditions may be prescribed, including:
- mannitol to decrease cerebral edema
- an anticonvulsant or a sedative to reduce restlessness

- acetaminophen to relieve headache and fever
- an analgesic, such as codeine, that doesn't mask neurologic symptoms.

Supportive therapy

Supportive measures commonly include:
- bed rest
- hypothermia
- fluids as ordered
- isolation until the causative microorganism is identified and, if the cultures are positive, for 24 hours more after the start of antibiotic therapy or according to hospital policy.

Additional therapies

Other therapies may be required for coexisting conditions, such as endocarditis, pneumonia, and neurologic complications.

- Advise all staff members that the patient is at high risk for injury.
- Maintain adequate nutrition by providing small, frequent meals. Alternatively, the patient may require parenteral feedings. Consult with a nutritionist if appropriate.
- To ensure the patient's comfort, keep his room peaceful and orderly and dim the lights to decrease photophobia, if appropriate. Provide a non-narcotic analgesic, such as acetaminophen, to relieve headache. Be sure not to flex the patient's neck because this can cause severe discomfort and elevate ICP.

- Organize patient care and activities to maximize rest periods.

Timesaving tip: Create and post a schedule of daily rest periods and plan your nursing care accordingly. Consult with the patient and his family about the best times for rest. Post the schedule where all can see it.

- Reassure the patient, who may be frightened by his illness and frequent diagnostic tests. Explain to the family that the disorientation, reduced attention span, or impaired memory caused by meningitis usually disappears.

Assessment TimeSaver

Early warning signs in meningitis

Prompt recognition of a meningitis patient's worsening condition and early intervention may prevent more serious consequences. Timely recognition will depend on your ability to detect subtle changes in the patient's baseline status. Look for:
• sudden restlessness
• subtle changes in behavior, speech, or orientation
• deterioration in Glasgow Coma Scale score
• fever above 101.5° F (38.6° C)
• sluggish pupil reaction

• unilateral hippus (abnormally exaggerated rhythmic contraction and dilation of pupil)
• seizures
• increased resistance to passive movement
• inability to stretch out arms, or arms that tremble when outstretched
• elevated blood pressure
• bradycardia
• widened pulse pressure
• decreased sensory function
• vomiting
• loss of mental function
• headache.

• If a severe neurologic deficit appears to be permanent, refer the patient to a rehabilitation program.

Patient teaching
• Explain the nature of meningitis and its treatment to the patient and family members.
• Anyone who has come in close contact with a patient with meningococcal meningitis needs antibiotic prophylaxis and immediate medical attention if fever or other signs of meningitis develop. If appropriate, direct the patient and family members to notify recent contacts.
• Teach the patient about all of his prescribed medications. Stress the importance of taking antibiotics on time and completing the entire course of therapy.
• Encourage the patient to keep follow-up appointments. (See *Ensuring continued care for the patient with meningitis,* page 152.)

EVALUATION

To evaluate the patient's response to your care, gather reassessment data and compare this information to the patient outcomes specified in your plan of care.

Teaching and counseling
Begin by evaluating the effectiveness of your teaching and counseling. Note statements by the patient indicating his understanding of the condition, including its progression and possible complications. Consider the following questions:
• Has the patient identified activities that intensify his pain?
• Has he identified activities that promote comfort and relaxation?
• After treatment, does he express a feeling of relief from pain?
• Is he willing to use support systems to help with coping?
• Does he report feeling less anxious?

Discharge TimeSaver

Ensuring continued care for the patient with meningitis

Review the following teaching topics, referrals, and follow-up appointments to make sure that your patient is adequately prepared for discharge.

Teaching topics
Make sure that the following topics have been covered and that your patient's learning has been evaluated:
☐ process, risk factors, and complications of meningitis
☐ prescribed medications and possible adverse effects
☐ signs and symptoms to report to the doctor immediately.

Referrals
Make sure that the patient has been provided with necessary referrals to:

☐ social services
☐ physical therapist if needed
☐ speech therapist if needed.

Follow-up appointments
Make sure that the necessary follow-up appointments have been scheduled and that the patient has been notified:
☐ doctor
☐ diagnostic tests.

Physical condition
Physical examination and diagnostic test results will also help to evaluate the effectiveness of care. If treatment has been effective, you should note the following:
• ICP less than or equal to 15 mm Hg
• a score of 11 to 15 on the Glasgow Coma Scale
• reactive pupils
• normal respiration
• systolic blood pressure that's within 20 mm Hg of acceptable baseline level
• normal pulse rate
• absence of vomiting or seizures
• absence of injuries
• adequate motor skills
• temperature below 101.6° F (38.7°C).

Encephalitis

An infection in the cerebral hemispheres, brain stem, or cerebellum, encephalitis is categorized as primary, postinfectious, or parainfectious. Primary encephalitis results from a single virus within the central nervous system. Postinfectious or parainfectious encephalitis occurs in combination with other viral illnesses. Incidence may be sporadic or epidemic.

Causes
Viruses, including the enteroviruses, herpes simplex virus type 1, and arboviruses, are the most common cause of encephalitis. Bacteria, fungi, or parasites may also cause the disorder.

Enteroviruses, the most common cause of epidemic encephalitis, include:
- coxsackievirus
- poliovirus
- echovirus
- viruses causing mumps and chicken pox.

Herpes simplex virus type 1 is the most common cause of sporadic encephalitis in North America. The infection may be fatal if the patient doesn't receive treatment before he becomes comatose.

Arboviruses are mosquito-borne or tick-borne and usually occur in rural areas. Common arboviruses include:
- Western equine encephalitis, which occurs throughout the entire Western Hemisphere
- California encephalitis, which occurs throughout the United States
- St. Louis encephalitis, which occurs in Florida and in the western and southern United States. (See *Complications of encephalitis*.)

ASSESSMENT

The different forms of viral encephalitis have similar clinical features. However, the severity of illness varies greatly, ranging from mild to rapidly fatal. Obtain a thorough history from the patient and family members. Support your findings by reviewing physical examination and diagnostic test results.

Health history
The patient may report the following signs and symptoms:
- headache
- muscle stiffness
- malaise
- sore throat
- confusion
- stupor
- hemiparesis

Complications of encephalitis

Potential complications associated with viral encephalitis include:
- bronchial pneumonia
- urine retention
- urinary tract infection
- pressure ulcers
- coma
- epilepsy
- parkinsonism
- mental deterioration
- cognitive deficits
- personality changes
- motor deficits
- dysphagia.

- upper respiratory tract symptoms
- altered level of consciousness (LOC) ranging from lethargy or drowsiness to stupor
- seizures (may be the only presenting sign of encephalitis)
- fever
- nausea
- vomiting.

Risk factors
Encephalitis may result from recent exposure to infectious disease, ulcerations of the oral cavity or cold sores, and a recent tick or mosquito bite.

Be sure to investigate all risk factors thoroughly when obtaining a health history. Because the patient may be unaware of an insect bite, inquire about any recent camping trips or other outdoor activities. Also, determine if he has been exposed to pets, such as dogs, that may carry ticks. These clues can aid early diagnosis.

Physical examination

Physical findings depend on the severity of the disease. Assessment of LOC typically reveals a patient who is confused, disoriented, hallucinating, or comatose. Cranial nerve examination may reveal ocular palsies, facial weakness, and dysphagia. Assessment of motor function may reveal hemiparesis or paralysis of the extremities and altered deep tendon reflexes.

Cerebral hemisphere involvement may result in focal deficits, such as involuntary movements, ataxia, disturbances of taste and smell, and poor memory. With meningeal irritation, the patient may demonstrate Kernig's or Brudzinski's signs and nuchal rigidity.

If intracranial pressure (ICP) is elevated, you'll note a change in vital signs and respiratory patterns.

Diagnostic test results

Epidemic encephalitis can normally be diagnosed from clinical findings and the patient history. However, sporadic encephalitis can be difficult to distinguish from other febrile illnesses, such as gastroenteritis or meningitis. The following tests can help diagnose encephalitis:

• Blood or cerebrospinal fluid (CSF) analysis can identify the virus and confirm the diagnosis. CSF analysis commonly reveals clear fluid, a slightly elevated white blood cell count and protein levels, and a normal glucose level.
• Serologic studies may show rising titers of complement-fixing antibodies in herpes encephalitis.
• Lumbar puncture discloses elevated CSF pressure in all forms of encephalitis.
• EEG reveals slow waveforms.
• Computed tomography (CT) scan may disclose temporal lobe lesions

that indicate herpes virus. However, magnetic resonance imaging provides more precise views of cerebral tissue than CT scanning.
• Brain biopsy can diagnose or confirm herpes simplex encephalitis.

NURSING DIAGNOSIS

Common nursing diagnoses for a patient with encephalitis include:
• Hyperthermia related to infection
• Altered thought processes related to increased ICP or cerebral edema
• Impaired physical mobility related to neurologic dysfunction
• Altered cerebral tissue perfusion related to increased ICP.

PLANNING

Based on the nursing diagnosis *hyperthermia,* develop appropriate patient outcomes. For example, your patient will:
• have an oral temperature below 101.6° F (38.7° C)
• report early warning signs of hyperthermia, such as fatigue, chills, and general malaise.

Based on the nursing diagnosis *altered thought processes,* develop appropriate patient outcomes. For example, your patient will:
• exhibit orientation to person, place, and time
• report his daily needs
• participate in decision making
• relate to others in an appropriate manner.

Based on the nursing diagnosis *impaired physical mobility,* develop appropriate patient outcomes. For example, your patient will:
• maintain maximum mobility within the limits of his neurologic impairment
• remain free of complications caused by immobility, such as con-

Treatments

Medical care of the patient with encephalitis

Treatment for encephalitis includes drug therapy and supportive measures.

Drug therapy
Drug therapy for encephalitis usually includes:
• acyclovir or vidarabine (these antiviral agents are effective only against herpes encephalitis and must be administered before coma)
• I.V. mannitol to reduce intracranial pressure (ICP)
• corticosteroids to reduce cerebral inflammation and edema
• I.V. phenytoin to reduce seizures
• antibiotics to prevent associated infections, such as pneumonia or sinusitis

• sedatives for restlessness
• acetaminophen to relieve headache and reduce fever.

Additional treatments
Other therapeutic measures include:
• maintaining fluid levels sufficient to prevent dehydration without increasing cerebral edema
• keeping an open airway
• maintaining normal arterial blood gas levels by administering oxygen
• providing mechanical ventilation to treat increased ICP or depressed level of consciousness
• maintaining nutrition, especially during a coma
• providing a rehabilitation program to deal with neurologic deficits.

tractures, venous stasis, thrombus formation, or skin breakdown.

Based on the nursing diagnosis *altered cerebral tissue perfusion,* develop appropriate patient outcomes. For example, your patient will:
• exhibit ICP less than or equal to 15 mm Hg
• demonstrate a score of 11 to 15 on the Glasgow Coma Scale
• exhibit reactive pupils
• exhibit normal respiration
• have a systolic blood pressure within 20 mm Hg of acceptable baseline level
• display a normal pulse rate
• experience no vomiting or seizures
• demonstrate acceptable motor skills.

IMPLEMENTATION

Medical treatment of encephalitis includes administration of antiviral agents and supportive measures. (See *Medical care of the patient with encephalitis.*)

Nursing interventions
• Monitor neurologic function often during the acute phase of the illness.
• Monitor for signs of increased ICP, especially early indications. (See *Warning signs of worsening encephalitis,* page 156.) Later signs of increased ICP include widened pulse pressure, vomiting, bradycardia, ataxic respirations, posturing, fixed and dilated pupils, and decreased LOC.

Assessment TimeSaver

Warning signs of worsening encephalitis

Use this list as a quick reference guide to warning signs of deterioration in your patient's condition:
• sudden restlessness or lethargy
• subtle changes in behavior, speech, or orientation
• deterioration in Glasgow Coma Scale
• fever above 101.5° F (38.6° C)
• sluggish or fixed and dilated pupils
• unilateral hippus (abnormally exaggerated rhythmic contraction and dilation of pupil)

• seizures
• increased resistance to passive movement
• worsening motor deficit
• inability to stretch out arms, or arms that tremble when outstretched
• ataxic respirations
• widened pulse pressure
• bradycardia
• headache
• vomiting.

• Maintain adequate fluid intake to prevent dehydration while avoiding cerebral edema.
• Administer acyclovir or vidarabine by slow I.V. infusion only if ordered.
• Monitor for adverse effects, such as tremor, dizziness, hallucinations, anorexia, nausea, vomiting, diarrhea, pruritus, rash, and anemia.
• Check infusion sites often to prevent infiltration and phlebitis.
• Give antipyretics and, if necessary, use a hypothermia blanket to control fever.
• Assess the patient's respiratory status frequently and maintain a patent airway to prevent atelectasis and pneumonia.
• Assess the patient's mobility.
• Be sure to turn the patient often, and support his affected extremities with pillows and adaptive devices. Assist him with range-of-motion exercises and position him to prevent joint stiffness, contractures, and neck pain.

• Assess for signs of thrombophlebitis, and apply compression boots if necessary.
• Provide skin care measures.

Patient management
• Ensure the patient's safety by keeping the bed's side rails up and padded.
• Have airway and suction equipment available.
• Reorient the patient if he's delirious or confused. Consider marking a calendar for him and providing a clock and familiar photographs.
• Always keep the patient informed, even if he is comatose.
• Consult with the occupational therapist about arranging meaningful activities for the patient.
• When speaking to the patient, use short, simple sentences. Always explain what you're going to do, then repeat yourself.
• Praise the patient when he demonstrates improved cognitive skills.
• Provide adequate nutrition by giving the patient small, frequent meals

Discharge TimeSaver

Ensuring continued care for the patient with encephalitis

Review the following teaching topics, referrals, and follow-up appointments to make sure that your patient is adequately prepared for discharge.

Teaching topics

Make sure that the following topics have been covered and that your patient's learning has been evaluated:

☐ process, risk factors, and complications of encephalitis

☐ prescribed medications, including dosage and possible adverse effects

☐ signs and symptoms to be reported to the doctor immediately.

Referrals

Make sure that the patient has been provided with necessary referrals to:

☐ social services

☐ rehabilitation center for physical therapy, occupational therapy, or speech therapy if needed.

Follow-up appointments

Make sure that the necessary follow-up appointments have been scheduled and that the patient has been notified:

☐ doctor

☐ diagnostic tests.

---

or providing nasogastric tube or parenteral feedings if necessary.

• Consult with the speech therapist if the patient's speech is impaired.

• Give the patient a mild laxative or stool softener to prevent constipation and minimize the risk of increased ICP resulting from straining during defecation.

• Maintain a quiet environment. Encourage normal sleep or rest patterns.

• Provide emotional support to the patient and family members.

Patient teaching

• Teach the patient and his family about encephalitis and its effects, diagnostic tests, and treatment measures, including any prescribed medications. Explain that behavior changes caused by the disease usually disappear.

• Refer the patient to a rehabilitation program if necessary for neurologic deficits.

Timesaving tip: Because the patient's attention span may be limited, keep your teaching sessions brief and make sure the environment is free of extraneous noise and activity. Schedule teaching when the family can be present. (See *Ensuring continued care for the patient with encephalitis.*)

EVALUATION

When evaluating the patient's response to your care, gather reassessment data and compare this information to the patient outcomes specified in your plan of care.

Teaching and counseling

Begin by evaluating the effectiveness of your teaching and counseling.

Note statements by the patient indicating his understanding of the condition, including its progression and possible complications. Consider the following questions:
- Is he willing to use support systems to help him cope?
- Does he report feeling less anxious?
- Does he report his daily needs?
- Does he relate to others in an appropriate manner?
- Is he willing to participate in decision making?
- Does he exhibit maximum mobility within the limits of his neurologic impairment?

Physical condition
Physical examination and diagnostic test results will also help to evaluate the effectiveness of care. If treatment has been effective, you should note the following:
- an oral temperature below 101.6° F (38.7° C)
- orientation to person, place and time
- freedom from complications of immobility, such as contractures, venous stasis, thrombus formation, or skin breakdown
- ICP less than or equal to 15 mm Hg
- score of 11 to 15 on the Glasgow Coma Scale
- reactive pupils
- normal respiration
- systolic blood pressure that's within 20 mm Hg of acceptable baseline level
- normal pulse rate
- absence of vomiting or seizures
- absence of injuries
- acceptable motor skills.

Brain abscess

Also called an intracranial abscess, this disorder occurs when disintegration of brain tissue leads to a free or encapsulated collection of pus in a cerebral cavity. The abscess occurs most commonly in the cerebellum and the frontal, parietal, temporal, or occipital lobes and, less commonly, in the basal ganglia.

Brain abscesses vary in size and may occur singly or in groups. Complications may include paralysis, altered mentation, seizures, and brain herniation. (See *Key points about brain abscess,* opposite, and *What happens in brain abscess,* page 160.)

Causes
Pyogenic bacteria, such as anaerobic streptococci and bacteroides, are the most common cause of brain abscess. Parasites or fungi may cause a brain abscess in immunosuppressed patients, such as those with acquired immunodeficiency syndrome.

ASSESSMENT
Accurate assessment requires a thorough history from the patient or family members, supported by physical examination and diagnostic test findings. (See *Correlating sites and signs of brain abscess,* page 161.)

Health history
Most patients seek treatment within 2 weeks. The patient (or a family member) typically reports such signs and symptoms as:
- headache
- stiff neck
- low-grade fever
- chills and malaise
- nausea and vomiting

• altered level of consciousness (LOC), including irritability, decreased alertness, drowsiness, and stupor.

Also ask about possible risk factors. (See *Risk factors for brain abscess,* page 162.)

Physical examination

Physical findings usually depend on the severity of the abscess. Neurologic examination typically reveals an altered LOC manifested by confusion or lethargy. Evaluation of motor skills normally reveals generalized weakness and sometimes hemiplegia.

Examination of the pupils may reveal a normal response early in the illness, but an increasingly sluggish response as intracranial pressure (ICP) rises. As ICP continues to rise, the patient's pupils will become fixed and dilated, his respiratory pattern will be altered, his pulse pressure will widen, and bradycardia may occur.

Diagnostic test results

The following tests can help diagnose a brain abscess:

• EEG, computed tomography scan, magnetic resonance imaging, arteriography, and brain biopsy can help locate the abscess.

• Cerebrospinal fluid analysis can confirm the infection.

• Other tests include cultures to identify the infection and X-rays, radioisotope scans, and ventriculography to further help identify the location.

NURSING DIAGNOSIS

Common nursing diagnoses for a patient with a brain abscess include:

• Altered cerebral tissue perfusion related to increased ICP

• Impaired physical mobility related to neurologic dysfunction

FactFinder

Key points about brain abscess

• *Incidence:* Although brain abscesses are rare, they can develop at any age. They occur most commonly between ages 10 and 35. Brain abscess occurs in about 2% of children with congenital heart disease.

• *Chief causes:* At least 40% of brain abscesses result from mastoid or ear infections and 10% result from sinus infections.

• *Prognosis:* The prognosis in a single brain abscess is fair. The prognosis in multiple, metastatic abscesses from systemic infection is poor. Left untreated, brain abscesses usually prove fatal. Mortality may be as high as 60%.

• *Chief diagnostic methods:* EEG, computed tomography scan, and magnetic resonance imaging.

• *Treatment:* Therapy consists of antibiotics to combat the underlying infection and surgical aspiration, drainage, or removal of the abscess (if encapsulated).

• *Complications:* Without treatment, empyema and meningitis may result. Hemiparesis, focal seizures, cranial nerve palsies, and visual deficits may occur even with treatment.

• High risk for injury related to sensory impairment

• Impaired verbal communication related to altered LOC or other neurologic deficit.

What happens in brain abscess

The illustrations below show the steps in the development of brain abscess.

Bacterial invasion
Bacteria invade the brain.

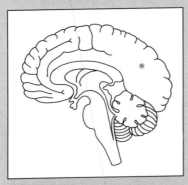

Inflammation
Inflammation occurs, causing tissue necrosis and pus formation. Associated vascular congestion leads to cerebral edema, and the necrotic tissue then liquefies.

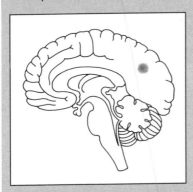

Capsule formation
Over a period of weeks, a fibroglial capsule forms and cavitates. This may lead to increased intracranial pressure.

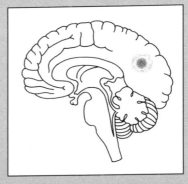

Rupture
Without treatment, the encapsulated abscess can rupture, causing additional abscesses and possibly empyema and meningitis.

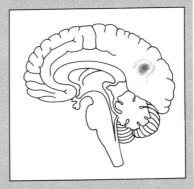

Correlating sites and signs of brain abscess

The patient's signs and symptoms correspond to the site of brain abscess. The most common sites are the frontal, parietal, occipital, and temporal lobes and the cerebellum. Refer to the illustration below for a quick review.

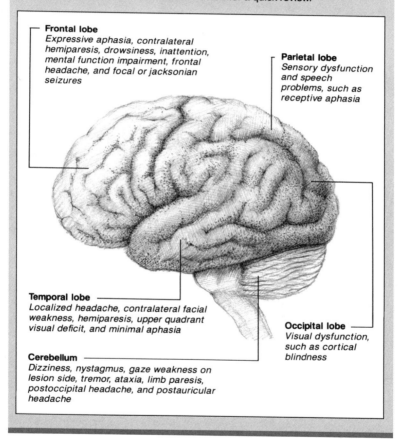

Frontal lobe
Expressive aphasia, contralateral hemiparesis, drowsiness, inattention, mental function impairment, frontal headache, and focal or jacksonian seizures

Parietal lobe
Sensory dysfunction and speech problems, such as receptive aphasia

Temporal lobe
Localized headache, contralateral facial weakness, hemiparesis, upper quadrant visual deficit, and minimal aphasia

Occipital lobe
Visual dysfunction, such as cortical blindness

Cerebellum
Dizziness, nystagmus, gaze weakness on lesion side, tremor, ataxia, limb paresis, postoccipital headache, and postauricular headache

PLANNING

Based on the nursing diagnosis *altered cerebral tissue perfusion*, develop appropriate patient outcomes. For example, your patient will:
• have an ICP less than or equal to 15 mm Hg

- demonstrate a score of 11 to 15 on the Glasgow Coma Scale
- exhibit reactive pupils
- exhibit normal respiration
- have a systolic blood pressure within 20 mm Hg of an acceptable baseline level
- display a normal pulse rate
- experience no vomiting or seizures

- demonstrate acceptable motor skills.

Based on the nursing diagnosis *impaired physical mobility,* develop appropriate patient outcomes. For example, your patient will:
- maintain maximum mobility within the limits of his neurologic impairment
- remain free of complications caused by immobility, such as contractures, venous stasis, thrombus formation, or skin breakdown.

Based on the nursing diagnosis *high risk for injury,* develop appropriate patient outcomes. For example, your patient will:
- remain free of injury
- demonstrate compliance with safety measures.

Based on the nursing diagnosis *impaired verbal communication,* develop appropriate patient outcomes. For example, your patient will:
- use methods other than speaking to report his needs
- confirm that his needs are consistently met
- display a consistent ability to follow directions
- demonstrate an improved ability to speak.

IMPLEMENTATION

Medical treatment for a brain abscess consists mainly of antibiotics to treat the underlying infection and, if necessary, surgery to remove the abscess once it encapsulates. (See *Medical care of the patient with brain abscess.*)

Nursing interventions
- Assess the patient frequently for signs of increasing ICP, such as altered LOC, vomiting, seizures, restlessness, abnormal pupil response, and worsening motor skills. Take note of a 2-point drop on the Glas-

Treatments

Medical care of the patient with brain abscess

Medical treatment for brain abscess includes drug therapy, surgery, and preventive or supportive measures.

Drug therapy
The patient with brain abscess usually receives antibiotics to combat the underlying infection.

Surgery
Although somewhat controversial, a craniotomy may be performed to remove the abscess, but only after it becomes encapsulated. Surgery is contraindicated in patients with congenital heart disease or other debilitating cardiac conditions.

Postoperative measures
Computed tomography scans are performed after surgery to make sure that the infection has been eliminated. Antibiotics, such as metronidazole, nafcillin, or high-dose penicilin G, begun at least 2 weeks before surgery and continued for at least 4 weeks after surgery, help reduce the risk of infection.

Preventive or supportive measures
During the acute phase, treatment measures can only provide relief. These include:
• mechanical ventilation
• I.V. diuretics
• corticosteroids to maintain intracranial pressure levels and avoid cerebral edema
• anticonvulsants to prevent seizures.
Treatment for multiple abscesses usually consists of antibiotic therapy alone.

gow Coma Scale score or reports from family members of peculiar behavior by the patient.
• To detect cerebral herniation, a possible complication of elevated ICP levels, check for fixed and dilated pupils, widened pulse pressure, tachycardia, and abnormal respiration. (See *Responding to impending brain herniation,* page 164.)
• Monitor vital signs.
• Maintain adequate fluid levels to avoid cerebral edema but prevent dehydration.
• Provide emotional support to the patient and family.
• Encourage the patient to use an alternative form of communication, if necessary, such as eye blinking or using a magic slate, a chalkboard, or an alphabet board.

Timesaving tip: If the patient has a speech deficit, give him a deck of cards on which common requests or statements are printed. He can then show you the card appropriate to his need. Consult with the speech therapist about the patient's speech deficits, and follow through as needed.
• Prevent joint stiffness, contractures, and neck pain by properly aligning the patient in his bed and turning him every 2 hours. Make certain that a turning schedule appears in the plan of care.
• Keep the call light near the patient, and check on him often. Ensure safe-

Treatments

Responding to impending brain herniation

If you suspect that brain herniation is imminent, you must act immediately. Perform the interventions in the following checklist:

☐ Notify the doctor at once.

☐ Make sure that the head of the bed is elevated 30 to 45 degrees and that the patient's head is aligned without neck flexion or head rotation. Check that his hips are not flexed more than 90 degrees.

☐ Begin a slow I.V. infusion at a keep-vein-open rate.

☐ If a ventriculostomy catheter is inserted, drain cerebrospinal fluid as directed.

☐ Administer an osmotic diuretic (such as mannitol) or a loop diuretic (such as furosemide), or both, as ordered.

☐ Administer corticosteroids as ordered.

☐ Check the patient's temperature, and treat fever if necessary.

☐ Maintain a calm environment.

☐ Prepare the patient for emergency computed tomography scan, magnetic resonance imaging, or neurosurgery.

☐ If the patient is being mechanically ventilated, use hyperventilation to keep his partial pressure of arterial carbon dioxide between 25 and 30 mm Hg.

• Support the patient's extremities with pillows and adaptive devices if necessary.

• Assist with range-of-motion exercises.

• Consult with the physical therapist about impaired mobility.

• Assess for signs of thrombophlebitis, and apply antiembolism stockings if necessary.

• Provide skin care.

• Administer prescribed medications and observe their effect.

Postoperative measures

• Monitor the patient's neurologic status and vital signs.

• Monitor the patient for increasing ICP and meningitis by checking for nuchal rigidity, headaches, chills, and sweating.

• Change the dressing as soon as it becomes damp.

• Prevent reaccumulation of the abscess by positioning the patient on the operative side to promote drainage.

• Provide the patient with meticulous skin care to prevent pressure ulcers, and align him properly in his bed to preserve joint function and prevent contractures.

• Help the patient ambulate to prevent complications of immobility.

• Encourage the patient to be independent. Point out actions that he can perform successfully.

• Consult with the social services department about the patient's discharge. If the patient has mild deficits, he is usually discharged home. If his deficits are more severe, he may need long-term rehabilitation or care.

Patient teaching

• Explain the nature of brain abscess to the patient and his family. Make sure they understand the diagnostic tests and treatments that will be per-

ty by keeping the side rails of his bed up and padded. Have airway and suction equipment available.

Ensuring continued care for the patient with brain abscess

Review the following teaching topics, referrals, and follow-up appointments to make sure that your patient is adequately prepared for discharge.

Teaching topics

Make sure that the following topics have been covered and that your patient's learning has been evaluated:

☐ nature of brain abscess, including its process, risk factors, and complications

☐ prescribed medications, including dosage and possible adverse effects

☐ signs and symptoms that should be reported to the doctor immediately

☐ importance of keeping follow-up appointments.

Referrals

Make sure that the patient has been provided with necessary referrals to:

☐ social services

☐ rehabilitation facility for physical or speech therapy, if needed.

Follow-up appointments

Make sure that the necessary follow-up appointments have been scheduled and that the patient has been notified:

☐ neurologist

☐ neurosurgeon

☐ diagnostic tests for reevaluation.

formed. Explain all procedures to the patient, even if he's comatose.

• If surgery is necessary, explain the procedure to the patient and answer his questions.

• If the patient requires isolation because of postoperative drainage, make sure he and his family understand why. Inform the family that infection can occur again even after treatment.

• Teach the patient and his family about prescribed medications. Explain that antibiotic and anticonvulsant drugs may still be necessary after discharge. Make certain the patient and his family understand the importance of taking all medications as prescribed.

• To prevent future brain abscesses, stress the need for prompt treatment

of otitis media, mastoiditis, dental abscess, and other infections.

• Encourage the patient to keep all follow-up appointments and to follow through on all recommended rehabilitation measures. (See *Ensuring continued care for the patient with brain abscess*.)

EVALUATION

When evaluating the patient's response to your care, gather reassessment data and compare this information to the patient outcomes specified in your plan of care.

Teaching and counseling

Begin by evaluating the effectiveness of your teaching and counseling. Note statements by the patient indicating his understanding of the con-

dition, including its progression and possible complications. Consider asking the following questions:
• Is the patient willing to use support systems to help him cope?
• Does he report feeling less anxious?
• Does he report his daily needs?
• Is he willing to use methods other than speaking to report his needs?
• Does he confirm that his needs are consistently met?
• Has he displayed a consistent ability to follow directions?
• Has he demonstrated an improved ability to speak?
• Has he exhibited maximum mobility within the limits of his neurologic impairment?
• Has he remained free of injuries?

Physical condition
Physical examination and diagnostic test results will provide additional evaluation information. If treatment has been successful, you should note the following outcomes:
• ICP less than or equal to 15 mm Hg
• score of 11 to 15 on the Glasgow Coma Scale
• reactive pupils
• normal respiration
• a systolic blood pressure within 20 mm Hg of acceptable baseline level
• normal pulse rate
• absence of vomiting or seizures
• acceptable motor skills
• absence of complications caused by immobility, such as contractures, venous stasis, thrombus formation, or skin breakdown.

Guillain-Barré syndrome

An acute, rapidly progressive, and potentially fatal form of polyneuritis, Guillain-Barré syndrome destroys

the myelin around the peripheral nerves, resulting in weakened and often paralyzed extremities and respiratory muscles, abnormal sensations, and the loss of reflexes. Commonly preceded by an upper respiratory tract infection, surgery, or vaccination, the syndrome is also known as infectious polyneuritis, Landry-Guillain-Barré syndrome, or acute idiopathic polyneuritis.

During the acute phase, the patient requires constant monitoring and support of vital functions. If he survives the acute phase, the patient usually recovers in several months, although he may need vigorous retraining, orthopedic adaptive devices, or corrective surgery to overcome residual deficits. (See *Key points about Guillain-Barré syndrome*, opposite, and *Nerve degeneration in Guillain-Barré syndrome*, page 168.)

Causes
Although the syndrome doesn't have an identified cause, it's thought to involve both cell-mediated and humoral immune responses to a virus. Research suggests that exposure to a virus causes either the production of myelinotoxic antibodies or a cell-mediated process of delayed hypersensitivity in genetically predisposed patients. Infection leads to destruction of the myelin cells that insulate the nerve fibers, disrupting the body's command system. Signs and symptoms commonly occur 4 to 21 days following infection.

Most patients seek treatment when the syndrome is in the acute phase. It progresses rapidly, often in 24 to 72 hours. Your assessment should include careful and rapid consideration of the patient's health history, physi-

FactFinder

Key points about Guillain-Barré syndrome

- *Incidence:* The syndrome strikes about 2 out of every 100,000 people and occurs equally in both sexes. People ages 30 to 50 are most commonly affected.
- *Chief sign:* Flaccid paralysis.
- *Risk factors:* Surgery, rabies and swine influenza vaccination, viral illness, Hodgkin's disease, and systemic lupus erythematosus.
- *Complications:* Thrombophlebitis, pulmonary embolus, pressure ulcers, contractures, muscle wasting, aspiration, respiratory infections, and cardiac disorders.
- *Course of illness:* The *acute phase* begins when the first definitive symptom develops and ends 1 to 3 weeks later, when no further deterioration is observed. The *plateau phase* lasts up to 2 weeks. The *recovery phase* normally extends from 4 to 6 months but can take up to 2 years in a severe case.
- *Chief diagnostic method:* Cerebrospinal fluid analysis.
- *Treatment:* Endotracheal intubation or tracheotomy; plasmapheresis for approximately 1 week. Mechanical ventilation may be necessary for respiratory difficulties.
- *Prognosis:* About 85% of patients with Guillain-Barré syndrome recover completely, though the recovery period can vary from weeks to years.

cal examination findings, and diagnostic test results.

Health history
Guillain-Barré syndrome is characterized by motor weakness and areflexia. Your assessment will depend on the specific type of syndrome affecting the patient. (See *Classifying Guillain-Barré syndrome*, page 169.)

Physical examination
Neurologic, respiratory, and cardiac assessments are essential parts of the examination for this syndrome.

Neurologic assessment
The neurologic examination primarily uncovers muscle weakness, often accompanied by motor loss beginning in the legs (ascending type). However, weakness sometimes develops in the arms first (descending type) or in the arms and legs simultaneously. (See *Testing for thoracic sensation,* page 170.) Cranial nerve involvement may result in facial weakness, diplopia, and difficulty talking, chewing, and swallowing.

The neurologic examination also may reveal a loss of position sense and diminished deep tendon reflexes.

Respiratory assessment
Your auscultation may reveal diminished breath sounds and congestion indicating that respiratory muscles are affected.

Cardiovascular assessment
Your assessment may reveal hypotension, hypertension, sinus tachycardia, sinus bradycardia, and other arrhythmias caused by autonomic instability.

Nerve degeneration in Guillain-Barré syndrome

In Guillain-Barré syndrome, the myelin sheath of peripheral nerves and of anterior and posterior roots at spinal segmental levels demyelinates and degenerates. Early in the disease, inflammation (with lymphocytes and macrophages) and edema of the myelin occur. Later, patchy demyelination causes Schwann's cell loss, leaving a widened node of Ranvier.

Because Guillain-Barré syndrome involves both dorsal and ventral nerve roots, nerve degeneration leads to sensory and motor impairment. Clinical signs include paresthesia and lower motor neuron paralysis with areflexia.

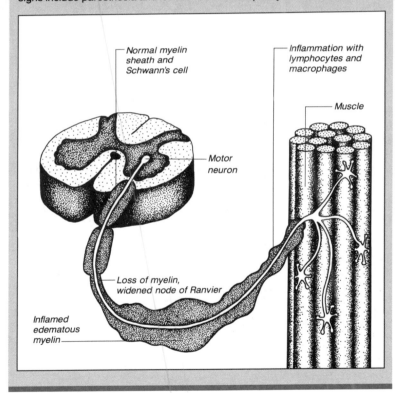

Diagnostic test results

• Cerebrospinal fluid (CSF) analysis may show a normal white blood cell count and an elevated protein count.
• Electromyography may demonstrate repeated firing of the same motor unit instead of widespread sectional stimulation.
• Electrophysiologic testing may reveal diminished nerve conduction velocities.
• Pulmonary function studies may exhibit decreased vital capacity and decreased tidal volume.
• Arterial blood gas (ABG) analysis may reflect decreased partial pressure of arterial oxygen (PaO_2) and increased partial pressure of arterial carbon dioxide ($PaCO_2$).

NURSING DIAGNOSIS

Common nursing diagnoses for a patient with the syndrome include:
• Impaired physical mobility related to paralysis
• Impaired gas exchange related to alveolar hypoventilation
• Ineffective airway clearance related to inability to cough effectively or take deep breaths
• Ineffective breathing pattern related to respiratory muscle paralysis
• Ineffective individual coping related to fear of disability or death
• High risk for injury related to sensory or motor dysfunction and autonomic instability
• Fatigue related to the disease process.

PLANNING

Based on the nursing diagnosis *impaired physical mobility,* develop appropriate patient outcomes. For example, your patient will:
• participate in an exercise regimen

Classifying Guillain-Barré syndrome

The four types of Guillain-Barré syndrome and their characteristics are discussed below.

Ascending type
• Weakness and numbness that begins in the legs and progresses upward to the trunk, arms, and cranial nerves
• Symmetrical motor deficits, from paresis to quadriplegia
• Sensory deficits, such as mild numbness that commonly affects the toes
• Diminished or absent reflexes
• Respiratory insufficiency in about 50% of patients

Descending type
• Motor deficits that begin with weakness in the brain stem cranial nerves and progress downward
• Sensory deficits, such as distal numbness that commonly affects the hands
• Diminished or absent reflexes
• Rapid respiratory involvement

Miller-Fisher variant type
• Ophthalmoplegia, areflexia, and pronounced ataxia
• Usually no sensory loss
• Rarely respiratory involvement

Pure motor type
• Identical to ascending type, except that sensory signs and symptoms are absent
• May be a mild form of ascending type
• Muscle pain generally absent

Testing for thoracic sensation

When Guillain-Barré syndrome progresses rapidly, check for ascending sensory loss every hour by touching the patient or pricking his skin lightly with a pin. Move systematically from the iliac crest (thoracic segment T12) to the scapula, occasionally switching to the blunt end of the pin to test the patient's ability to discriminate between sharp and dull sensations.

Mark the level of diminished sensation with indelible ink. If diminished sensation ascends to T8 or higher, the patient's respiratory function will probably be impaired.

As the syndrome subsides, sensory and motor weakness descend to the lower thoracic segments, allowing the intercostal and extremity muscles to recover.

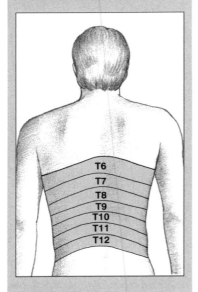

- remain free of complications caused by immobility, such as contractures, venous stasis, thrombus formation, or skin breakdown
- maximize his muscle strength
- remain free of atrophy.

Based on the nursing diagnosis *impaired gas exchange,* develop appropriate patient outcomes. For example, your patient will:
- exhibit PaO_2 greater than or equal to 75 mm Hg
- exhibit $PaCO_2$ of 35 to 45 mm Hg
- display Ph of 7.35 to 7.42.

Based on the nursing diagnosis *ineffective airway clearance,* develop appropriate patient outcomes. For example, your patient will:
- exhibit clear breath sounds
- produce thin, clear mucus.

Based on the nursing diagnosis *ineffective breathing pattern,* develop appropriate patient outcomes. For example, your patient will:
- exhibit vital capacity greater than 15 ml/kg
- show symmetrical chest excursion
- display normal ABG levels
- display acceptable vital signs.

Based on the nursing diagnosis *ineffective individual coping,* develop appropriate patient outcomes. For example, your patient will:
- speak about his illness
- identify personal strengths and coping mechanisms
- seek and accept help
- participate in his own care.

Based on the nursing diagnosis *high risk for injury,* develop appropriate patient outcomes. For example, your patient will:
- remain free of injury
- discuss safety measures with his caregiver after discharge.

Based on the nursing diagnosis *fatigue,* develop appropriate patient outcomes. For example, your patient will:

Treatments

Medical care of the patient with Guillain-Barré syndrome

Treatment is primarily supportive, requiring endotracheal intubation or tracheotomy and mechanical ventilation in case of respiratory failure. It may also involve drug therapy or investigational treatments.

Supportive therapy
The following treatments may be used to relieve symptoms:
• anticoagulant therapy and anti-embolism stockings to prevent thrombophlebitis and pulmonary embolism
• plasmapheresis to temporarily reduce the number of circulating antibodies (reserved for the most severely affected patients).

Drug therapy
The following drugs may be used to treat respiratory and cardiovascular problems resulting from the syndrome:
• propranolol to treat tachycardia and hypotension
• atropine to treat bradycardia
• nifedipine and labetalol to treat hypertensive crises
• esmolol to treat severe tachyarrhythmia
• corticosteroids to suppress the inflammatory response.

Investigational treatments
Alternative therapies may include:
• anti-T-cell monoclonal antibodies
• immunosuppressants, such as azathioprine and cyclophosphamide.

• explain how fatigue relates to disease process and activity level
• identify measures to reduce fatigue
• incorporate measures to prevent fatigue as part of his daily activities
• report increased energy.

IMPLEMENTATION

Treatment consists primarily of supportive measures aimed at limiting the complications of the illness. (See *Medical care of the patient with Guillain-Barré syndrome*.)

Nursing interventions
• Assess the patient's respiratory status during the acute phase, and take serial vital capacity recordings at least every 8 hours (every 4 hours in the acute phase). Use a respirometer with a mouthpiece or a face mask for bedside testing.
• Check for signs of respiratory distress, such as restlessness, confusion, dyspnea, tachypnea, diminished chest excursion, and a weak cough.
• Listen for clear breath sounds, and obtain ABG measurements as ordered.
• Be prepared to assist with endotracheal intubation and mechanical ventilation in case respiratory status deteriorates.
• Turn the patient at least once every 2 hours, and perform postural drainage and chest percussion to maintain a patent airway and help prevent pneumonia and atelectasis.
• Assist the patient with controlled coughing and incentive spirometry.

• Suction the patient if necessary, and ensure adequate hydration to help thin secretions and facilitate airway clearance as ordered.

• Prevent aspiration by first testing the patient's gag reflex. If his gag reflex is absent, feed him by nasogastric tube. Otherwise, elevate the head of the bed before giving him anything to eat.

• Monitor the patient's motor and sensory functions once every 2 hours.

• Apply splints to affected limbs.

• Inspect the patient's legs regularly for signs of thrombophlebitis, such as localized pain, tenderness, erythema, edema, and positive Homans' sign.

• To prevent thrombophlebitis, apply antiembolism stockings and give prophylactic anticoagulants as ordered.

• Check for postural hypotension by monitoring blood pressure and pulse rate. Apply toe-to-groin elastic bandages or an abdominal binder if necessary.

• Monitor the patient's blood pressure and heart rate and rhythm for complications caused by autonomic dysfunction.

• Help the patient with transfers, positioning, and assistive devices. Keep his room free of clutter. Place a call light near his bed.

• Provide meticulous skin care to prevent breakdown and contractures. Pay special attention to the sacrum, heels, and ankles. Use alternating pressure pads at points of contact. Use air bed therapy as necessary.

• Provide eye and mouth care every 4 hours for the patient with facial paralysis. Protect the corneas with eye ointments and tape.

• Perform passive range-of-motion exercises. Remember that the thighs, shoulders, and trunk will cause the most pain on passive movement and turning. When the patient's condition stabilizes, change to gentle stretching and active assistance exercises.

• Monitor for urine retention by measuring and recording intake and output every 8 hours. Offer the bedpan every 3 to 4 hours, and encourage adequate fluid intake (2,000 ml/day) unless contraindicated. If urine retention develops, begin intermittent catheterization as ordered. If necessary, use Credé's maneuver (pressure applied over the symphysis pubis) to expel urine from the bladder.

• Prevent constipation by offering prune juice and a high-fiber diet. Give suppositories (glycerin or bisacodyl) or enemas as ordered.

• Encourage the patient to use an alternative form of communication, if necessary, such as eye blinking or using a magic slate, a chalkboard, or an alphabet board.

• Provide the patient with daily periods of uninterrupted rest.

• Provide activities for the patient, such as television, family visits, and listening to tapes.

• Provide emotional support to the patient and his family by listening to their concerns and helping to identify positive coping mechanisms. Remember that the patient with Guillain-Barré syndrome will usually feel isolated and helpless, especially at first, so offering hope in a realistic and appropriate manner will be an important part of your support. Also, encouraging the patient to participate in decisions concerning his own care can decrease his feeling of helplessness.

• Administer medications as ordered, and monitor their effects.

• Consult with the social services department about the patient's discharge needs.

Ensuring continued care for the patient with Guillain-Barré syndrome

Review the following teaching topics, referrals, and follow-up appointments to make sure that your patient is adequately prepared for discharge.

Teaching topics

Make sure that the following topics have been covered and that your patient's learning has been evaluated:

☐ nature of Guillain-Barré syndrome, including its progression, risk factors, and complications

☐ prescribed medications, including dosage and possible adverse effects

☐ signs and symptoms that should be reported to the doctor immediately

☐ importance of keeping follow-up appointments

☐ importance of a mobility program

☐ need for skin care

☐ guidelines for home safety

☐ importance of independent activity.

Referrals

Make sure that the patient has been provided with necessary referrals to:

☐ social services department for assistance with home health care or with placement in long-term care facility

☐ rehabilitation center for physical therapy or speech therapy if needed

☐ psychologist

☐ support groups.

Follow-up appointments

Make sure that the necessary follow-up appointments have been scheduled and that the patient has been notified:

☐ neurologist

☐ respiratory specialist

☐ plasmapheresis.

Patient teaching

• Explain the nature of Guillain-Barré syndrome to the patient and his family. Be sure they understand the diagnostic tests and treatments that will be performed. Explain all procedures to the patient, even if he's comatose.

• Explain the reason for all diagnostic tests and treatments. For example, if the patient loses his gag reflex, explain why tube feedings are necessary to maintain nutritional status.

• Provide information about all prescribed drugs.

• Teach the family to help the patient maintain mental alertness, fight boredom, and avoid depression. Suggest that they plan frequent visits, read books to the patient, or borrow library books on tape for him.

• Prepare a home care plan, and teach the patient and family about management and safety, including transfer techniques, using a walker or cane, eating methods, skin care, a bowel and bladder elimination program, scheduled rest periods, and home safety measures, such as grab bars and removal of throw rugs.

• Encourage the patient to be as independent and active as possible after discharge. (See *Ensuring continued care for the patient with Guillain-Barré syndrome.*)

EVALUATION

When evaluating the patient's response to your care, gather reassessment data and compare this information to the patient outcomes specified in your plan of care.

Teaching and counseling

Begin by evaluating the effectiveness of your teaching and counseling. Note statements by the patient indicating his understanding of the condition, including its progression and possible complications. Consider the following questions:
• Is he willing to participate in a mobility program?
• Has he remained free of complications related to immobility?
• Does he maximize his muscle strength?
• Has he remained free of injuries?
• Does he participate in his own care as much as possible and display positive coping mechanisms?
• Has he incorporated measures to prevent or reduce fatigue into his daily activities?

Physical condition

Physical examination and diagnostic test results will also help to evaluate the effectiveness of your care. If treatment has been effective, you should note:
• PaO_2 greater than or equal to 75 mm Hg
• $PaCO_2$ between 35 and 45 mm Hg
• pH of 7.35 to 7.42
• clear breath sounds
• thin, clear mucus and effective coughing
• vital capacity above 15 ml/kg
• symmetrical chest excursion
• normal ABG levels
• vital signs within the normal range.

CHAPTER 6

Caring for patients with cerebrovascular disorders

Transient ischemic attacks

Sudden, brief episodes of neurologic deficits caused by focal cerebral ischemia, transient ischemic attacks (TIAs) usually last 5 to 20 minutes and are followed by a rapid clearing of neurologic deficits (typically within 24 hours). Recurrent attacks are common.

TIAs may herald a cerebrovascular accident (CVA). Early recognition and treatment of TIAs may prevent a CVA. (See *Understanding TIAs.*)

Causes
Causes of TIAs include:
• *vascular disorders*, such as extensive extracranial atherosclerosis, arteritis, and fibromuscular dysplasia
• *blood disorders,* such as hypercoagulability, polycythemia, and recurrent embolism
• *cerebrovascular insufficiency* from diminished cardiac output, mechanical obstruction of one of the neck's major vessels, or subclavian steal syndrome (decreased supply of blood to the subclavian artery). (See *Key points about TIAs*, page 178.)

ASSESSMENT

Because a TIA usually resolves itself by the time the patient reaches the hospital, focus your assessment on obtaining a thorough health history, including previous medical conditions.

Timesaving tip: To save assessment time, ask the patient about recent falls. A patient is less likely to forget about or minimize frequent falls than other signs of a TIA.

Health history
If the patient experienced a *vertebrobasilar ischemic attack*, he may have the following signs and symptoms:
• dizziness
• diplopia, dark or blurred vision, visual field deficits, or ptosis
• dysarthria
• dysphagia
• unilateral or bilateral weakness and numbness in the fingers, arms, or legs (or all three sites)
• staggering gait or a veering to one side.

If the patient experienced a *carotid ischemic attack,* he may have the following signs and symptoms:
• transient blindness in one eye
• altered level of consciousness (LOC)
• numbness of the tongue
• unilateral or bilateral weakness and numbness in the fingers, arms, or legs (or in all three sites)
• seizures.

Ask how long the signs and symptoms lasted and whether or not the patient experienced them before.

Review the patient's history for cerebrovascular disease, seizures, arrhythmias, myocardial infarction, hypertension, diabetes mellitus, atherosclerosis, hyperlipoproteinemia, and collagen vascular disorders. Note also a history of cigarette smoking, lack of exercise, obesity and, for the female patient, use of oral contraceptives. Review the medical histories of family members as well.

Physical examination
A neurologic examination usually reveals varied deficits, which are transient and brief. A cardiac examination may reveal heart or vascular disease. For example, auscultation of the carotid artery may detect bruits. Palpation may detect faint peripheral

Understanding TIAs

There are two types of transient ischemic attacks (TIAs) — vertebrobasilar and carotid.

Vertebrobasilar TIAs
This type of TIA results from inadequate blood flow from the vertebral arteries. The two vertebral arteries (on either side of the head) extend from the subclavian artery, through the upper six cervical vertebrae, then enter the skull through the foramen magnum and join to form the basilar artery. A vertebrobasilar TIA may occur secondary to occluded blood flow from the subclavian artery, which supplies blood to the vertebrobasilar arterial pathway.

Carotid TIAs
This type of TIA results from inadequate blood flow from the carotid artery. Inadequate blood flow may be caused by a narrowing or partial occlusion at the bifurcation of the common carotid artery where it branches into the internal and external carotid arteries.

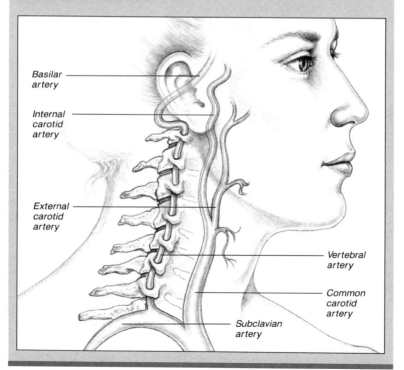

Basilar artery

Internal carotid artery

External carotid artery

Vertebral artery

Common carotid artery

Subclavian artery

pulses. A blood pressure check may reveal hypertension.

Diagnostic test results

Findings may or may not reveal changes related to the TIA's underlying cause.

• Oculoplethysmography may indicate carotid occlusive disease by revealing delayed pulse arrival in one eye.

• Carotid Doppler or transcranial Doppler studies may detect blood flow disturbances.

• Cerebral angiography may be needed to confirm carotid stenosis or occlusion.

• Digital subtraction angiography may reveal carotid occlusion or severe carotid stenosis.

• Magnetic resonance imaging and magnetic resonance arteriography may provide additional information.

NURSING DIAGNOSIS

Common nursing diagnoses for a patient with TIAs include:

• High risk for injury related to temporarily impaired LOC, balance, and motor and sensory functions

• Anxiety related to impending surgery or impending CVA

• Knowledge deficit related to treatment and the need to decrease risk factors

• Altered cerebral tissue perfusion related to transient decrease in blood flow supplied by extracranial vessels.

PLANNING

Based on the nursing diagnosis *high risk for injury*, develop appropriate patient outcomes. For example, your patient will:

• modify his environment and activity to minimize injury

• remain free of serious injury.

Based on the nursing diagnosis *anxiety*, develop appropriate patient outcomes. For example, your patient will:

• discuss feelings of anxiety

• identify the source of his anxiety

• identify and use effective coping mechanisms

• report feeling less anxiety.

Based on the nursing diagnosis *knowledge deficit*, develop appropriate patient outcomes. For example, your patient will:

• describe the upcoming surgery, including preoperative and postoperative risks

• state the purpose, action, dosage, possible adverse effects, and precautions for all prescribed drugs

Treatments

Medical care of the patient with TIAs

Therapy for transient ischemic attacks (TIAs) may include drugs, surgery, or other treatments.

Drug therapy
Aspirin is the preferred drug for treating a TIA and is probably most helpful when the TIA is caused by emboli resulting from atherosclerotic plaque. Warfarin may be prescribed, but prolonged therapy increases the risk of hemorrhagic complications. Short-term I.V. heparin may be ordered for patients suspected of having carotid or vertebrobasilar stenosis from thrombus formation. Dipyridamole and sulfinpyrazone are now only occasionally prescribed.

Surgery
If the patient doesn't respond to drug therapy and is at high risk for a cerebrovascular accident (CVA), surgery may be considered. Presently, however, surgery is used primarily to treat carotid artery obstruction resulting from atherosclerosis or stenosis. Surgery for vertebrobasilar TIAs is rarely performed since only the proximal vertebrobasilar arteries are surgically accessible, and these arteries usually don't lead to a CVA. Current surgical procedures include carotid endarterectomy and extracranial-intracranial (EC-IC) bypass. However, the EC-IC bypass is considered controversial.

Additional treatments
Lifestyle changes to reduce risk factors may include weight loss, smoking cessation, hypertension and diabetes management, and daily exercise. Women taking oral contraceptives should seek other birth-control options.

• identify lifestyle changes that will help reduce the risk of TIAs and CVA
• describe a plan to make lifestyle changes.
  Based on the nursing diagnosis *altered cerebral tissue perfusion*, develop appropriate patient outcomes. For example, your patient will:
• remain alert and oriented to time, person, and place
• retain bilaterally equal motor function
• experience no sensory deficits
• show normal bilateral pupillary reaction in response to light

• demonstrate blood pressure within normal range for his age
• be free of speech or memory deficits.

IMPLEMENTATION
Treatment for TIAs focuses on drug therapy. If the patient doesn't respond to such therapy, he may require surgery. Lifestyle modifications may help reduce the risk of CVA. (See *Medical care of the patient with TIAs*.)

Nursing interventions

• Prepare the patient for diagnostic tests. After invasive tests, monitor for complications.

• Administer ordered medications, and assess for bleeding. Monitor the results of laboratory tests, including prothrombin time in patients receiving oral anticoagulants and partial thromboplastin time in patients receiving heparin. Also monitor the patient's hemoglobin level, hematocrit, and platelet count.

• Monitor neurologic status and vital signs to detect TIA recurrence or progression to CVA.

• Keep the call button near the patient and instruct him to use it if he experiences any symptoms.

• Keep the bed's side rails raised at night and at other times if warranted. Keep the patient's room free of clutter.

• If the patient fears a CVA, offer emotional support. Allow him to express his fears and concerns. Explain clearly the goals of treatment.

• If the patient requires surgery, prepare him physically and emotionally. Following surgery, assess his neurologic status to detect early signs of complications, especially increased intracranial pressure and cerebral ischemia. Also assess vital signs. Expect to maintain the patient's systolic blood pressure at 120 to 170 mm Hg to ensure cerebral perfusion. Assess for airway obstruction, which may be related to excessive swelling in the neck, hematoma formation, or faulty head positioning.

Patient teaching

• Explain the nature of the disorder and the need for prompt treatment to help prevent a CVA.

• Explain the purpose of diagnostic tests.

• Inform the patient about the prescribed drugs, including their purpose, action, dosage, route, possible adverse effects, and precautions. Tell the patient to be sure to notify the doctor if bleeding occurs. Explain the importance of keeping follow-up laboratory appointments.

• To prevent falls, instruct the patient to sit down and rest immediately if he experiences dizziness, disturbed balance, or weakness. Ask the doctor if the patient can drive or operate dangerous equipment. To help prevent falls at home, advise the patient on making minor changes, such as installation of a grab bar in the tub area.

• Educate the patient about planned surgery. Clarify his risks, and explain preoperative, postoperative, and follow-up home care.

• Help the patient plan to reduce TIA risk. Begin by working with him on a program for moderate exercise. If needed, refer him to a smoking cessation or weight loss program. Discuss the need to comply with all treatments, which may include taking prescribed medications to control blood pressure or diabetes mellitus.

• Tell the patient to report any neurologic symptoms, especially those lasting longer than 24 hours.

• Stress the need for keeping follow-up appointments. (See *Ensuring continued care for the patient with TIAs*.)

EVALUATION

When evaluating the patient's response to your nursing care, gather reassessment data and compare this information with the patient outcomes specified in your plan of care. Consult with other members of the health care team as necessary.

Discharge TimeSaver

Ensuring continued care for the patient with TIAs

Review the following teaching topics, referrals, and follow-up appointments to make sure that your patient is adequately prepared for discharge.

Teaching topics
Make sure that the following topics have been covered and that your patient's learning has been evaluated:
□ explanation of a TIA and its risk factors and associated complications
□ risk reduction measures
□ drug therapy
□ home safety measures
□ warning signs and symptoms to report to the doctor.

Referrals
Make sure that the patient has been provided with necessary referrals to:
□ dietitian

□ weight-loss support group
□ smoking cessation program
□ physical therapist
□ occupational therapist
□ speech therapist.

Follow-up appointments
Make sure that the necessary follow-up appointments have been scheduled and that the patient has been notified:
□ doctor
□ surgeon
□ diagnostic tests for reevaluation
□ physical rehabilitation center.

Teaching and counseling
Talk to the patient to determine the effectiveness of teaching and counseling. Consider the following questions:
• Does the patient demonstrate an adequate understanding of TIAs?
• Does he understand medical treatments, including their risks?
• Can he state the purpose, action, dosage, possible adverse effects, and precautions for all prescribed drugs?
• Can the patient identify lifestyle changes that will help reduce the risk of TIAs and CVA?
• Has he discussed feelings of anxiety?
• Does he appear less anxious about his condition?

Include family members in your evaluation. Consider the following questions:
• Do the patient and family members adequately understand the need for modifications in the home to help prevent falls?
• Do they understand the need to modify the patient's lifestyle to reduce the risk of further TIAs?

Physical condition
A physical assessment and diagnostic tests will also help you to evaluate the effectiveness of your plan of care. Note whether or not your patient has achieved the following conditions:
• absence of serious injury
• adequate cerebral tissue perfusion
• absence of deterioration in LOC
• bilaterally equal motor function

• bilaterally normal pupillary reaction to light
• normal blood pressure
• absence of speech and memory deficits.

Cerebrovascular accident

Also called a stroke, a cerebrovascular accident (CVA) occurs when impaired circulation in the brain disrupts the supply of oxygen. Recovery from a CVA depends on how quickly and completely circulation is restored. However, almost half of all patients who survive a CVA are permanently disabled and will suffer a recurrent attack. (See *Key points about CVA*.)

Complications of a CVA include:
• unstable blood pressure from loss of vasomotor control
• fluid imbalances
• malnutrition
• infection, such as encephalitis, brain abscess, and pneumonia
• depression
• contractures
• pulmonary emboli.

Causes

Impaired cerebral circulation may result from thrombosis, embolism, or hemorrhage. (See *Causes of CVA*, pages 184 and 185.)

ASSESSMENT

If you suspect that a patient is having a CVA or has had one, contact the doctor immediately. Make certain that the patient has an unobstructed airway and is adequately ventilated. Assess his vital signs and perform as complete a neurologic examination as the situation allows. If the patient doesn't appear to be in immediate danger, obtain a health history.

Health history

While obtaining the history, observe the patient for altered level of consciousness (LOC) and for cognitive and emotional problems. When speaking with the patient, you may note communication problems, such as dysarthria or aphasia.

Ask the patient, or his family if necessary, whether he experienced the following signs and symptoms:
• headache
• vomiting
• seizures
• altered LOC
• sensory or motor changes
• intellectual, emotional, or memory impairment
• visual problems
• bowel or bladder incontinence.

Risk factors

Determine whether the patient has any risk factors associated with CVA, including:
• head injury
• atherosclerosis, hypertension, arrhythmias, myocardial infarction, rheumatic heart disease, postural hypotension, or cardiac hypertrophy
• previous heart surgery
• emboli
• diabetes mellitus or gout.

Other risk factors include obesity; high serum cholesterol, lipoprotein, or triglyceride levels; lack of exercise; smoking; recent pregnancy; or a family history of cerebrovascular disease.

Medication history

Ask if the patient is taking any medications, especially anticoagulants, aspirin, or oral contraceptives. Check for I.V. drug abuse.

Psychosocial history
Obtain a psychosocial history, noting the patient's level of independence before the CVA, his living arrangements, family relationships, employment and financial status, and social and leisure activities. This information may prove helpful when planning outpatient care.

Physical examination
The effects of a CVA vary with the part of the brain affected, the severity of the episode, and the extent that collateral circulation develops to help the brain compensate for its decreased blood supply.

Cerebral function
Assessing LOC and cognition with a standard tool, such as the Glasgow Coma Scale, may reveal the following:
• unconsciousness (most likely with a hemorrhagic CVA)
• disorientation
• restlessness
• decreased attention span
• difficulties with comprehension
• forgetfulness
• impaired judgment
• lack of motivation.

The patient may also exhibit emotional difficulties such as anxiety or mood swings.

Cranial nerve function
Impairment of cranial nerves IX and X, which control swallowing, gagging, and coughing, may place the patient at risk for aspiration and inadequate nutrition. Damage to cranial nerves II and III may result in visual field deficits and in loss of the pupillary reflex. Remember, a failure of the pupils to react to light or a unilateral and sluggish pupillary response may indicate increased intracranial pressure (ICP). Impairment of cranial

FactFinder
Key points about CVA

• *Morbidity and mortality:* Cerebrovascular accident (CVA) is the third leading cause of death and the most common cause of neurologic disability in North America. It strikes more than 500,000 people each year, killing more than 250,000.
• *Populations at risk:* Though CVA can strike people of any age, it mostly affects men over age 65. Blacks face an especially high risk.
• *Epidemiologic trends:* Improved control of hypertension, the main risk factor for CVA, and improved treatment for transient ischemic attacks seem to have helped reduce the incidence of CVA over the past 30 years. However, CVA among young people is increasing, caused possibly by emboli from I.V. drug abuse.

nerves V and VII may result in loss of the corneal reflex.

Timesaving tip: If time is critical, limit your assessment of cranial nerves to II, III, V, VII, IX, and X.

Cerebellar and motor functions
Assessing the patient's cerebellar and motor functions helps determine which cerebral hemisphere is affected. Left hemiparesis or hemiplegia means the right hemisphere is affected, whereas right hemiparesis or hemiplegia means the left hemisphere is affected. Note any problems with balance and gait.

Causes of CVA

A cerebrovascular accident (CVA) results from impaired circulation in one or more of the brain's blood vessels. Impairments are usually caused by thrombosis, embolism, or hemorrhage.

Thrombosis
The most common cause of CVA is thrombosis, which is usually related to atherosclerosis. Plaque and atheromatous deposits gradually occlude the artery.

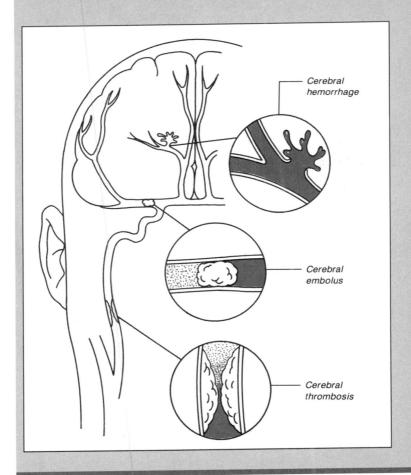

Cerebral hemorrhage

Cerebral embolus

Cerebral thrombosis

Occlusion leads to ischemia and infarction of brain tissue, followed by edema and necrosis. Thrombosis usually occurs in the extracerebral vessels but sometimes occurs in the intracerebral vessels.

Embolism
Embolism may cause a CVA. Usually, fragments break off from a mural thrombus in the left atrium or ventricle or from bacterial vegetations affecting heart valves. These emboli travel through the carotid artery and typically lodge in the smaller cerebral vessels, most often the left middle cerebral artery. Ischemia may occur quite suddenly, often followed by necrosis and edema. However, if the embolus breaks apart, enters and is absorbed by a smaller vessel, the symptoms may subside.

Hemorrhage
The most devastating cause of CVA, hemorrhage occurs when a cerebral vessel ruptures and bleeds into brain tissue or the subarachnoid space. Hemorrhagic CVAs usually result from a rupturing arteriosclerotic vessel caused by exposure to prolonged hypertension, a cerebral aneurysm, or an arteriovenous malformation. Effects may be severe. More than 50% of patients die within the first 3 days from brain herniation.

Sensory function
Assessing the patient's sensations may reveal losses, ranging from slight impairment of touch to the inability to perceive the position and motion of body parts.

The patient may be unaware of one side of his body (neglect syndrome) due to disruption of the nondominant (usually right) cerebral hemisphere. If paralyzed, the patient may actually deny any motor impairment. Visual-spatial problems may also exist.

The patient also may have difficulty interpreting visual, tactile, and auditory stimuli. A visual examination may reveal diplopia or visual field deficits. For example, he may exhibit hemianopia (blindness in half of the visual field), caused by damage to the optic tract or the occipital lobe.

Deep tendon reflexes
Assessing the patient's muscle tone may initially reveal flaccid paralysis with decreased deep tendon reflexes. Later, these reflexes usually return to normal, whereas muscle tone and, sometimes, spasticity increases. Bowel and bladder incontinence may result from impaired muscle control and altered LOC and cognition. (See *Neurologic deficits in CVA*, pages 186 and 187.)

Cardiovascular system
Checking for cardiovascular signs, such as murmurs or bruits, may reveal possible causes of CVA.

Diagnostic test results
The following tests may help identify causes of CVA:
• Cerebral angiography detects disruption or displacement of the cerebral circulation by occlusion or hemorrhage.
• Digital subtraction angiography evaluates the patency of cerebral ves-

Neurologic deficits in CVA

A cerebrovascular accident (CVA) can cause neurologic deficits ranging from mild hand weakness to complete unilateral paralysis. Such functional loss results from damaged brain tissue normally perfused by the occluded or ruptured artery. Most CVAs occur in the anterior cerebral circulation and result in damage to the middle cerebral artery, internal carotid artery, or anterior cerebral artery. CVAs can also occur in the posterior cerebral circulation and cause damage to the vertebral or basilar artery and the posterior cerebral artery. The list below correlates CVA symptoms with anatomic sites.

Middle cerebral artery
When a CVA occurs in the middle cerebral artery, the patient may experience:
- aphasia
- dysphasia
- reading difficulty (dyslexia)
- writing inability (dysgraphia)
- visual field deficits
- contralateral hemiparesis (more severe in the face and arm than in the leg)
- altered level of consciousness (LOC)
- contralateral sensory deficit.

Internal carotid artery
When a CVA occurs in the internal carotid artery, the patient may experience:
- headaches
- weakness, paralysis, numbness, sensory changes, and visual deficits, such as blurring, on the affected side
- altered LOC
- bruits over the carotid artery
- aphasia
- dysphasia
- ptosis.

Anterior cerebral artery
When a CVA occurs in the anterior cerebral artery, the patient may experience:
- confusion, weakness, and numbness on the affected side
- paralysis of the contralateral foot and leg
- footdrop
- incontinence
- loss of coordination
- impaired sensory functions
- personality changes.

Vertebral or basilar artery
When a CVA occurs in the vertebral or basilar artery, the patient may experience:

sels and identifies their position. It also detects and evaluates lesions and other vascular abnormalities.
• Computed tomography (CT) scan, commonly used for patients with transient ischemic attacks, detects structural abnormalities, edema, and lesions, such as nonhemorrhagic infarction and aneurysms.
• Positron emission tomography evaluates cerebral metabolism and cerebral blood flow changes, which is

- numbness around the lips and mouth
- dizziness
- weakness on the affected side
- visual deficits, such as color blindness, lack of depth perception, and diplopia
- poor coordination
- dysphagia
- slurred speech
- amnesia
- ataxia
- coma or confusion
- impaired gag reflex
- headache.

Posterior cerebral artery
When a CVA occurs in the posterior cerebral artery, the patient may experience:
- visual field deficits
- sensory impairment
- dyslexia
- coma
- cortical blindness from ischemia in the occipital area
- "locked-in" syndrome during which the patient is in a state of complete paralysis, except for some form of voluntary eye movement.

especially useful in an ischemic CVA.
- Single-photon emission tomography identifies cerebral blood flow and helps diagnose cerebral infarction.

- Magnetic resonance imaging (MRI) evaluates the location and size of lesions. Although not as useful as a CT scan for distinguishing among hemorrhage, tumor, and infarction, MRI proves more useful for examining the cerebellum and brain stem.
- Transcranial Doppler studies examine the size of intracranial vessels and the direction and velocity of cerebral blood flow.
- Cerebral blood flow studies measure blood flow to the brain and help detect abnormalities.
- Ophthalmoscopic examination detects hypertension and atherosclerotic changes in retinal arteries.
- EEG detects reduced electrical activity in an area of cortical infarction. Especially useful when the CT scan is inconclusive, it can also differentiate seizure activity from CVA.
- Neuropsychological tests evaluate mental and verbal abilities and sometimes personality traits.
- Electrocardiography reveals abnormalities caused by a cardiac-induced CVA.

Additional diagnostic tests
Establish a baseline for the following laboratory tests:
- urinalysis
- coagulation studies
- complete blood count
- serum osmolality
- serum electrolytes, glucose, triglycerides, and creatinine levels
- blood urea nitrogen.

NURSING DIAGNOSIS

Common nursing diagnoses for a patient with CVA include:
- Altered cerebral tissue perfusion related to impaired cerebral blood flow, increased ICP, and hypoxia

• Impaired physical mobility related to decreased LOC and damage to the motor cortex or pathways
• Impaired verbal communication related to impaired cognitive functioning, weakness (dysarthria), or damage to speech centers in the dominant cerebral hemisphere (aphasia)
• Sensory or perceptual alterations (visual, auditory, kinesthetic, gustatory, tactile, olfactory) related to damaged sensory pathways and cortex
• High risk for injury related to sensory, motor, and cognitive impairments.

PLANNING

The effects of CVAs can range from moderate to severe and usually are irreversible. Direct your care toward controlling the consequences of altered cerebral tissue perfusion and helping the patient cope with sensory and perceptual difficulties and physical limitations. Remember, the prognosis for each patient will vary depending on the cause of the CVA, its location and severity, and the patient's age, health, motivation, and support.

Based on the nursing diagnosis *altered cerebral tissue perfusion*, develop appropriate patient outcomes. For example, your patient will:
• be alert and aware of time, place, and person
• exhibit normally reactive pupils
• maintain an ICP that's less than or equal to 15 mm Hg
• maintain a cerebral perfusion pressure that's greater than 60 mm Hg
• report an absence of headache, nausea, and vomiting
• show stable, normal vital signs.

Based on the nursing diagnosis *impaired physical mobility*, develop appropriate patient outcomes. For example, your patient will:
• demonstrate prescribed exercises and positioning, transfer, and assisted ambulation techniques with help from family members
• plan with family members for continued physical rehabilitation following discharge
• demonstrate adequate mobility and absence of contractures and pressure ulcers
• perform activities of daily living (ADLs) independently.

Based on the nursing diagnosis *impaired verbal communication*, develop appropriate patient outcomes. For example, your patient will:
• use alternative methods to communicate needs
• communicate more frequently despite difficulties with speech
• follow simple directions consistently.

Based on the nursing diagnosis *sensory or perceptual alterations*, develop appropriate patient outcomes. For example, your patient will:
• remain injury-free
• adapt to sensory loss sufficiently to perform ADLs.

Based on the nursing diagnosis *high risk for injury*, develop appropriate patient outcomes. For example, your patient will:
• remain safe while in the hospital
• discuss home safety with family members.

IMPLEMENTATION

Acute care measures may be needed to sustain the patient's life. A special diet and drug regimen may help reduce the risks of future CVAs. In some cases, surgery may help the patient adapt to physical deficits. (See *Medical care of the patient with CVA*.)

Treatments

Medical care of the patient with CVA

Therapy for a cerebrovascular accident (CVA) may include acute care, surgery, drugs, and other measures.

Acute care measures

Acute care for a CVA may include mechanical ventilation, intracranial pressure (ICP) and cardiac monitoring, administration of I.V. fluids and electrolytes, and nasogastric intubation.

Surgery

The need for and type of surgery required for a CVA depend on its cause and extent, and may include a craniotomy to remove a hematoma, endarterectomy to remove atherosclerotic plaque from the inner arterial wall, or a bypass to circumvent an artery blocked by occlusion or stenosis. Ventricular shunts may be necessary to drain cerebrospinal fluid.

Drug therapy

Drug therapy for a CVA may include:

- anticonvulsants, such as phenytoin or phenobarbital, to treat or prevent seizures
- stool softeners, such as dioctyl sodium sulfosuccinate, to avoid straining, which increases ICP
- corticosteroids, such as dexamethasone, to reduce associated cerebral edema
- analgesics, such as codeine, to relieve headache
- anticoagulants to prevent thrombotic or embolic CVAs and to treat a thrombotic CVA in progress
- antihypertensives to lower blood pressure
- vasodilators to treat ischemia.

Additional measures

Besides drug therapy, physical rehabilitation and a special diet help decrease risk factors. Other care measures may help the patient adapt to specific deficits, such as speech impairment and paralysis.

Nursing interventions

- Maintain an open airway, ventilate adequately, and administer supplementary oxygen. Assist with endotracheal intubation and mechanical ventilation if necessary. Continue monitoring the patient's airway, breathing, and circulation (ABCs). Remember, if the patient's LOC deteriorates, his respirations may deteriorate as well.
- Monitor vital and neurologic signs as needed. Compare the results with baseline findings. Report any deterioration immediately.

- During the first 72 hours, watch especially for signs of increased ICP; altered LOC is the most important sign. Also look for delayed response to verbal suggestion, slowed speech, and increasing restlessness and confusion. Monitor ICP if LOC deteriorates significantly. (See *Recognizing increased ICP,* page 190.)
- Continue to assess sensory function, speech, skin color, and temperature. Note the presence of nuchal rigidity or headache. Remember, when a CVA is impending, blood pressure increases suddenly, pulse rate be-

comes rapid and bounding, and the patient may complain of a headache. When rising ICP accompanies a CVA, blood pressure increases but pulse rate decreases.

Treating increased ICP

- Implement measures to prevent increased ICP. Elevate the head of the bed 30 to 45 degrees and maintain the head in a midline neutral position to encourage venous return. Avoid extreme hip flexion and, if the patient is alert, instruct him to avoid isometric muscle contractions and Valsalva's maneuver. Hyperoxygenate and hyperventilate the patient. Remove secretions by continual suctioning for no more than 10 seconds at a time. Proceed deliberately, allowing the patient time to rest between interventions.
- Consult with the doctor concerning the desired blood pressure range. Give medications such as vasopres-
sors or antihypertensives if prescribed.
- Maintain fluid and electrolyte balance. If the patient can take liquids orally, offer them as often as fluid limitations permit. Administer I.V. fluids as ordered, but never give too much too fast because this can increase ICP. Monitor the patient's fluid intake and output.

Additional interventions

- Repeatedly explain to the patient what is happening and why.
- Offer the urinal or bedpan every 2 hours. If the patient is incontinent, consider using an indwelling urinary catheter, but remember that this device increases the risk of infection.
- Establish a bowel training program if needed. Watch for signs that the patient is straining during defecation since this increases ICP. Provide a high-fiber diet, and administer stool softeners as ordered. Offer prune juice or apple juice.

Timesaving tip: To help prevent bowel incontinence and thus save valuable nursing care time, determine the patient's usual time for elimination, and consistently offer the bedpan or encourage use of the bedside commode. Give laxatives only if necessary.

- Consult with the dietitian about proper nutrition and with the speech pathologist about managing the impaired swallowing and gag reflex. When feeding the patient, place the food tray within his sight. Have him sit upright, and tilt his head slightly forward to eat. If the patient has dysphagia or one-sided facial weakness, give him semisoft foods and tell him to chew on the unaffected side of his mouth. Stay with the patient who may aspirate food. If oral feedings aren't possible, insert a nasogastric feeding tube as ordered.

• Clean and irrigate the patient's mouth carefully. Care for his dentures as needed.
• Care for the patient's eyes by removing secretions with a cotton ball moistened with 0.9% sodium chloride solution. For loss of corneal reflex, apply eyedrops or ointment as ordered.
• Give medications as ordered. Watch for and report any adverse reactions.
• Report signs of deep venous thrombosis, such as calf pain, or signs of pulmonary emboli, such as chest pain, dyspnea, dusky color, tachycardia, fever, and changed sensorium. To prevent thrombosis and emboli, apply antiembolism stockings, frequently change the patient's position, and help him ambulate. For the immobile patient, use continuous pneumatic compression sleeves.
• Align the patient appropriately. Avoid footdrop and contractures by using such devices as cradle boots, footboards, or high-topped sneakers. Avoid pressure ulcers by using a convoluted foam mattress, flotation pads, or a pulsating mattress. Avoid pneumonia by turning the patient at least every 2 hours. Control dependent edema by elevating the affected hand and arm and placing the hand in a functional position. After consulting with the physical therapist, plan a rehabilitation schedule with the patient and his family. Coordinate the rehabilitation plan with the nursing staff.
• Ask the physiotherapist about using proprioceptive neuromuscular facilitation to help restore function and prevent disability. (See *Restoring neurologic and reflex functions after CVA.*)
• Assist the patient with passive range-of-motion exercises for both the affected and unaffected sides at

---

Restoring neurologic and reflex functions after CVA

Proprioceptive neuromuscular facilitation (PNF) techniques use reflexes and patterning methods that are similar to range-of-motion exercises to help restore neurologic and reflex functions after a cerebrovascular accident (CVA) and to help prevent disability. Examples of PNF techniques follow.

Hip bridging and logrolling
• Have the patient lie in bed supine with his knees flexed and feet flat. Then lift his hips up off the bed and lower them again. Repeat this several times. Later, teach the patient to do it himself. This technique, known as "hip bridging," strengthens trunk muscles, causes the legs to bear weight, and decreases leg spasticity.
• Then have the patient logroll from side to side. This reeducates postural reflex and heightens awareness of two sides of the body.

Rocking
• For the patient able to sit in a rocking chair, sit him with his hips and knees aligned at right angles. Place his feet on a firm surface, such as a rubber footstool. Each time the patient rocks, he will bear weight. This exercise helps put the limbs through basic functional motions.

least four times each day while he is unconscious or immobilized.

Timesaving tip: To help shorten the patient's rehabilitation time and to save you time, encourage the conscious or mobile patient to participate in his own rehabilitation, while ensuring that his efforts don't cause recurrence of hemorrhage. Teach him to use his unaffected side to exercise his affected side. Encourage him to raise his hands over his head by clasping them together in front and then raising his arms.

• Apply pressure splints to the arms or legs with sensory loss. Alternate inflation and deflation to help restimulate sensory function.

• If the patient has a limited field of vision, encourage him to turn his head and look in the affected direction.

• If unilateral neglect occurs, encourage him to look at the affected side and to exercise it with his unaffected hand.

• With the patient, family, and speech therapist, help the patient develop an effective means of communicating. Be sure that the nursing staff knows of any communication problem the patient may have.

Timesaving tip: To help save valuable time for the entire nursing staff, post a sign above the patient's bed to inform the health care team and visitors of alternative communication methods.

• If the patient has receptive (Wernicke's) aphasia, speak slowly, using simple sentences. Use supplementary gestures or pictures when necessary.

• If the patient has expressive (Broca's) aphasia or dysarthria, he'll have difficulty speaking. Allow such patients enough time to speak.

Timesaving tip: To help the patient with Broca's aphasia and save time spent in trying to understand him, create a communication board displaying pictures of common needs, such as a bedpan or a glass of water. Or create conversation cards by printing simple messages on index cards, such as "I am thirsty" or "Please raise my bed." Punch holes in the cards, and attach them to a large key ring. The patient can express his needs by showing you the appropriate card.

• Encourage the patient to express himself, but remember that mood changes from brain damage and resentment over dependency may make establishing rapport difficult.

• Discuss realistic short-term goals with the patient and his family, and involve them in his care. Help the patient and his family find effective means to cope with his condition and care. If necessary, refer them for counseling.

• Protect the patient from injury by keeping the bed's side rails raised at all times and padding them as needed. Place a call button on his unaffected side, and have him call you before he gets out of bed. When he's out of bed, supervise his activities, including the use of ambulation aids.

• Encourage the patient to be as independent as possible. Consult with an occupational therapist for help with teaching self-care techniques. Develop a consistent daily routine for performing ADLs, allowing sufficient time for completion.

• Before surgery, monitor the patient's vital signs, fluid and electrolyte balance, and intake and output.

• After surgery, dress the incision area, provide analgesics, and monitor for surgical complications, including further neurologic deficits, infection, hemorrhage, and fluid and electrolyte imbalance. Also monitor the patient's vital signs, fluid and electrolyte balance, and intake and output.

Patient teaching

• Teach the patient and his family about CVA. Explain diagnostic tests, treatments, and the patient's rehabilitation program.

• If surgery is scheduled, make sure that the patient and his family understand the procedure and any associated consequences.

• After consulting an occupational therapist and a physical therapist, teach the patient self-care skills. If speech therapy is necessary, encourage the patient to begin as soon as possible. Devise a discharge plan with the patient and his family. Provide the patient with appropriate home safety equipment, such as grab bars for the toilet and ramps. Involve the patient's family with his rehabilitation program. (See *Making eating easier,* pages 194 and 195.)

• When describing self-care skills to patients with sensory or cognitive impairment, demonstrate each component of the activity. Then recombine the components into the complete skill. Be sure to give the patient time to understand.

• Explain the importance of following the prescribed exercise program to the patient and his family. Make certain that they can perform the exercises. Emphasize the importance of wearing slings, splints, or other prescribed devices to prevent complications. Also make sure that the patient and his family understand transfer techniques and the use of ambulatory aids.

• If a special diet is required, such as a weight loss diet for an obese patient or semisoft foods for the patient with dysphagia, have the dietitian explain it to the patient. If appropriate, explain the danger of aspiration to the patient's family, and teach preventive measures. Be sure family members are skilled in the abdominal thrust maneuver.

• Urge the patient and his family to report any signs of an impending CVA, such as a severe headache, drowsiness, confusion, and dizziness. Emphasize regular follow-up visits.

• Teach the patient and, if necessary, a family member about the purpose, dosage, mechanism of action, and possible adverse effects of all prescribed medications. Make sure that the patient taking aspirin realizes that he mustn't substitute acetaminophen.

• Teach the patient and his family about the importance of home safety measures, such as installing grab bars near the toilet and bathtub, removing throw rugs, and securing carpets to the floor.

• Counsel the patient and his family about lifestyle changes that may reduce the risk of another CVA. For example, discuss smoking cessation and measures to control diseases such as diabetes or hypertension. Explain the importance of following a low-cholesterol, low-salt diet; increasing activity; avoiding prolonged bed rest; and minimizing stress.

• Encourage the patient and his family to contact a local support group and to obtain information from the National Institute of Neurological Disorders and Stroke. Refer them to a local home health care agency if necessary. (See *Ensuring continued care for the patient with CVA,* page 196.)

EVALUATION

When evaluating the patient's response to your nursing care, gather reassessment data and compare this information with the expected outcomes documented in your plan of care.

(Text continues on page 196.)

Making eating easier

Special glasses, cups, plates, and utensils can make eating easier and more enjoyable for the patient who's had a cerebrovascular accident and can save you time by allowing the patient to feed himself.

Glasses and cups

If your patient has trouble holding a glass, suggest that he use a plastic tumbler. Plastic is lighter and less slippery than glass. Or he might try placing terry cloth sleeves over glasses to make them easier to grasp.

Also tell the patient about specially designed cups. For example, he can use a cup with two handles, a pedestal or a T-handle, or a weighted base that may be easier to hold.

A cup with a V-shaped opening on its rim may be helpful for the patient with a stiff neck. He can easily empty this cup without bending his neck backward.

If the patient's hands are unsteady, he may find it easier to hold a cup with a large handle or drink from a lidded cup with a lip to help reduce spills. If the patient has decreased sensation or feeling in his hands, an insulated cup or mug can prevent him from being burned.

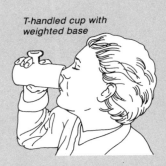

T-handled cup with weighted base

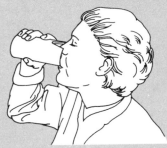

Cup with V-shaped opening

Drinking straws

Inform the patient that flexible or rigid straws, either disposable or reusable, come in several sizes. Some straws are wide enough for drinking soups and thick liquids. If the patient has trouble holding the straw in place, suggest he use a snap-on plastic lid with a slot for the straw.

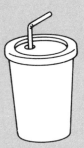

Straw secured by slotted lid

Dishes

Advise the patient to use only unbreakable dishes, if possible. To keep a plate from sliding, tell him to place a damp sponge, washcloth, paper towel, or rubber disk under it. Consider using a plate with a nonskid base or place mats made of dimpled rubber or foam. Suction cups attached to the bottom of a plate or bowl also help prevent slipping.

A plate guard is a helpful device that blocks food from falling off the plate, allowing it to be picked up easily with a fork or spoon. Tell family members to attach the guard to the side of the plate opposite the hand that the patient uses to feed himself.

A scooper plate has high sides that provide a built-in surface for pushing food onto the utensil. A sectioned plate or tray may also be convenient.

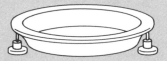

Dish with sides and suction cups

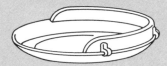

Plate guard

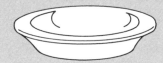

Scooper plate

Flatware

If the patient's hand is weak, explain that ordinary flatware with ridged wood, plastic, or cork handles is easier to grasp than smooth metal handles. Handles can also be built by taping the utensil to a bicycle handlebar or by wrapping a foam curler pad or tape around the utensil (this also works for holding pens, pencils, toothbrushes, or razors). Family members may also try taping the utensil directly to the patient's hand.

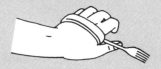

Utensil with strap

Discharge TimeSaver

Ensuring continued care for the patient with CVA

Review the following teaching topics, referrals, and follow-up appointments to make sure that your patient is adequately prepared for discharge.

Teaching topics
Make sure that the following topics have been covered and that your patient's learning has been evaluated:
☐ explanation of CVA and its complications
☐ ways to reduce risk of complications or of recurrent CVAs
☐ prescribed medications, including precautions and possible adverse effects
☐ guidelines for positioning and transfer techniques, exercise, and activity
☐ guidelines for performing activities of daily living within limitations imposed by illness
☐ nutritional guidelines and eating techniques
☐ use of assistive devices
☐ communication techniques
☐ home safety measures
☐ bowel and bladder elimination program

☐ sources of information and support
☐ recognizing and reporting warning signs and symptoms.

Referrals
Make sure that the patient has been provided with necessary referrals to:
☐ social services for equipment, medication, and home health care
☐ dietitian
☐ psychologist
☐ physical therapist
☐ speech therapist
☐ occupational therapist.

Follow-up appointments
Make sure that the necessary follow-up appointments have been scheduled and that your patient has been notified:
☐ doctor
☐ diagnostic tests for reevaluation
☐ physical rehabilitation center.

Teaching and counseling
Begin by determining the effectiveness of teaching and counseling. Consider the following questions:
• Have the patient and his family demonstrated prescribed exercises and positioning, transfer, and assisted ambulation techniques?
• Have they made plans for continued physical rehabilitation following discharge?
• Have they discussed home safety measures?

• Has the patient demonstrated adequate mobility and absence of contractures and pressure ulcers?
• Is he able to perform ADLs independently?
• Has he learned to use alternative methods to communicate needs?
• Does he make more frequent efforts to communicate despite the difficulties?
• Is he able to consistently follow simple directions?
• Is he free of injuries?

• Is he able to adapt to sensory loss as evidenced by performance of ADLs?

Physical condition
Note whether or not the patient:
• exhibits alertness and awareness of time, place, and person
• exhibits normally reacting pupils
• maintains an ICP that's less than or equal to 15 mm Hg
• maintains cerebral perfusion pressure that's greater than 60 mm Hg
• reports an absence of headache, nausea, and vomiting
• shows stable, normal vital signs.

Cerebral aneurysm

In this disorder, the wall of a cerebral artery or vein weakens and dilates to form a sac. In the most common form of cerebral aneurysm — a saccular or berry aneurysm — a saclike outpouching forms in the cerebral artery wall. (See *Key points about cerebral aneurysm*, at right, and *Common sites of cerebral aneurysm*, page 198.)

Rupture of a cerebral aneurysm usually results in a subarachnoid hemorrhage. Less often, the aneurysm may rupture into other areas of the brain, leading to an intracranial hematoma. A ruptured cerebral aneurysm may cause cerebral vasospasms or a life-threatening increase in intracranial pressure (ICP). About 40% of aneurysm patients experience cerebral vasospasms, usually 4 to 10 days after the initial bleeding. Vasospasms may lead to cerebral ischemia and infarction, further neurologic deficits, or death.

Another possible complication is rebleeding, which usually develops 24 to 48 hours after the initial bleeding and again 7 to 10 days later. If blood obstructs the flow and resorp-

FactFinder
Key points about cerebral aneurysm

• *Incidence:* Cerebral aneurysms occur more commonly in adults than in children and slightly more commonly in women than in men (especially women in their late 40s or early to middle 50s).
• *Frequency:* Cerebral aneurysm is the fourth most common cerebrovascular disorder.
• *Prognosis:* Almost half of all patients with a ruptured cerebral aneurysm die from the initial bleeding.
• *Complications:* Rebleeding occurs in about 50% of patients who survive the initial bleeding. Multiple aneurysms occur in about 20% of all patients with a cerebral aneurysm.

tion of the cerebrospinal fluid (CSF), hydrocephalus may develop months later.

The prognosis for a patient with a ruptured cerebral aneurysm depends on the extent and location of the aneurysm, the patient's age, his general health, and his neurologic condition. Approximately 50% of patients who suffer a subarachnoid hemorrhage die immediately. However, with new and better treatments, life expectancy is improving.

Causes
A cerebral aneurysm may result from congenital defects or from preexisting conditions, such as hypertensive vascular disease, atherosclerosis, or head injury.

Common sites of cerebral aneurysm

Cerebral aneurysms usually occur at arterial bifurcations in the circle of Willis and its branches. The illustration below shows the most common sites.

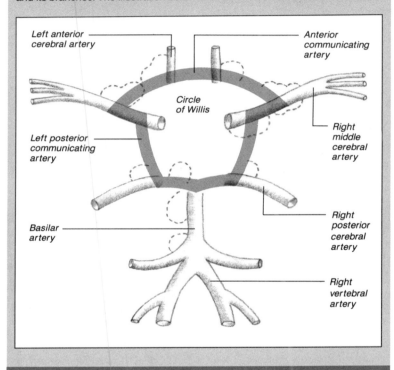

Left anterior cerebral artery

Anterior communicating artery

Circle of Willis

Left posterior communicating artery

Right middle cerebral artery

Basilar artery

Right posterior cerebral artery

Right vertebral artery

Most patients with a cerebral aneurysm are asymptomatic until a rupture occurs. If you suspect that a patient has had a cerebral aneurysm rupture or is in danger of a rupture, contact the doctor immediately. Make certain that the patient has an unobstructed airway and is adequately ventilated. Assess his vital signs.

Health history
If the patient is unconscious or has severe neurologic impairments, you will have to obtain information from a family member. Before an aneurysm ruptures, the patient may experience the following symptoms:
• a sudden, unusually severe headache
• nausea and vomiting
• loss of consciousness.

The patient or family member may report that an activity, such as exercise or sexual intercourse, preceded the cerebral aneurysm. Sometimes, the patient has a history of seizures.

When a cerebral aneurysm leaks rather than ruptures, the patient may report premonitory symptoms such as a headache, a stiff back and legs, or intermittent nausea. Symptoms may last for several days.

Determine if the patient has had any disorders or experiences that increase the risk of cerebral aneurysm, including head injury, hypertension, atherosclerosis, a previously ruptured cerebral aneurysm, or chronic use of cocaine.

Physical examination
Findings will depend on the location of the cerebral aneurysm and the severity of the hemorrhage, if present.

Neurologic assessment
Assess the patient's level of consciousness (LOC) and record baseline findings on a standard form such as the Glasgow Coma Scale. Your findings may vary from a brief loss of consciousness to a deep coma. Restlessness and irritability may occur from meningeal irritation or hypoxia.

Motor functions
Check for focal deficits, most commonly hemiparesis. If the patient is unconscious, check both sides of his body, watching for spontaneous movement and body position.

Sensory functions
When assessing sensory functions, watch for various unilateral deficits, such as neglect syndrome, which may occur if the right parietal lobe is involved.

Cranial nerves
Assess for focal deficits caused by compression of the cranial nerves. The deficits listed below occur much more commonly than other cranial nerve deficits (unless brain herniation develops).
• Visual field deficits, such as homonymous hemianopia, may result from compression of cranial nerve II.
• Ptosis, pupillary dilation, and divergent strabismus may result from compression of cranial nerve III.
• Gaze palsies may result from compression of cranial nerves III, IV, or V.

Additional neurologic findings
Additional assessment may reveal signs of meningeal irritation, including nuchal rigidity, fever, photophobia, seizures, and positive Kernig's and Brudzinski's signs.

Once you've completed the neurologic assessment, grade the severity of the subarachnoid hemorrhage. This will help you plan treatment and establish outcomes. (See *Classifying subarachnoid hemorrhage,* page 200.)

Diagnostic test results
After a cerebral aneurysm rupture, the following tests can help confirm the diagnosis:
• Cerebral angiography, the definitive test, can show the aneurysm's location and structure and the presence of any vasospasm or intracerebral clot.
• Computed tomography scan can locate the clot and identify hydrocephalus, areas of infarction, and the extent of hemorrhage within the cisterns around the brain.
• Lumbar puncture can detect blood in the CSF. Don't use this test if the patient shows signs of increased ICP.
• Skull X-rays can show calcification in the walls of a large aneurysm.

Classifying subarachnoid hemorrhage

Hunt's classification system, shown below, classifies symptoms of subarachnoid hemorrhage according to the grade of bleeding involved.

Grade	Symptoms
I (minimal bleeding)	• Alert • No neurologic deficit • Slight headache • Minimal nuchal rigidity
II (mild bleeding)	• Alert • Minimal neurologic deficits • Mild to severe headache • Nuchal rigidity
III (moderate bleeding)	• Confused or drowsy • Severe headache • Mild focal deficit • Nuchal rigidity
IV (moderate to severe bleeding)	• Stuporous • Mild to severe hemiparesis • Nuchal rigidity
V (severe bleeding)	• Comatose with decerebrate posturing (if nonfatal)

NURSING DIAGNOSIS

Common nursing diagnoses for a patient with a cerebral aneurysm include:
• Altered cerebral tissue perfusion related to increased ICP, hypoxia, subarachnoid hemorrhage, or vasospasm
• Pain (head, neck, or back) related to subarachnoid hemorrhage
• High risk for injury related to altered LOC and focal and sensory deficits
• Impaired physical mobility related to decreased LOC and damage to the motor cortex.

PLANNING

If a cerebral aneurysm ruptures, the consequences are often severe. Direct your nursing care toward controlling the effects of altered cerebral tissue perfusion, minimizing pain, and helping the patient avoid injury and cope with impaired physical mobility.

Based on the nursing diagnosis *altered cerebral tissue perfusion,* develop appropriate patient outcomes. For example, your patient will:
• be alert and oriented to time, place, and person
• exhibit normally reacting pupils
• maintain ICP that's less than or equal to 15 mm Hg
• report an absence of headache, nausea, and vomiting

• show stable vital signs within his normal or prescribed range
• demonstrate bilaterally equal motor function
• comply with precautions to avoid subarachnoid hemorrhage
• comply with precautions to prevent another cerebral aneurysm.

Based on the nursing diagnosis *pain*, develop appropriate patient outcomes. For example, your patient will:
• report the early warning signs of a severe headache
• describe specific remedies that provide pain relief
• express understanding of the need to report promptly early warning signs of a severe headache to his doctor following discharge from the hospital.

Based on the nursing diagnosis *high risk for injury*, develop appropriate patient outcomes. For example, your patient will:
• remain free of injury throughout his hospitalization
• discuss effective ways to promote safety at home with family members.

Based on the nursing diagnosis *impaired physical mobility*, develop appropriate patient outcomes. For example, your patient will:
• demonstrate prescribed exercises, positioning, transfer, and assisted ambulation techniques with help from family members
• plan with help from family members for continued physical rehabilitation following discharge
• demonstrate freedom from the complications of immobility
• perform activities of daily living (ADLs) independently.

IMPLEMENTATION

The patient with a ruptured cerebral aneurysm may need emergency care, frequent assessment of neurologic and vital signs, and close monitoring for rebleeding and increased ICP. Surgical repair may also be necessary to reduce the risk of rebleeding. (See *Medical care of the patient with cerebral aneurysm*, page 202.)

Nursing interventions

• Maintain an open airway, provide adequate ventilation, and administer supplementary oxygen. Assist with endotracheal intubation and mechanical ventilation if necessary.
• Institute precautions to reduce the risk of rebleeding and to avoid increasing ICP. Such precautions should include enforcing absolute bed rest, limiting visitation, and helping the patient avoid stimulants, such as caffeine, and strenuous physical activity, including extreme hip or neck flexion and Valsalva's maneuver. When suctioning is necessary, hyperoxygenate and hyperventilate before and after the procedure, and suction in intervals of 15 seconds or less.
• Since ICP will probably be high because of cerebral edema, intracranial hematoma, or hydrocephalus, administer prescribed corticosteroids and osmotic diuretics. Increased partial pressure of carbon dioxide in arterial blood ($PaCO_2$) may cause vasodilation and increased ICP; therefore, try to maintain the patient's $PaCO_2$ between 25 and 30 mm Hg. If a ventriculostomy is necessary, monitor CSF output hourly or as prescribed.
• Monitor the patient's vital signs and check his neurologic signs as needed. Compare these measurements with baseline assessment data and report deterioration immediately.

Timesaving tip: Keep baseline assessment data at the patient's bedside for quick reference.

Treatments

Medical care of the patient with cerebral aneurysm

In most cases, medical care focuses on a cerebral aneurysm that has already ruptured. Therapy may include emergency treatment, surgery, or other more conservative treatments.

Emergency treatment
Initial emergency treatment may include oxygenation and mechanical ventilation, which can restore deteriorating respiration or reduce intracranial pressure.

Surgery
To reduce the risk of rebleeding, the doctor may attempt to surgically repair the aneurysm by clipping, ligating, or wrapping the aneurysm neck with muscle. Most hospitals now attempt surgery within 2 days after the hemorrhage.

Other treatments
Aneurysm precautions, drug therapy, or hypertensive-hypervolemic therapy may be initiated instead of surgery if the patient is too weak, if the aneurysm is in a dangerous location, or if vasospasm occurs.

Aneurysm precautions
Precautions commonly instituted to prevent rebleeding include:
• rest in a quiet, darkened room for up to 4 to 6 weeks if immediate surgery isn't possible
• use of antiembolism stockings or sequential compression boots (to decrease the risk of deep vein thrombosis and pulmonary emboli)
• avoidance of coffee, other stimulants, and aspirin.

Drug therapy
Drugs commonly prescribed include:
• analgesics, such as codeine, to control pain
• an antihypertensive drug, such as hydralazine, to control hypertension
• a vasoconstrictor to maintain blood pressure at the optimum level (20 to 40 mm Hg above normal).
• corticosteroids to reduce cerebral edema
• anticonvulsants to prevent seizures
• sedatives to relax the patient
• aminocaproic acid for fibrinolytic inhibition (rarely used because of the risk of rebleeding and deep vein thrombosis)
• a calcium channel blocker, such as nimodipine, to reduce cerebral vasospasm by preventing calcium influx into the cells of cerebral vessels (despite secondary adverse effects).

Hypertensive-hypervolemic therapy
Hypertensive-hypervolemic therapy, also known as hypervolemic hemodilution, may be ordered to control vasospasm. This therapy uses I.V. fluids, plasma volume expanders, and vasopressors to increase the volume and decrease the viscosity of the blood, enabling the blood to more easily perfuse past the narrowed vessel. Pulmonary artery wedge pressure, hemoglobin level, hematocrit, cardiac output, central venous pressure, and blood pressure are monitored carefully if this therapy is used.

Also monitor cerebral blood flow either daily or continuously as ordered.
• Watch for danger signs that may indicate rebleeding, vasospasm, or increased ICP. These include a decreasing LOC, pupils that react sluggishly and separately in response to light, a fixed dilated pupil, the start of or worsening of hemiparesis or motor deficit, increased blood pressure, slowed pulse rate, sudden beginning or worsening of a headache, renewed or persistent vomiting, and renewed or worsened nuchal rigidity.
• Give the patient a mild sedative and analgesic if necessary. Keep his room as quiet as possible.
• Monitor blood pressure frequently, since hypertension may lead to rebleeding. Remember, however, that if vasospasm is present, the blood pressure must be sufficient to push the blood through the narrowed vessels.
• Institute hypertensive and hypervolemic therapy as ordered. Administer I.V. fluids and medications as prescribed to control vasospasm. Monitor the patient's pulmonary artery wedge pressure, carbon dioxide, and hematocrit levels. Auscultate the lungs for crackles, and watch for pulmonary edema on chest X-rays. Monitor the patient's intake and output carefully, and continue to monitor his blood pressure and apical rate. Usually, your goal will be to perfuse blood past the vasospasm by increasing systolic blood pressure to 150 to 160 mm Hg. When hypertensive and hypervolemic therapy is ordered, pulmonary edema is a risk, so monitor the patient's pulmonary status closely.
• Notify the doctor immediately if the patient fails to maintain blood pressure — especially, systolic pressure — in the desired range.

• Monitor the patient for seizures, and administer prescribed anticonvulsants.
• Maintain the patient's temperature within a normal range. Use prescribed measures, such as a hypothermia blanket, as needed. Remember not to use a rectal thermometer, which may cause Valsalva's maneuver and thus increase ICP.
• Administer a continuous infusion of aminocaproic acid I.V. in dextrose 5% in water, as prescribed, adjusting the dosage in patients with renal insufficiency. Be sure to monitor the patient for adverse reactions, such as phlebitis, which is common with I.V. administration, and nausea and diarrhea, which are more common with oral administration. Reduce the risk of deep vein thrombosis by applying antiembolism stockings, and administer calcium channel blockers as prescribed.
• Provide emotional support to the patient and his family. Minimize stress by encouraging the patient to relax and to express his concerns.
• Help the patient and his family find effective coping strategies. For example, they may find a visit from their clergyman very supportive.
• Position the patient appropriately to prevent injury or contractures. Turn him often to protect his skin, making sure that he relaxes his muscles. Assist the patient with passive range-of-motion (ROM) exercises. Don't permit active ROM or isometric exercises during the acute period.
• Help the patient eat if necessary. Consult with a speech pathologist to evaluate the patient's swallowing and gag reflexes. Closely monitor a patient who is at risk for aspiration, making sure you have suctioning equipment available.
• If the patient can't swallow, insert a nasogastric tube, as ordered, and ad-

minister tube feedings. Tape the tube so it doesn't press against the nostril and irritate the skin. Provide nose and mouth care frequently.

• If the patient can eat solids, a high-fiber diet, such as bran, salads, and fruit, will prevent straining during defecation, which may result in increased ICP. Administer a stool softener, such as dioctyl sodium sulfosuccinate, or a mild laxative as prescribed. Begin a bowel elimination program based on the patient's usual habits. If the patient is receiving corticosteroids, check the stool for occult blood.

• If the patient has palsy of cranial nerve V, administer artificial tears or a lubricant to the affected eye as ordered.

• To protect the patient from injury, raise the bed's side rails. Try to avoid using restraints, which may agitate the patient and raise ICP.

• Prepare the patient for surgery if necessary.

• Perform postcraniotomy care if necessary. Inspect the patient's head dressing for bleeding and CSF drainage. Position the patient so that his neck is straight and flexing it won't interfere with cerebral drainage. Monitor ICP as ordered, and maintain adequate respiratory function and brain oxygenation by using supplementary oxygen and mechanical ventilation as ordered.

• Monitor the patient for postoperative complications, including increased neurologic deficits resulting from cerebral hemorrhage or vasospasm, increased ICP resulting from cerebral ischemia or cerebral edema, sudden hemiplegia, fluid and electrolyte disturbances, and GI bleeding. Also monitor for mental status changes, such as disorientation or amnesia.

• When the danger of rebleeding has passed, plan a rehabilitation program for the patient with the doctor, physical therapist, speech therapist, and occupational therapist. Encourage the patient and his family to participate.

• Plan the patient's discharge with the social services department, and make sure that he receives any equipment necessary for home health care. (See *Ensuring continued care for the patient with cerebral aneurysm.*)

Patient teaching
• Teach the patient and his family about his condition. Encourage family members to be realistic, and answer their questions honestly, but never discourage hope.

• Explain all tests, neurologic examinations, treatments, and procedures to the patient.

• Explain necessary cerebral aneurysm precautions and their purpose to the patient and his family.

• If surgery becomes necessary, be sure that the patient and his family understand the procedure and possible complications.

• Make sure that the patient and his family understand the physical rehabilitation plan. Let them know whether the patient will be an inpatient or an outpatient at the rehabilitation center.

• Provide nutritional guidelines to the patient and his family. If the patient is at risk for aspiration, explain appropriate safety measures, such as consulting with a speech pathologist for swallowing evaluations and other suggestions specific to the patient's needs.

• Explain to the patient and his family how to continue the bowel and bladder elimination program.

• Explain to the patient and his family the purpose, mechanism of action,

Ensuring continued care for the patient with cerebral aneurysm

Review the following teaching topics, referrals, and follow-up appointments to make sure that your patient is adequately prepared for discharge.

Teaching topics
Make sure that the following topics have been covered and that your patient's learning has been evaluated:
☐ explanation of cerebral aneurysm and its complications
☐ prescribed medication, including its purpose, dosage, and possible adverse effects
☐ postsurgical care
☐ dietary guidelines
☐ plans for physical rehabilitation
☐ home safety measures
☐ bowel and bladder elimination program
☐ sources of information and support
☐ need for follow-up care
☐ warning signs and symptoms to report to the doctor.

Referrals
Make sure that the patient has been provided with necessary referrals to:
☐ social services for equipment, medication, home health care, and transportation
☐ dietitian
☐ psychologist
☐ physical therapist
☐ speech therapist
☐ occupational therapist.

Follow-up appointments
Make sure that the necessary follow-up appointments have been scheduled and that the patient has been notified:
☐ doctor
☐ diagnostic tests for reevaluation
☐ physical rehabilitation center.

dosage, possible adverse effects, and precautions for all prescribed medications.

• Teach family members to recognize and immediately report signs of rebleeding, such as headache, nausea, vomiting, and changes in LOC, including irritability and restlessness.

• If the patient will be going home, make sure that he and his family are adept at transfer techniques and understand the need for home safety measures.

• Provide sources of information and support.

EVALUATION

When considering the patient's response to your nursing care, gather reassessment data and compare this information with the patient outcomes specified in your plan of care. Consult with other members of the health care team as necessary.

Teaching and counseling
Talk to the patient to determine the effectiveness of teaching and counseling. Consider the following questions:

• Does the patient observe precautions to prevent subarachnoid hemorrhage or other complications of cerebral aneurysm?

• Does he express an understanding of the need to report promptly early warning signs, such as a severe headache, to his doctor?

• Can he describe specific remedies that provide pain relief?

• Has he discussed home safety strategies with family members?

• Can he perform prescribed exercises, positioning, transfer, and assisted ambulation techniques with help from family members?

• Does he understand the purpose and possible adverse effects of prescribed medications?

• Has he planned with family members for continued physical rehabilitation following discharge?

• Is he willing to contact recommended sources of information and support?

• Does the patient demonstrate freedom from the complications of immobility?

• Does he perform ADLs independently?

Physical condition

A physical assessment and diagnostic tests will also help you to evaluate the effectiveness of your plan of care. Note whether or not your patient has achieved the following parameters:

• alertness and orientation to person, place, and time

• normally reacting pupils

• ICP that's less than or equal to 15 mm Hg

• absence of headache, nausea, and vomiting

• stable vital signs within his normal or prescribed range

• bilaterally equal motor function

• absence of injury.

Caring for patients with degenerative disorders

Alzheimer's disease

A chronic condition characterized by declining intellectual capacity, Alzheimer's disease is the most common dementia. It causes gradual loss of memory accompanied by loss of at least one other cognitive function, such as language, abstraction, or spatial orientation.

A progressive loss of neurons in the brain, especially the cerebral cortex, causes increasingly severe symptoms. Over time, the patient loses memory, language, and motor function. Eventually, he loses the capacity to regulate basic body functions. (See *Understanding pathologic changes in Alzheimer's disease,* opposite, and *Key points about Alzheimer's disease,* page 210.)

Alzheimer's disease can prove taxing for family members, who may feel guilty for not doing enough for the patient or exhausted from doing too much. Family members are vulnerable to depression and severe stress.

Causes

Researchers are investigating several possible causes of Alzheimer's disease. Neither environmental nor viral causes have been identified, but some evidence suggests a genetic basis for the disorder. In particular, the early-onset form of the disorder appears to be linked to an autosomal dominant gene. Patients with Down's syndrome also appear to have an increased susceptibility to Alzheimer's disease. Closed-head trauma, producing a period of unconsciousness, also increases the risk of developing Alzheimer's disease later in life.

Other possible causes include:
• serum protein abnormalities

• viruses
• nerve cell defects.

ASSESSMENT

Assessment focuses on the patient's health history and physical examination findings, with diagnostic tests used to rule out other forms of dementia. One assessment goal is to differentiate Alzheimer's disease from other neurologic or psychiatric disorders, especially other forms of dementia.

Health history

The patient may initially experience subtle changes, such as forgetfulness and mild memory loss without loss of social skills or changes in behavior patterns. However, as the disorder progresses, the patient exhibits increasing loss of short-term memory, making it difficult for him to learn and remember new information.

Make careful observations of the patient during the interview. Look for evidence of the following changes in the patient's condition:
• deterioration in personal hygiene and appearance
• an inability to concentrate
• difficulty with abstract thinking and activities that require judgment
• difficulty in communicating (may progress to an inability to speak or write)
• repetitive actions or speech
• restlessness or aimless wandering
• negative personality changes, such as irritability, depression, paranoia, hostility, and combativeness
• nocturnal awakenings
• disorientation.

In early stages, Alzheimer's disease may be almost imperceptible, with symptoms resembling ordinary forgetfulness. Once the illness becomes more advanced, the patient

Understanding pathologic changes in Alzheimer's disease

Researchers have identified a number of pathologic brain changes that characterize Alzheimer's disease.

Neurofibrillary tangles
These twisted clumps of protein are found in damaged nerve cells, especially in the hippocampus and cerebral cortex.

Neuritic plaques
Clusters of dying neurons and abnormal nerve terminals form plaques. These occur most densely in the hippocampus but are also found in the cerebral cortex. Generally, the more plaques and tangles found in the brain, the more severe the symptoms of Alzheimer's disease.

Beta amyloid
This dense, starch-like protein forms the core of neuritic plaques. Some beta amyloid appears in all aging brains, but not in the pattern characteristic of Alzheimer's disease and usually not accompanied by dying neurons.

Loss of neurotransmitters
As neuronal death occurs in the cortex, hippocampus, and hypothalamus, these regions also experience a significant decline in the neurotransmitters acetylcholine and norepinephrine.

Abnormal cerebral circulation
Oxygen metabolism and blood flow in the brain decline in Alzheimer's disease. Also, researchers have noted thickening of capillary walls in the blood-brain barrier. This thickening may inhibit perfusion across the blood-brain barrier.

---

may no longer be able to provide a reliable health history. Therefore, interviewing caregivers is essential for understanding changes in the patient's behavior and thought patterns.

Common caregiver observations
Caregivers may report that the patient:
• feels suspicious and fearful of imagined people and situations
• fails to identify his environment, objects, or people
• complains of stolen or misplaced objects
• seems overly dependent on others

• has difficulty finishing thoughts and following directions
• has trouble using correct words and may often substitute words
• exhibits emotional lability, such as laughing or crying inappropriately, mood swings, or sudden angry outbursts.

As the disorder progresses, caregivers may report:
• eating irregularities such as eating voraciously or forgetting to eat meals
• frequent falls
• language problems, such as aphasia and dysarthria.

In the final stages, the caregiver may report that the patient:

Key points about Alzheimer's disease

- *Incidence:* About 4 million North Americans have Alzheimer's disease. Most of them are over age 65. And nearly half of all North Americans over age 85 have Alzheimer's disease.

  Alzheimer's disease is the fourth leading cause of death in adults in the United States, ranking behind heart disease, cancer, and stroke. It's also a major cause of death in Canada, where it kills nearly twice as many women as men. (This ratio, however, may be due to men's shorter lifespan.)
- *Prognosis:* Most patients die 2 to 15 years after onset of symptoms. The average duration of the illness before death is 8 years.
- *Treatment:* Because no cure exists, treatment aims to support the patient and caregiver. Various experimental therapies have attempted to slow the disease's course but so far with little success.
- *Leading complications:* Patients may incur self-inflicted injuries or accidents. The disease may lead to pneumonia or other infections, and to aspiration, dehydration, or malnutrition.

- has lost the ability to care for himself and is totally dependent on the caregiver
- has bowel and bladder incontinence
- experiences mobility problems and is more prone to falls

- is uncommunicative and unable to recognize close friends and family members
- experiences seizures. (See *Correlating sites and signs of Alzheimer's disease.*)

Medication history
Because drug toxicity is the leading cause of reversible dementia-like states in older patients, you should obtain a complete list of all the patient's prescription and nonprescription drugs.

Additional findings
Explore the family and medical history. For example, ask if any other family members have been diagnosed with Alzheimer's disease. The patient's medical history may help rule out other causes of dementia.

Assess the caregiver's response to the patient's illness. Caregivers are at high risk for depression, so ask about a history of insomnia, loss of appetite or weight, drug or alcohol abuse, and related factors.

Physical examination
Physical findings depend on the stage of illness. Assessment of the patient's level of consciousness typically shows alertness, but with distinct abnormalities in cognitive function. Note the presence or absence of the following:
- memory deficits
- diminished perception and judgment
- loss of attention and concentration
- communication and language problems
- slowed information processing.

Timesaving tip: To test for delayed recall, instruct the patient to listen to and try to remember a list of familiar words. Ask him to repeat this list at established intervals.

Correlating sites and signs of Alzheimer's disease

Progressive and degenerative, Alzheimer's disease destroys brain cells over 5 to 20 years. In the early stages of the disease, the brain's nerve cells become twisted, forming neurofibrillary tangles. Plaques develop around the neurons. Sometimes called senile plaques, they are made of degenerating nerve tissue mixed with beta amyloid.

Destruction begins in the hippocampus, a component of the limbic system, and spreads to the surface of the brain. The patient's signs and symptoms correspond to the area of brain lesions.

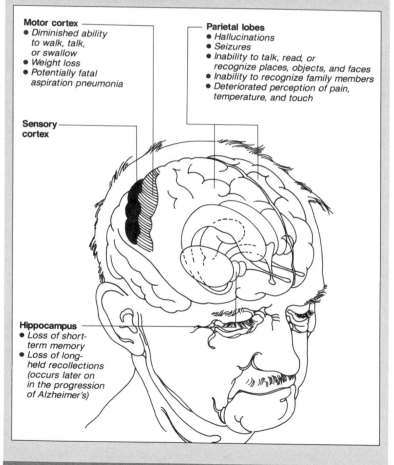

Motor cortex
- *Diminished ability to walk, talk, or swallow*
- *Weight loss*
- *Potentially fatal aspiration pneumonia*

Sensory cortex

Parietal lobes
- *Hallucinations*
- *Seizures*
- *Inability to talk, read, or recognize places, objects, and faces*
- *Inability to recognize family members*
- *Deteriorated perception of pain, temperature, and touch*

Hippocampus
- *Loss of short-term memory*
- *Loss of long-held recollections (occurs later on in the progression of Alzheimer's)*

Even in the first 15 seconds to 2 minutes, a patient in early-stage Alzheimer's disease will show substantial memory loss. Healthy older people usually preserve the capacity for delayed recall. (For another quick assessment tool, see *Clock-drawing test.*)

If the patient's disease has progressed past the early stages, you may note signs of motor deterioration, such as gait disturbances, myoclonus, and tremors. In the final stages, the patient may have urinary or fecal incontinence, muscle twitching, and seizures.

Diagnostic test results

A diagnosis of Alzheimer's disease can't actually be confirmed until death, when pathologic findings are revealed at autopsy. The following tests may help evaluate the patient's condition and rule out other disorders:

• Positron emission tomography shows decreased metabolic activity of the cerebral cortex.

• Computed tomography may show excessive, progressive brain atrophy as well as enlarged ventricles.

• Magnetic resonance imaging may reveal brain atrophy and rule out intracranial lesions as the cause of dementia.

• EEG evaluates the brain's electrical activity and may show slowing of the brain waves, which occurs with dementia.

• Cerebrospinal fluid analysis may help to determine if the patient's signs and symptoms stem from a chronic neurologic infection.

• Laboratory tests may help to rule out other causes of dementia, especially drug toxicity and endocrine and metabolic disorders.

NURSING DIAGNOSIS

Common nursing diagnoses for a patient with Alzheimer's disease include:

• Altered thought processes related to neuronal degeneration

• High risk for injury related to impaired cognition, seizures, and gait disturbances

• Altered nutrition: Less than body requirements related to forgetfulness and inadequate support systems.

You may also need to develop nursing diagnoses for the patient's caregiver, such as:

• High risk for caregiver role strain related to responsibility for a family member with significant home care needs.

PLANNING

Focus your plan of care on making life more tolerable for the patient and his caregivers and promoting a supportive environment.

Based on the nursing diagnosis *altered thought processes*, develop appropriate patient outcomes. For example, your patient will:

• perform activities of daily living (ADLs) independently for as long as possible

• participate in structured physical and social activities for as long as possible

• remain safe and protected from injury.

Based on the nursing diagnosis *high risk for injury*, develop appropriate patient outcomes. For example, your patient will:

• remain injury-free throughout hospitalization.

The patient's caregiver will:

• describe plans to meet the patient's safety needs at home.

Assessment TimeSaver

Clock-drawing test

This test provides a quick and simple method to evaluate impairment of visuo-spatial skills in Alzheimer's disease.

Performing the test
• Ask the patient to draw a clock with all the numbers on it. Then ask him to draw hands on the face of the clock to make it read 2:45.
• Repeat your instructions, using exactly the same wording, as often as necessary. However, don't give the patient any other instructions.
• Don't cover any clocks or other timepieces in the room.

Evaluating results
• Observe the patient's drawing carefully. Are the circle and the numbers generally intact? Are the hands in the correct position, as in the illustration?

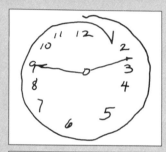

• If the hands don't point to the correct numbers and the rendering of the clock is distorted, as in the second illustration, suspect a visuospatial impairment.

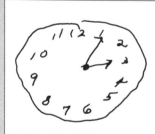

• Suspect severe visuospatial impairment if the hands aren't used to indicate the time or are left out altogether; if the numbers are crowded together, missing, or reversed; or if the clock face is highly distorted, as in the third illustration.

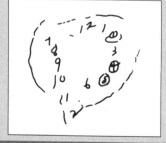

Based on the nursing diagnosis *altered nutrition: less than body requirements*, develop appropriate patient outcomes. For example, your patient will:
• agree to consume an adequate number of calories daily
• maintain body weight in an acceptable range for age, sex, and height.

Based on the nursing diagnosis *high risk for caregiver role strain*, develop appropriate outcomes. For example, the caregiver will:
• express feelings about his responsibilities as a caregiver
• identify and use effective coping mechanisms
• agree to use available support systems and other resources, such as an Alzheimer's support group.

IMPLEMENTATION

Treatment · may address specific symptoms or attempt to slow disease progression. (See *Medical care of the patient with Alzheimer's disease.*)

Nursing interventions

Target your interventions to the stage of the patient's disorder.
• Establish an effective communication system with the patient and his family to help them adjust to the patient's altered cognitive abilities.
• If the patient has early-stage Alzheimer's disease, teach him to use memory aids.
• Provide emotional support to the patient and his family. Encourage them to talk about their concerns. Listen to them and answer their questions honestly. Encourage the caregiver to vent feelings of frustration, anger, and guilt. Help them identify sources of support.
• Establish and follow a daily patient routine. Patients tend to be more

comfortable and less confused with familiar, predictable routines.
• When the patient enters the hospital, expect his symptoms to get worse, at least temporarily. Away from the familiar home environment, the patient may become more disoriented and confused. To decrease the patient's adjustment time and cause a minimum of disruption, ask the caregiver to describe the patient's usual routine at home. Use this information to plan a schedule of daily activities for his hospital stay.
• Use a soft tone, a slow, calm manner, and simple sentences when speaking to the patient. If he doesn't understand you, repeat yourself using the same words. Because the patient's thought processes are slow, make sure that you allow him sufficient time to answer. Be supportive when the patient expresses his feelings.
• Prevent excessive stimulation and keep familiar objects and pictures at the patient's bedside. If the patient can still follow directions and read, leave memory aids, such as notes or pictures.
• Administer ordered drugs and note their effects. If the patient has trouble swallowing, crush tablets and open capsules and mix them with a semi-soft food. Always check with the pharmacist before crushing tablets or opening capsules.
• Protect the patient from injury by providing a safe, structured environment.

Timesaving tip: Because most falls occur during the daytime hours when the nursing staff is busiest, try bringing high-risk patients to one central location, such as the unit lounge. There, one staff member can supervise several patients, freeing the rest of the staff for other duties. Because the patient has

Treatments

Medical care of the patient with Alzheimer's disease

No cure or definitive treatment exists for Alzheimer's disease. However, several therapies may be prescribed in an attempt to prolong or enhance cerebral function.

Drug therapy
• Tacrine hydrochloride (Cognex), a potent centrally acting anticholinesterase agent, helps treat memory deficits.
• Cerebral vasodilators, such as ergoloid mesylates, isoxsuprine, and cyclandelate, can enhance cerebral circulation.

• Psychostimulators, such as methylphenidate, can enhance the patient's mood.
• Antidepressants are used if depression seems to exacerbate the patient's dementia.

Oxygen therapy
Hyperbaric oxygen increases cerebral oxygenation.

Experimental therapies
New drug therapies include choline salts, lecithin, physostigmine, enkephalins, and naloxone.

---

a short attention span, provide purposeful activity.
• Discourage frequent daytime naps, which may alter nighttime sleeping patterns.
• Encourage the patient to exercise, as ordered, to help maintain mobility.
• Promote patient independence and allow ample time for him to perform tasks.
• Isolate tasks so that the patient can complete them more easily.
• Emphasize the need for sufficient fluid intake and adequate nutrition. Consult with the dietitian as needed, and plan necessary caloric intake. Provide a well-balanced diet with adequate fiber, and avoid stimulants, such as coffee, tea, cola, and chocolate. Promote independence by encouraging the patient's input in menu selection, and by providing finger foods.
• Monitor the patient's weight.
• If the patient has dysphagia, provide semisolid foods. Nasogastric or gastrostomy tube feedings may be an ethical choice in the terminal stage of illness.
• Because the patient may be disoriented or his neuromuscular functioning may be impaired, take the patient to the bathroom at least every 2 hours. Place a picture of a toilet on the bathroom door to cue the patient.
• Assist the patient with hygiene, dressing, and grooming as necessary. Isolate tasks. For example, hand the patient a toothbrush, demonstrate its use, and say, "Brush your teeth."

Patient teaching
• Teach the patient's family about Alzheimer's disease. Explain that the cause of the disease is unknown. Review its signs and symptoms with them. Be gentle and supportive; however, make it clear that the disease progresses at an unpredictable rate and that the patient will eventually suffer complete memory loss and total physical deterioration. (See *Ensur-*

Discharge TimeSaver

Ensuring continued care for the patient with Alzheimer's disease

Review the following teaching topics, referrals, and follow-up appointments to make sure that your patient is adequately prepared for discharge.

Teaching topics
Make sure that the following topics have been covered and that your patient's learning has been evaluated:
☐ explanation of the disease, its progressive nature, and its major symptoms
☐ medications, including any adverse effects
☐ dietary adjustments
☐ need for activity, exercise, and rest
☐ home care planning, including safety measures, establishing a daily routine, and avoiding overstimulation
☐ communication techniques
☐ measures to maintain independence and self-esteem
☐ sources of information and support for the patient and caregiver

☐ information about placement in a nursing home or long-term care facility.

Referrals
Make sure that the patient has been provided with necessary referrals to:
☐ social services
☐ dietitian
☐ psychologist
☐ speech therapist.

Follow-up appointments
Make sure that the necessary follow-up appointments have been scheduled and that the patient has been notified:
☐ doctor or clinic
☐ diagnostic tests for reevaluation, if appropriate.

ing continued care for the patient with Alzheimer's disease.)
• Review the diagnostic tests that will be performed and the treatment the patient will require.
• Advise the family to have the patient exercise. Suggest physical activities such as walking. Explain that purposeful tasks, such as folding towels, sweeping, or indoor bicycle riding, may be helpful.
• Stress the importance of diet. Instruct the family to limit the number of foods on the patient's plate and limit utensils so he won't have to make decisions. If he has coordination problems, tell the family to cut

his food and to provide finger foods, such as fruit and sandwiches.
• Encourage the family to allow the patient as much independence as possible while ensuring his and others' safety. Provide information about home safety needs. Teach measures to prevent falls. Explain the importance of removing potential safety hazards, such as scissors, knobs from the stove, medications, and cleaning solutions. Tell them to keep the environment simple and uncluttered and not to change it. Explain the importance of identifying important locations using signs with large letters or, if the patient can't understand that,

Evaluation TimeSaver

Assessing safety risks

Use this checklist to evaluate safety risks for the patient with Alzheimer's disease. During your evaluation, review your hospital's policy and consult with the patient, caregiver, and members of the health care team. You also may want to consult the hospital's risk manager.

Factors enhancing home safety
☐ Clear, written instructions about safety measures
☐ Effective teaching of safety measures
☐ Effective home supervision
☐ Inclusion of caregiver in teaching sessions
☐ Willingness of family members to recognize the patient's declining cognitive functioning
☐ Proper drug use
☐ Adequate lighting
☐ Water heater set to never exceed a temperature of 120°F (48.8°C)
☐ Removal of dangerous objects or potential poisons from patient's reach
☐ Smoking cessation (patient and family members)
☐ No low or broken furniture, unpadded sharp edges on furniture, or changes in furniture arrangement
☐ Clean, spare traffic patterns, no throw rugs, and no steps without barricades
☐ Safe use of stove and other appliances
☐ Durable, nonbreakable fixtures, decorations, and kitchenware
☐ Sturdy door locks
☐ Moderate stimulation
☐ Identification bracelet
☐ Low bed
☐ Sufficient, effective memory aids
☐ Stair markings
☐ Safety rails in bathroom, stairways, or halls

Factors enhancing hospital safety
☐ Clear policy regarding use of physical restraints or sedatives
☐ Adherence to established safety policies
☐ Identification of the patient's high risk for injury
☐ Effective communication of the patient's high-risk status to staff members
☐ Adequate staffing and effective use of available staff members
☐ Staff members well educated in safety measures, such as transfer techniques
☐ Use of wheelchairs for no other purpose than transportation
☐ Absence of clutter
☐ Raised toilet seats
☐ Bed at proper height
☐ Properly functioning equipment
☐ Seating with high backs and armrests
☐ Adequate lighting in rooms and hallways
☐ Absence of dangerous items, such as scissors or disinfectant, in patient's room
☐ No wheels on overbed table. If patient uses it for support, table could slide out from under him.
☐ Appropriate use of side rails (may hinder safety if improperly used)
☐ Adequate paging system
☐ Familiar environment
☐ Moderate stimulation
☐ No smoking (patient and staff)
☐ Floors dried after cleaning

using pictures, such as a picture of a toilet on the bathroom door. Tell them to barricade stairways with high gates if the patient begins wandering or develops motor problems. Encourage them to install additional locks. Provide an identification bracelet for the patient.

• Advise the caregiver to create a routine for all the patient's activities, which will avoid confusion. If the patient becomes upset, tell the family to remain calm and to try redirecting him after his feelings are validated.

• Before discharge, set up an appointment with the social services department, which will help the family assess its home care needs.

• Refer the family to support groups, such as the Alzheimer's Association.

EVALUATION

When evaluating a patient's response to your care, gather reassessment data and compare this information with the patient outcomes specified in your plan of care. Consider the following questions:

• Does the patient participate in exercise programs and social activities?

• Is he oriented to time, place, and person?

• Is he able to perform ADLs independently?

Physical condition
A physical examination also will help to evaluate the effectiveness of care. Consider the following questions:

• Has the patient remained injury-free throughout his hospitalization? (See *Assessing safety risks,* page 217.)

• Does he consume an adequate number of daily calories?

• Has the patient maintained an appropriate weight for his age, sex, and height?

Caregiver response to illness
Evaluate the caregiver's response to the patient's disease. Take note of statements by the caregiver indicating his:

• feelings about his responsibilities as a caregiver

• intention to use support systems

• willingness to use safety measures at home

• willingness to identify and use effective coping mechanisms.

Parkinson's disease

One of the most common cripplers, Parkinson's disease is a slow, chronic degenerative condition. It characteristically causes progressive muscle rigidity, postural instability, bradykinesia, and resting tremors.

As the patient loses mobility, he may experience injury from falls and skin breakdown. Deterioration progresses for an average of 10 years, culminating in death, which usually results from aspiration pneumonia or some other infection. (See *Who's at risk for Parkinson's disease.*)

Causes
Parkinson's disease results from a deficiency of the neurotransmitter dopamine. What causes dopamine deficiency is unknown. Parkinsonism may occur after epidemic encephalitis. Trauma or ischemia may produce parkinsonian symptoms, as may long-term administration of certain drugs, such as phenothiazines and reserpine. Rarely, parkinsonian symptoms stem from exposure to toxins, such as manganese dust or carbon monoxide. (See *Understanding Parkinson's disease,* pages 220 and 221.)

ASSESSMENT

Symptoms are often subtle and occur in varying combinations. They also change as the disease progresses. Early symptoms, such as fatigue and generalized slowness, may be mistaken for normal aging. Therefore, assessment requires consideration of the patient's health history, physical examination findings, and diagnostic test results. You should also inquire about past medical conditions and obtain a thorough medication history to uncover possible causes of parkinsonian symptoms.

Health history

The patient or his family may report gait, balance, and posture disturbances. They may also mention slow movements or difficulty initiating movements. Ask when symptoms began and if they've gotten progressively worse.

Find out if the patient has experienced tremors, which typically begin in the fingers. Although the patient may not be able to pinpoint when tremors began, he may report they increase with stress or anxiety and decrease with purposeful movement and sleep.

Initially, the patient may complain of fatigue when performing activities of daily living (ADLs). He also may report muscle cramps in his legs, neck, and trunk. Constipation, urine retention, and dysphagia may eventually occur.

Find out if the patient has symptoms secondary to autonomic nervous system involvement, including oily skin, increased perspiration, lacrimation, heat sensitivity, and postural hypotension. Family members may report that the patient has rapid mood swings or experiences depression.

FactFinder

Who's at risk for Parkinson's disease

- Parkinson's disease occurs throughout the world in all racial and ethnic groups.
- Parkinson's disease primarily affects adults over age 50, although it occasionally occurs before the age of 40. It affects men more than women.
- The disease strikes 1 in every 100 persons over the age of 60.
- Because the population is aging, the incidence of Parkinson's disease is growing—roughly 60,000 new cases are diagnosed annually in the United States alone.

Physical examination

If Parkinson's disease is suspected, focus on the following four areas: rigidity, bradykinesia, postural instability, and tremors.

Rigidity

A cardinal sign of parkinsonism, rigidity can involve any or all of the striated muscles. Inspection may reveal a masklike facial expression, with fixed, wide-open eyes. Drooling may be apparent. Vocal cord rigidity may lead to dysarthria and hypophonia. Passive movement of the extremities may reveal "cogwheel" or "lead-pipe" rigidity.

Bradykinesia

If this sign is present, you'll note that the patient takes a long time to perform a purposeful action, such as sitting down, rising, or walking to the door.

Understanding Parkinson's disease

Parkinson's disease results from deterioration of dopaminergic neurons in the substantia nigra, a part of the basal ganglia.

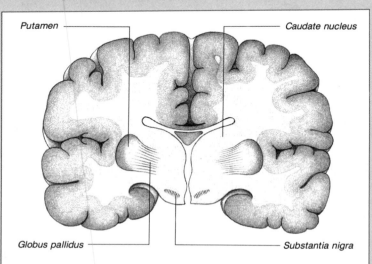

Dopamine pathway
Deterioration of dopaminergic neurons in the substantia nigra causes an interruption in the dopamine pathway.

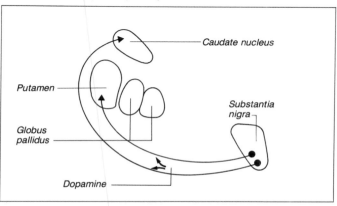

Normal function of the basal ganglia

The basal ganglia play an important role in the extrapyramidal motor system. The ganglia control complex motor activities, including posture, balance, locomotion, and associated movements. The major basal ganglia include the corpus striatum (caudate nucleus, putamen, and globus pallidus), the substantia nigra, and the subthalamic nuclei.

Normally, the function of the basal ganglia is controlled by two neurotransmitters, dopamine and acetylcholine. Dopamine, which is produced in the substantia nigra, has an inhibitive effect on the basal ganglia. Acetylcholine has an excitative effect. Together, these two neurotransmitters counterbalance each other, producing coordinated voluntary movement.

Effects of Parkinson's disease

For unknown reasons, neurons in the substantia nigra that project into the corpus striatum degenerate. This causes a dopamine deficiency in the basal ganglia. As a result, the excitative effect of acetylcholine is unchecked, causing the patient to experience symptoms of cholinergic excess, such as rigidity, tremors, bradykinesia, and postural instability.

The illustration at left shows the location of the basal ganglia in the brain. The inset shows the dopamine pathway — the neuronal pathway that degenerates in Parkinson's disease.

Timesaving tip: To rapidly assess the patient for bradykinesia, ask him to quickly alternate his hands from a palms-up to a palms-down position. If he has bradykinesia, he will not be able to perform this task.

You may also observe akinesia — an inability to initiate and carry out simple motor movements. For example, the patient may not be able to stand up when you ask him to do so.

Postural instability

Assess the patient's posture as he stands and walks. You may note a stooped posture. His gait often lacks normal parallel motion. It may be propulsive (the tendency to take rapid steps forward), following slow initiation of movement. At times, he may take rapid steps backward instead of going forward, which places him in danger of falling. You may also note that he has difficulty pivoting and seems to lose his balance if he moves suddenly.

In some patients, the combined effects of rigidity, bradykinesia, and postural instability result in the characteristic slow, shuffling gait of Parkinson's disease. This gait is associated with short steps and the absence of accompanying swinging of arms.

Tremors

Observe the patient's fingers while his hands are at rest. Look for the classic "pill-rolling" tremor, in which the thumb moves against the distal second and third fingers of the hand. (See *Key characteristics of Parkinson's disease*, page 222.)

Additional findings

Rarely, oculogyric crisis (eyes fixed upward, with involuntary tonic movements) or blepharospasm (contraction of the orbicular muscle of the

Key characteristics of Parkinson's disease

You may shorten your assessment time by focusing on the key characteristics of Parkinson's disease.

Distinguishing between types of rigidity

Patients with Parkinson's disease almost always exhibit rigidity, which results from increased muscle tone at rest. Use the following techniques to help you distinguish cogwheel from lead-pipe rigidity. Keep in mind that rigidity may be unilateral or bilateral.

Cogwheel rigidity
As you perform passive range-of-motion (ROM) exercises on the patient's joints, assess for cogwheel rigidity.

Lead-pipe rigidity
In other patients, passive ROM exercises may reveal lead-pipe rigidity — total resistance over the range of motion.

Recognizing the characteristic gait
Characteristically, the patient walks in a stooped-over position with small shuffling steps. Once movement is begun, he frequently accelerates almost to a trot.

Recognizing pill-rolling tremors
Observe for the characteristic pill-rolling tremor when the patient's hands are at rest. The thumb moves across the palm, giving it a pill-rolling characteristic. Usually, the tremor is exaggerated with rest, relieved with movement, and disappears during sleep.

---

eye) occurs. Parkinson's disease doesn't usually affect the patient's intellect. However, you may note cognitive disturbances, such as memory deficits or confusion in the patient with severe Parkinson's disease. Usually, these symptoms result from drug toxicity or another form of dementia.

Diagnostic test results
A computed tomography scan or magnetic resonance imaging may be performed to rule out other disorders, such as intracranial tumors.

Although urinalysis may reveal reduced dopamine levels, it usually has little value in identifying Parkinson's disease. Like Alzheimer's disease, a dopamine deficiency is only evident at autopsy.

NURSING DIAGNOSIS

Common nursing diagnoses for a patient with Parkinson's disease include:
• Impaired physical mobility related to abnormal motor functioning
• Altered nutrition: Less than body requirements related to dysphagia, tremors, and depression
• Impaired verbal communication related to dysarthria and hypophonia
• High risk for injury related to gait disturbances, rigidity, and tremors

• Knowledge deficit related to the disease, its treatment, and the patient's quality of life.

PLANNING

Focus your nursing care on helping the patient maintain his mobility, avoid falls and other complications, communicate effectively, and identify sources of support.

Based on the nursing diagnosis *impaired physical mobility*, develop appropriate patient outcomes. For example, your patient will:
• ambulate independently for as long as possible
• use assistive devices to maintain mobility
• remain free of contractures.

Based on the nursing diagnosis *altered nutrition: less than body requirements,* develop appropriate patient outcomes. For example, your patient will:
• state intention to consume an adequate number of calories daily
• state intention to maintain body weight in an acceptable range for age, sex, and height.

Based on the nursing diagnosis *impaired verbal communication,* develop appropriate patient outcomes. For example, your patient will:
• make an effort to communicate effectively, using alternate communication strategies if necessary
• express plans to use appropriate resources to maximize communications skills.

Based on the nursing diagnosis *high risk for injury,* develop appropriate patient outcomes. For example, your patient will:
• remain injury-free throughout hospitalization
• identify effective strategies to promote safety at home, with the caregiver.

Based on the nursing diagnosis *knowledge deficit,* develop appropriate outcomes for the patient and caregiver. For example, your patient and his caregiver will:
• communicate an understanding of Parkinson's disease and its symptoms
• demonstrate how to perform physical therapy techniques and self-care skills, including how to use assistive devices
• describe measures to prevent complications related to progressive disability
• agree to comply with follow-up care program.

IMPLEMENTATION

Treatment focuses on helping the patient maintain his mobility and independence and remain free of complications. (See *Medical care of the patient with Parkinson's disease*, page 224.)

Nursing interventions
• Provide emotional and psychological support to the patient and his family. Listen to their specific concerns and answer their questions. Encourage the patient to use coping skills. Help him identify social activities that he can continue to participate in. Encourage participation to help bolster self-esteem and prevent depression.
• Encourage independence by asking the patient to participate in care-related decisions. Help him identify ADLs that he can perform and teach him necessary self-care skills.
• Counsel the patient to help himself as much as possible. Provide positive reinforcement. Make certain that all caregivers are aware of the patient's capabilities. Allow sufficient time for the patient to complete his care.

Treatments

Medical care of the patient with Parkinson's disease

No cure exists for Parkinson's disease, so medical care aims to relieve symptoms and keep the patient mobile and functioning independently as long as possible. Treatment focuses on a medication regimen, physical therapy and, rarely, neurosurgery.

Drug therapy

The medication regimen usually includes levodopa, a dopamine replacement that is most effective during the first few years it's prescribed. The drug is given in increasing doses until signs and symptoms are relieved or adverse reactions appear.

Because adverse effects can be serious, levodopa is frequently given in combination with carbidopa (a dopa-decarboxylase inhibitor) to halt peripheral dopamine synthesis. The patient may also receive bromocriptine to reduce the levodopa dose.

Selegiline may be administered with carbidopa and levodopa, especially when their combined effectiveness decreases. This drug probably acts by inhibiting monamine oxidase type B, an enzyme that breaks down dopamine. Some neurologists now initiate selegiline therapy as a first-line therapy in early-stage Parkinson's disease because evidence suggests that this drug slows the destruction of dopaminergic neurons in the substantia nigra.

Other medications

• Anticholinergics, such as trihexyphenidyl or benztropine, and antihistamines, such as diphenhydramine, are alternative therapies. These drugs may be prescribed when levodopa proves ineffective or too toxic.
• Anticholinergics may be used to control tremors and rigidity. They may also be used in combination with levodopa.
• Antihistamines may help decrease tremors because of their central anticholinergic and sedative effects.
• Amantadine, an antiviral agent, is used early in treatment to reduce rigidity, tremors, and akinesia.
• Tricyclic antidepressants may be given to decrease the depression that often accompanies the disease.

Physical therapy

Physical therapy helps the patient maintain normal muscle tone and function. Appropriate physical therapy includes both active and passive range-of-motion exercises, routine daily activities, walking, and baths and massage to help relax muscles.

Neurosurgery

Stereotaxic surgery, aimed at destroying areas within the globus pallidus and ventrolateral thalamus in order to reduce tremors and rigidity, is rarely performed today, since the advent of more effective drug therapy.

More recently, experimental attempts at surgical implantation of the patient's own adrenal medulla cells into the corpus striatum have been made; however, generally these attempts have not been successful. Other experimental surgeries involve transplantation of fetal substantia nigra tissue.

• Provide assistive devices as appropriate. For example, to help the patient turn himself in bed, tie a rope to the foot of the bed and extend it to the patient so that he can grasp it and pull himself to a sitting position.

• Assist the patient with self-care in later stages of illness when disability is more profound.

• Monitor drug treatment and report any adverse reactions or failure to relieve symptoms. (See *Monitoring response to levodopa.*)

• Because fatigue may make the patient more dependent on others, provide rest periods between activities.

• Assess the patient's nutritional status. Monitor his body weight. Observe for conditions that can hinder adequate nutritional intake, such as difficulty swallowing or difficulty feeding secondary to tremors or depression.

• Consult with the dietitian, physical therapist, doctor, and occupational therapist, as needed, to plan an effective nutritional program.

• To decrease the risk of aspiration, instruct the patient to sit in an upright position when eating. Keep suction equipment available. Offer semisolid foods if he has difficulty swallowing. Consider providing supplementary feedings or small, frequent meals to increase caloric intake if needed.

• Help establish a regular bowel elimination routine by encouraging the patient to drink at least 2,000 ml of liquids daily (unless contraindicated) and to eat high-fiber foods. Encourage daily exercise and establishment of a regular time for elimination. Also make sure he has an elevated toilet seat to assist him from a standing to a sitting position.

• Work with the physical therapist to develop a program of daily exercises to increase muscle strength, decrease muscle rigidity, prevent contractures,

Assessment TimeSaver

Monitoring response to levodopa

Monitor the patient receiving levodopa carefully and adjust the dosage according to his response to therapy and his tolerance level. Overmedication can be toxic, whereas undermedication fails to ameliorate symptoms.

To help you assess the patient quickly, review the brief list of adverse effects listed below. Consider using a simple mnemonic device: *Too much, think FISH; too little, think BART.*

Excessive levodopa

High doses of levodopa over an extended period can lead to major complications, such as:
• Fluctuations in motor function
• Involuntary movements
• Sleep disturbances
• Hallucinations.

Insufficient levodopa

Inadequate dosage or failure to take the medication as prescribed may cause a recurrence of parkinsonian symptoms, such as:
• Bradykinesia
• Ambulation difficulties
• Rigidity
• Tremors.

and improve coordination. The program should include stretching exercises, swimming, use of a stationary bicycle, and postural exercises.

• If the patient experiences depression that isn't easily resolved without drug therapy, discuss the problem with the doctor, who may prescribe antidepressants.

Teaching TimeSaver

Encouraging alternative methods of communication

As the patient weakens, his speech may become impaired and he'll need new ways to communicate, such as lipreading, using a communication board, or using a talking computer.

Lipreading
Although lipreading is one of the most effective ways to communicate without speech, it will take the patient time and effort to learn. The following tips will help him and his family members to communicate:
• Instruct the patient to pause after forming each word with his lips. Then, repeat the word aloud, to make sure others understand him.
• Encourage family members to ask simple questions that require a yes-or-no answer. Instruct them to give the patient the opportunity to express himself in his own way, even if it takes more time.

Communication boards
A communication board allows the patient to express his thoughts by pointing to words, letters, pictures, or phrases on the board. Communication boards come in various forms, including manual and computerized versions. Offer these tips:
• Make sure the entire board is clearly visible when the patient is using it.
• If the patient can't lift his arm to point, perhaps family members can point for him. The patient may want to use a special pointer that requires only slight hand or arm movement.

Talking computers
If the patient owns or wishes to purchase a home computer, he may want "talking software." These programs provide a mechanical voice for the patient, who controls the program through a computer keyboard.

• Provide frequent warm baths and massage to help relax muscles and relieve cramps.
• Protect the patient from injury by raising the bed's side rails and assisting him as necessary when he walks. To minimize gait problems, teach him to use a wide-based stance. Keep his environment free of clutter that could result in falls. Make certain he sits in chairs with armrests and back supports. Also be sure that the patient and caregiver demonstrate proper use of any assistive devices, such as a walker or cane.
• If the patient's speech is affected, consult with the speech therapist.

(See *Encouraging alternative methods of communication*.)

Patient teaching
• Teach the patient and his family about the disorder, its progressive nature, and all ordered treatments. Explain the purpose, dosage, possible adverse effects, and precautions for all prescribed drugs. Tell the patient to notify the doctor if any drugs lose their effectiveness or cause adverse reactions. Explain that the doctor may need to adjust the dosage or change medications.
• If appropriate, show the family how to prevent pressure ulcers and contractures by proper positioning.

Discharge TimeSaver

Ensuring continued care for the patient with Parkinson's disease

Review the following teaching topics, referrals, and follow-up appointments to make sure that your patient is adequately prepared for discharge.

Teaching topics

Make sure that the following topics have been covered and that your patient's learning has been evaluated:
☐ explanation of Parkinson's disease, its progressive nature, and its major symptoms
☐ medications, including possible adverse effects
☐ nutritional needs
☐ physical therapy
☐ home safety
☐ communication techniques
☐ bowel elimination program
☐ measures to maintain independence and self-esteem
☐ sources of information and support for the patient and his family.

Referrals

Make sure that the patient has been provided with necessary referrals to:
☐ social services, regarding equipment, medications, need for home health care services, or transfer to a long-term care facility
☐ dietitian
☐ psychologist or counselor
☐ physical therapist
☐ speech therapist
☐ occupational therapist.

Follow-up appointments

Make sure that the necessary follow-up appointments have been scheduled and that the patient has been notified:
☐ doctor or clinic.

• Explain household safety measures to the patient and caregiver. For example, suggest installing or using side rails in bathrooms, halls, and stairs. Instruct them to remove throw rugs from frequently traveled floors to prevent patient injury. Also instruct the patient to rise slowly to a sitting position and to change any position slowly.

• Explain the importance of daily bathing to the patient with oily skin and increased perspiration.

• To make dressing easier, teach the patient to wear clothing fitted with zippers or Velcro fasteners rather than buttons.

• If appropriate, advise the patient how to eat. Tell him to place food on the tongue, close the lips, chew first on one side and then the other, then lift the tongue up and back and make a conscious effort to swallow. Instruct family members to allow plenty of time for meals.

• Encourage the patient to exercise daily and to follow the planned physical therapy program.

• Before discharge, explain the importance of keeping follow-up appointments. (See *Ensuring continued care for the patient with Parkinson's disease.*)

• Refer the patient and his family to the National Parkinson Foundation, the American Parkinson Disease Association, or the United Parkinson Foundation.

When evaluating the patient's response to your care, gather reassessment data and compare this information with the outcomes specified in your plan of care.

Teaching and counseling

Begin by determining the effectiveness of your teaching and counseling. Consider the following questions:
- Does the patient understand the causes of Parkinson's disease and its treatment?
- Is he willing to comply with drug, physical, speech, and occupational therapy programs?
- Has the patient maintained self-care skills to the greatest extent possible?
- Does he demonstrate competence in using assistive devices?
- Has he contacted appropriate sources of support?
- Have the patient and caregiver implemented strategies to promote home safety?
- Have the patient and his family taken steps to enhance social interaction? Does the patient participate in meaningful daily activities?

Physical condition

If the patient complies with treatment, your ongoing assessment should indicate:
- maximal mobility within the limits of his disease
- freedom from injury resulting from immobility
- absence of contractures
- consumption of an adequate number of calories daily
- maintenance of normal bowel elimination routine
- maintenance of body weight in the target range

- absence of complications related to progressive disability.

Myasthenia gravis

This disorder is marked by sporadic, but progressive, weakness of skeletal or voluntary muscles. Usually, myasthenia gravis affects muscles innervated by the cranial nerves (the muscles in the face, lips, tongue, neck, and throat), but it can affect any muscle group.

Myasthenia gravis follows an unpredictable course of recurring exacerbations and remissions. At worst, it may cause severe weakness leading to acute respiratory failure, a life-threatening emergency known as myasthenic crisis. (See *Key points about myasthenia gravis,* opposite, and *Distinguishing myasthenic from cholinergic crisis,* page 230.)

Causes

Myasthenia gravis is thought to be an autoimmune disorder. The patient's blood cells and thymus gland produce antibodies that block, destroy, or weaken neuromuscular receptors for acetylcholine. This, in turn, causes a failure in transmission of nerve impulses at the neuromuscular junction.

In addition, thymic abnormalities are extremely common in myasthenia gravis, with up to 15% of patients having thymomas and 80% having thymic hyperplasia. However, the relationship between thymic dysfunction and disease etiology is unclear.

Assessment findings vary. Symptoms often begin subtly and occur intermittently. Findings also depend on the muscles involved and the severity of the disease. Therefore, assessment requires a careful evaluation of the patient's health history, physical examination findings, and diagnostic test results.

Health history

The most common complaints are ptosis and diplopia. The patient will usually report muscle weakness and fatigue. She may describe the onset of symptoms as gradual or sudden. She may also describe episodes of remission and exacerbation.

Ask the patient about difficulty chewing and swallowing, and associated weight loss or choking episodes. Find out if the patient has trouble holding her head erect. She may report that she must tilt her head back to see properly. The patient may also report weakness of arm or hand muscles and, rarely, leg weakness, especially after even minimal exercise.

 Timesaving tip: To assess myasthenia gravis rapidly, look for evidence that weakness in the extremities is more proximal (closer to the body) than distal (further from it). For example, a patient with lower extremity proximal weakness may have difficulty getting out of a chair but can usually walk safely.

Fine-motor coordination in the hands may also be affected. This will be evident if the patient has difficulty sewing, writing, or buttoning her clothes.

When respiratory involvement occurs, the patient may complain of intermittent or worsening dyspnea. Complaints of vague apprehension or insomnia may provide the earliest clues to respiratory involvement. Pay attention if the patient expresses fear of an impending myasthenic crisis.

The patient usually reports that symptoms are milder on awakening and worsen as the day progresses or

---

> *FactFinder*
> ## Key points about myasthenia gravis
>
> • *Incidence:* Myasthenia gravis can occur at any age, but the incidence is highest in women ages 18 to 25 and in men ages 50 to 60. About three times as many women as men develop this disease.
> • *Prognosis:* Although no cure is known, drug treatment allows most patients to lead normal lives, except during exacerbations.
> • *Common signs and symptoms:* Ptosis and diplopia
> • *Chief diagnostic method:* Tensilon test
> • *First-line treatment:* Anticholinesterase drugs
> • *Life-threatening complications:* Myasthenic or cholinergic crisis
> • *Other complications:* Weight loss resulting from chewing or swallowing difficulties; pressure ulcers resulting from immobility; and breathing difficulties or lung infection resulting from respiratory muscle involvement

---

during activity. Short rest periods temporarily restore muscle function. Factors that trigger the onset or exacerbation of symptoms include menses, emotional stress, prolonged exposure to sunlight or cold, or infections. Inquire about past psychiatric disorders; mental health problems often are associated with emotional stress, a precipitating factor.

Physical examination

On inspection, the patient may have a sleepy, masklike expression (caused by involvement of the facial muscles) and a drooping jaw if she's tired. You

Distinguishing myasthenic from cholinergic crisis

In patients with myasthenia gravis, crisis refers to a rapid onset of severe muscle weakness and an exacerbation of skeletal muscle weakness. Because crisis involves the respiratory muscles, it can quickly lead to respiratory failure. Use the list below to quickly distinguish between myasthenic and cholinergic crises.

Myasthenic crisis
This form of crisis occurs when the patient is undermedicated with anticholinesterase drugs. Signs and symptoms include:
- increased blood pressure
- restlessness
- tachycardia
- absent cough reflex
- dysarthria
- dysphagia
- dyspnea
- cyanosis (possible).

If the patient responds positively to the Tensilon test, management of the crisis includes increasing the dosage of anticholinesterase drugs. Mechanical ventilation may be ordered for acute respiratory muscle paralysis.

Cholinergic crisis
This crisis results from overmedication with anticholinesterase drugs. Excessive accumulation of acetylcholine at the neuromuscular junction results in muscle weakness, because of prolonged depolarization or desensitization of the postsynaptic membrane. Main signs and symptoms are:
- apprehension
- nausea, vomiting, and diarrhea
- abdominal cramps
- increased secretions and saliva
- blurred vision
- dysarthria
- dysphagia
- dyspnea
- cyanosis (possible)
- pallor
- sweating
- bradycardia.

The patient will not react positively to the Tensilon test. Treatment consists of discontinuing all anticholinesterase drugs until toxic effects subside. Other therapies include possible mechanical ventilation and 1 mg atropine I.V. to counteract the cholinergic reaction.

---

may also note ptosis of the eyelids, especially on prolonged upward gaze. With progressive involvement, you may observe dysarthria, dysphonia, and swallowing and chewing difficulties.

Timesaving tip: The patient may have difficulty describing diplopia. To save time in identifying this symptom, ask her to cover one eye. If vision is clear, it suggests diplopia. A facial droop can be quickly picked up by asking the patient to show you her teeth — a smile may appear as a snarl.

Evaluate the patient's motor function. If the patient reports extremity weakness, assess her grip strength, which may be decreased. There may also be weakness of the neck muscles, which causes the patient's head to fall forward. Test each muscle group only once — putting a patient through a strenuous neurologic examination can cause unnecessary weakness and potential respiratory distress. Because respiratory muscle involvement is possible, you must also assess respiratory functioning.

If respiratory muscles are involved, you may note a weak, ineffective cough and diminished chest excursion. Lung auscultation may reveal hypoventilation and congestion. Apnea may occur suddenly.

A neurologic examination will usually not reveal coordination abnormalities or pathologic reflexes. Pupillary responses are usually preserved. Level of consciousness and cognition also are not impaired, unless myasthenia gravis is complicated by respiratory failure. (See *Clinical findings in myasthenia gravis.*)

Diagnostic test results

A positive Tensilon test confirms a diagnosis of myasthenia gravis. This test shows temporarily improved muscle function after an I.V. injection of edrophonium (Tensilon) or, occasionally, neostigmine. Muscle function improves in 30 to 60 seconds and lasts for up to 30 minutes. However, long-standing ocular muscle dysfunction often fails to respond to such testing.

Timesaving tip: Have atropine readily available when performing the Tensilon test. You may need atropine (an anticholinergic) to rapidly reverse any untoward effects of Tensilon (an anticholinesterase).

The following tests may also help establish the diagnosis or evaluate the patient's condition:
- Electromyography measures the electrical potential of muscle cells and reveals progressive diminution of muscle action potentials with repeti-

Assessment TimeSaver
Clinical findings in myasthenia gravis

As you assess the patient, focus on the signs and symptoms listed below:
- ptosis or diplopia
- facial weakness
- dysphagia
- dysarthria
- neck flexor weakness
- shoulder girdle weakness
- respiratory muscle weakness
- hand weakness
- lower extremity weakness.

tive stimulation in myasthenia gravis patients
- Chest X-rays, computed tomography, and magnetic resonance imaging may identify a thymoma
- Serum studies typically reveal elevated levels of acetylcholine-receptor antibodies.

NURSING DIAGNOSIS

Common nursing diagnoses for a patient with myasthenia gravis include:
- Ineffective airway clearance related to respiratory muscle weakness and impaired cough
- High risk for aspiration related to muscle weakness, and chewing and swallowing difficulties
- Altered nutrition: Less than body requirements related to weakness of muscles affecting chewing and swallowing
- Activity intolerance related to muscle fatigue
- Ineffective coping related to acute or chronic disease
- Knowledge deficit of the disease, its treatment, and quality of life issues.

Develop a plan of care that will help the patient avoid complications, obtain adequate rest, and maintain body weight. Also help her understand the nature of the disease and its treatments.

Based on the nursing diagnosis *ineffective airway clearance*, develop appropriate patient outcomes. For example, your patient will:
• demonstrate clear or markedly less congested breath sounds on auscultation
• exhibit productive coughing and expectoration of thin, clear secretions
• maintain arterial blood gas (ABG) levels within the normal range or at acceptable baseline levels.

Based on the nursing diagnosis *high risk for aspiration*, develop appropriate patient outcomes. For example, your patient will:
• not aspirate throughout hospitalization
• discuss measures to prevent aspiration.

Based on the nursing diagnosis *altered nutrition: less than body requirements*, develop appropriate patient outcomes. For example, your patient will:
• agree to consume an adequate number of calories daily
• maintain body weight in the target range for her age, sex, and height.

Based on the nursing diagnosis *activity intolerance*, develop appropriate patient outcomes. For example, your patient will:
• perform self-care measures to the best of her abilities
• coordinate daily activities, rest periods, and the timing of peak drug effects with the time of day that she is at her best

• agree to comply with daily scheduled rest periods and to avoid undue fatigue
• report improved activity tolerance.

Based on the nursing diagnosis *ineffective coping*, develop appropriate patient outcomes. For example, your patient will:
• express feelings concerning her disease and necessary lifestyle changes
• identify effective coping mechanisms
• agree to use available support systems.

Based on the nursing diagnosis *knowledge deficit*, develop appropriate patient outcomes. For example, your patient will:
• communicate an understanding of the disease process, its signs and symptoms, and its treatment
• communicate an understanding of prescribed medications, including their purpose, dosage, possible adverse effects, and precautions
• identify impending signs of a myasthenic crisis (due to inadequate medication or exacerbation of the disease) or a cholinergic crisis (due to excessive medication or a remission of the disease), and describe plans to obtain immediate assistance
• identify sources of support and attend myasthenia gravis support group meetings
• communicate an understanding of measures to prevent complications related to muscle weakness.

Treatment for myasthenia gravis reflects the patient's age and general health, as well as the disorder's severity. Focus your care on providing psychological support and patient teaching, as well as on identifying and preventing complications. (See

Treatments

Medical care of the patient with myasthenia gravis

Anticholinesterase therapy is the main treatment for myasthenia gravis, but other therapies, such as thymectomy or plasmapheresis, may be ordered in some patients.

Drug therapy
Commonly used anticholinesterase drugs include neostigmine (Prostigmin), pyridostigmine (Mestinon), and ambenonium chloride (Mytelase Caplets). These drugs counteract fatigue and muscle weakness and allow about 80% of normal muscle function. However, they become less effective as the disease worsens.

Corticosteroids also may be administered as an adjunct to therapy, especially when anticholinesterase medications lose their effectiveness. The doctor may order other immuno-

suppressive agents, such as azathioprine (Imuran). Cyclophosphamide (Cytoxan) may be used in severe cases.

Additional therapies
The patient may undergo plasmapheresis during exacerbations of the disease or if medications prove ineffective. This procedure removes acetylcholine-receptor antibodies and temporarily lessens the severity of symptoms.

Eighty percent of patients have thymic hyperplasia (a proliferation of thymus gland cells). Patients with thymic hyperplasia or thymomas (a benign tumor on the thymus gland) require thymectomy (removal of the thymus gland). In other patients, thymectomy is controversial.

Medical care of the patient with myasthenia gravis.)

Nursing interventions
• Provide psychological support. Listen to the patient's concerns and answer questions honestly. Encourage the patient to participate in her own care. Help her identify and use positive coping mechanisms, including identifying sources of support. Refer the patient for additional psychological counseling if indicated.
• Establish an accurate neurologic and respiratory baseline. Thereafter, regularly monitor neurologic status and, as warranted, respiratory rate, breath sounds, tidal volume, vital capacity, and ABG levels.

• Be alert for signs of an impending myasthenic crisis. The patient may need a ventilator and frequent suctioning to remove accumulating secretions.
• If the patient demonstrates a decreased ability to cough effectively, consider using the assisted coughing technique. Push inward and upward on the abdomen toward the diaphragm, while the patient exhales. Consult with the respiratory therapist as needed.
• Administer medications at evenly spaced intervals, and give them on time, as ordered, to prevent relapses. Giving medication on time is crucial — some patients who are given

their medication 5 minutes late may not be able to swallow it at that time.

Timesaving tip: If your patient is taking an anticholinesterase drug, have atropine readily available to prevent a critical time delay in an emergency. Be prepared to give atropine for anticholinesterase overdose or toxicity. Some patients take atropine routinely to combat the negative adverse effects of anticholinesterase therapy.

• Assess muscle strength 30 minutes before and 1 hour following administration of medications to note drug effectiveness. Usually, improvement in muscle weakness peaks 1 hour after drug administration. Weakness tends to worsen again within 4 hours after drug administration.

• Plan exercise, meals, care measures, and activities to make the most of the patient's energy peaks. For example, administer her medication about 30 minutes before meals to facilitate chewing or swallowing. Plan activities following rest periods or in the early morning. Encourage maximal self-care.

Timesaving tip: With the patient's help, write a daily schedule with time periods established for rest and activities. If you don't know the patient's schedule, you may overtire her and have to wait until she's rested to perform important tasks, such as range-of-motion exercises, getting her meal tray ready, or feeding her. Post the schedule so that family members and staff quickly become familiar with the routine and follow it. However, be aware that every day is different, and the patient may have to adjust her schedule accordingly.

• Consult with the dietitian, doctor, speech therapist, and physical therapist, as needed, to plan an effective nutritional program.

• When swallowing is difficult, give soft, semisolid foods (applesauce, mashed potatoes) instead of thin liquids to lessen the risk of choking. Offering small, frequent meals may also help. Have suction equipment available.

• Recommend a high-calorie diet if the patient has lost weight. Monitor the patient's daily caloric intake and weight.

• After a severe exacerbation, encourage the patient to increase social activity as soon as possible.

• If surgery is scheduled (thymectomy to remove thymoma, if present; and plasmapheresis to remove acetylcholine-receptor antibodies and temporarily lessen the severity of symptoms), prepare the patient according to hospital policy.

Patient teaching

• Educate the patient about the nature of the illness and its management. Help her determine the best means of maintaining quality of life. Vocational rehabilitation may be helpful. An occupational therapist may suggest assistive devices to be used in the home (for example, grab bars in the shower).

• Help the patient plan daily activities to coincide with medication peaks and rest periods. (See *Ensuring safe drug therapy.*)

• Stress the need for frequent rest periods throughout the day. Emphasize that periodic remissions, exacerbations, and day-to-day fluctuations are common.

• Teach the patient how to recognize signs of a crisis. Tell the patient to notify the doctor immediately if signs and symptoms of a myasthenic crisis occur.

• Warn the patient to avoid strenuous exercise, exposure to people with upper respiratory tract infections, and

exposure to the sun or cold weather. All of these factors may worsen signs and symptoms. Remind the patient to seek prompt medical attention and treatment if infection occurs.
• Because stress may also be a precipitating factor, teach the patient effective coping strategies.
• If the patient has diplopia, advise her that wearing an eye patch or glasses with one frosted lens may help.
• Tell the patient to avoid using aerosols and cleaners because they may aggravate respiratory symptoms.
• Warn the patient to avoid very hot water when showering or bathing, and to use the low setting when drying her hair.
• Advise the patient to wear a medical identification tag.
• Teach the patient with swallowing difficulties to eat semisolid foods and to avoid alcohol. Tell her that eating warm (not hot) foods can help ease swallowing. Advise ingestion of small, frequent meals, and the use of dietary supplements, as needed. Instruct the patient to cut food into small pieces and to chew thoroughly and eat slowly.
• If surgery is scheduled, provide preoperative teaching. Explain to the patient that before surgery, her chest will be cleaned and she'll receive a general anesthetic. (Explain to a male patient that his chest will be shaved.) Tell her that depending on where the surgeon makes the incision, she may awaken from surgery with a chest tube or a drain in place. Also tell her that she may require intubation and mechanical ventilation after surgery and that she'll have antimyasthenic drugs administered I.V. or I.M. until she can take them orally. Explain that these medications will be tapered so that the doctor can assess her muscle strength after surgery.

Teaching TimeSaver

Ensuring safe drug therapy

Teach the patient with myasthenia gravis to:
☐ use an alarm, if necessary, to remind her to take her medication
☐ have extra medication on hand at all times, particularly when going on a trip
☐ familiarize family, coworkers, and friends regarding the disease and medication schedule
☐ consult her doctor before taking any over-the-counter drugs.

• If the patient is scheduled for plasmapheresis, explain the treatment and answer any questions the patient may have.
• Before discharge, emphasize the need for regular follow-up care. (See *Ensuring continued care for the patient with myasthenia gravis*, page 236.)
• Refer the patient to the Myasthenia Gravis Foundation.

EVALUATION

When evaluating a patient's response to your nursing care, gather reassessment data and compare this information with the patient outcomes specified in your plan of care.

Teaching and counseling

Begin by determining the effectiveness of teaching and counseling. During the course of the evaluation, observe the patient's actions. Consider the following questions:
• Does the patient perform self-care activities to the best of her ability?

Discharge TimeSaver

Ensuring continued care for the patient with myasthenia gravis

Review the following teaching topics, referrals, and follow-up appointments to make sure that your patient is adequately prepared for discharge.

Teaching topics

Make sure that the following topics have been covered and that your patient's learning has been evaluated:
☐ explanation of the disease process, its symptoms, treatment, and impact on life
☐ medications, including possible adverse effects
☐ nutritional needs
☐ need for rest
☐ planning of activities to coincide with medication peak effectiveness
☐ signs of myasthenic or cholinergic crisis and the need for immediate intervention
☐ avoidance of precipitating factors
☐ measures to maintain independence and self-esteem
☐ sources of information and support.

Referrals

Make sure that the patient has been provided with necessary referrals to:
☐ social services, regarding equipment, medications, and the need for home health care services
☐ dietitian
☐ psychological counseling
☐ physical therapist
☐ speech therapist
☐ occupational therapist
☐ vocational rehabilitation.

Follow-up appointments

Make sure that the necessary follow-up appointments have been scheduled and that the patient has been notified:
☐ doctor
☐ physical therapist
☐ speech therapist
☐ occupational therapist.

• Has the patient learned to modify her lifestyle, balance activity with rest, and avoid precipitating factors?
• Does the patient report an increased tolerance for activity?
• Does the patient demonstrate improved coping skills?
• Does the patient express an understanding of the disease process, symptoms, and treatment?
• Does she know the signs of complications and when to seek emergency care?
• Does she express an understanding of her medication regimen and safety precautions?

• Has she agreed to comply with follow-up care?
• Has she made plans for maintaining her quality of life?

Physical condition

A physical examination and diagnostic tests also will help to evaluate the effectiveness of your care. Note whether or not your assessment findings indicate the following:
• clear or markedly less congested breath sounds
• absence of thick, copious sputum
• ABG values within a normal range or back to acceptable baseline levels

• no aspiration throughout hospitalization
• body weight within the acceptable range for age, sex, and height.

Amyotrophic lateral sclerosis

Also known as Lou Gehrig's disease, amyotrophic lateral sclerosis (ALS) is characterized by progressive degeneration of the anterior horn cells of the spinal cord, cranial nerves, and motor nuclei in the cerebral cortex and corticospinal tract. A chronic and debilitating disorder, ALS leads to death from complications such as respiratory failure or aspiration pneumonia. (See *Key points about ALS*.)

Causes

The exact cause of ALS is unknown. Possible causes include viral infections and immune complexes formed by autoimmune disorders. Factors that lead to acute deterioration include severe stress, which may result from myocardial infarction, traumatic injury, or physical exhaustion.

ASSESSMENT

Symptoms of ALS depend on the location of the affected motor neurons and the severity of the disease. The disease may begin in any muscle group, but eventually, all muscle groups become involved. Your assessment will focus on a health history and physical examination, supported by a review of diagnostic test findings.

Because the disorder may be inherited, ask the patient if other family members have developed ALS. To assist with the development of nursing diagnoses, ask the patient about

FactFinder

Key points about ALS

• *Incidence:* In North America, more than 30,000 people are estimated to have amyotrophic lateral sclerosis (ALS); about 5,000 more are newly diagnosed each year. ALS is about three times more common in men than in women and commonly affects more whites than blacks.
• *Age of onset:* Generally, ALS affects people ages 40 to 70.
• *Complications:* ALS interferes with the patient's ability to communicate and causes loss of mobility, which leads to pressure ulcers and contractures.
• *Prognosis:* Most patients with ALS die about 3 years after onset of symptoms, but some may live as long as 10 to 15 years.

his ability to perform activities of daily living and how he copes with his condition.

If ALS is known or suspected, perform a complete neurologic assessment, focusing on motor functions. Keep in mind that weakness, atrophy, and fasciculations are the principal signs of ALS. The patient usually retains mental status, eyelid movement, sensation, and bowel and bladder control.

Health history

In early-stage ALS, the patient may report asymmetrical weakness in one limb. The patient usually complains of fatigue and easy cramping in the affected muscles. He may frequently drop items and may experience difficulty performing tasks requiring use of affected muscles. As the disease progresses, he may report progressive weakness in muscles of the arms, legs, and trunk, as well as muscle wasting and fasciculations.

As the disease worsens, the patient may report difficulty talking, chewing, swallowing and, ultimately, breathing. The patient or his caregiver may disclose an accompanying history of uncontrollable emotional outbursts due to frontal lobe involvement.

Physical examination

On inspection, you may observe fasciculations and atrophy in the affected muscles. Fasciculations are most obvious in the feet and hands.

Testing muscle strength confirms muscle weakness. The patient may also exhibit brisk and overactive stretch reflexes. You may note a positive Babinski's sign.

The muscles of speech, chewing, and swallowing may be affected, and you may notice dysarthria, dysphagia, and drooling. In addition, the patient will have difficulty supporting his head and arms. When respiratory muscles are affected, you may observe shortness of breath. Auscultation may reveal decreased breath sounds.

In end-stage ALS, the patient has flaccid quadriplegia and bulbar paralysis with an inability to swallow and communicate. Consequently, the disease may progress rapidly and symptoms can worsen on a daily basis. In the final stages of illness, he is unable to breathe on his own.

Diagnostic test results

The following tests may aid in diagnosis:

• Electromyography will show fibrillations, which indicate muscle wasting or atrophy.

• Muscle biopsy may disclose atrophic fibers interspersed among normal fibers.

• Nerve conduction studies are usually normal.

• Cerebrospinal fluid analysis reveals increased protein content in one-third of patients with ALS.

• Computed tomography, magnetic resonance imaging, and EEG may help rule out other disorders, including multiple sclerosis, spinal cord neoplasms, syringomyelitis, myasthenia gravis, and progressive muscular dystrophy.

• Blood creatine kinase level is elevated.

NURSING DIAGNOSIS

Common nursing diagnoses for a patient with ALS include:

• Impaired physical mobility related to progressive muscle weakness and fatigue

• Impaired verbal communication (dysarthria, dysphonia) related to involvement of muscles of speech, chewing, and swallowing

• Anticipatory grieving related to terminal illness

• High risk for caregiver role strain related to needs of family member.

PLANNING

Develop a plan of care to help the patient communicate effectively and maintain his independence and mobility for as long as possible. Also plan measures to reduce stress for the caregiver.

Based on the nursing diagnosis *impaired physical mobility*, develop appropriate patient outcomes. For example, your patient will:

• state his intention to maintain maximum mobility within limitations of his illness, for as long as possible

• remain free of the complications of immobility.

Based on the nursing diagnosis *impaired verbal communication*, develop appropriate patient outcomes. For example, your patient will:

• make an effort to communicate effectively with others
• use alternative methods, when needed, to communicate needs.

Based on the nursing diagnosis *anticipatory grieving*, develop appropriate patient outcomes. For example, your patient will:

• express feelings concerning his terminal illness
• participate in decisions about his care
• identify resources, such as support groups, to enhance coping.

Based on the nursing diagnosis *high risk for caregiver role strain*, develop appropriate outcomes for the caregiver. For example, the caregiver will:

• describe his emotional response to stress
• use effective coping mechanisms
• identify and use available resources and support systems.

IMPLEMENTATION

Treatment for ALS is tailored to the patient's condition, particularly his muscular capacity. Implement a program that includes appropriate exercise, use of assistive devices, and psychological support. (See *Medical care of the patient with ALS*.)

Nursing interventions

• Because mental status remains intact while progressive physical degeneration takes place, the patient acutely perceives every change in his condition. Provide emotional and psychological support to the patient and his family. Allow them to express

Treatments

Medical care of the patient with ALS

Because amyotrophic lateral sclerosis (ALS) has no cure, treatment is supportive and based on the patient's symptoms.

Drug therapy

• Diazepam may be prescribed for spasticity.
• Quinine may relieve painful muscle cramps that occur in some patients.
• I.V. or intrathecal administration of thyrotropin-releasing hormone temporarily improves motor function in some patients but has no long-term benefits.

Other treatments

• Rehabilitative measures can help patients function effectively for a longer period. Occupational and physical therapy, specifically, may help maintain activities of daily living and optimize respiratory function.
• Mechanical ventilation can help prolong life.
• A feeding tube may be used for patients who are unable to chew or swallow.

their feelings. Stay with the patient during periods of severe stress. Help the patient and his caregiver to identify and use effective coping mechanisms. Refer the patient and his family for additional counseling and support groups, as needed.

• Implement a palliative care program to alleviate major physical problems.

• Have the patient perform active exercises and range-of-motion exercises on unaffected muscles to help strengthen these muscles. Stretching exercises are also helpful.

• As the patient's muscular capacity diminishes, assist with bathing, personal hygiene, grooming, toileting, and transfers from wheelchair to bed. Help establish a regular bowel and bladder elimination routine.

• When the patient's mobility decreases, take measures to prevent skin breakdown. Turn him often, keep his skin clean and dry, and use pressure-reducing devices, such as air mattress therapy.

• Arrange for the patient to get a walker or wheelchair before he is forced to use one; this will conserve muscle energy and strength.

• If the patient can't talk, provide an alternate means of communication, such as a message board, eye blinks for yes and no, or a computer.

• Administer ordered medications, as necessary. When appropriate, crush tablets and mix them with semisolid food for the patient with dysphagia.

• If the patient experiences breathing difficulty, encourage deep-breathing and coughing exercises. Suctioning, chest physiotherapy, and incentive spirometry may also prove helpful.

• If the patient chooses to use mechanical ventilation to assist his breathing, provide necessary care. Carefully assess the patient with respiratory involvement for infection because respiratory complications may be fatal.

Timesaving tip: To prevent prolonged or unnecessary treatment, become familiar with the patient's advanced directives, if such documents exist. Note that federal law now requires hospitals that participate in Medicare and Medicaid to inform patients of their right (under state law) to refuse treatment if they become incapacitated. The hospital is required to note in the medical record whether the patient has, in writing, rejected life support. Make sure that members of the health care team are aware of the patient's documented wishes before the decision to use life-prolonging therapy becomes urgent.

• If the patient has trouble swallowing, give him soft, semisolid foods and position him upright during meals. Have suctioning equipment available to prevent aspiration.

• If the patient has difficulty holding his head upright, use a soft cervical collar. Gastrostomy and nasogastric tube feedings may be necessary if he can no longer swallow.

Patient teaching

• Teach the patient and his family about ALS. Tell them honestly that this is a progressive, incurable disease. However, explain to the patient that treatments exist to make him more comfortable and to help him stay independent as long as possible.

• Teach the patient who has difficulty chewing to cut his food into smaller pieces or to use a blender or food processor to mince food. Suggest adding baby cereal to minced foods to help thicken them.

• Caution the patient against eating foods that stick in the mouth, such as peanut butter and chocolate. If the patient has drooling problems, suggest that he avoid foods such as grapefruit and fluids such as milk that increase salivation.

• Teach the family how to administer gastrostomy feedings if necessary.

• To help the patient handle increased accumulation of secretions and dysphagia and to reduce fear of choking, teach him to suction himself with a suction machine at home. If the patient is incapable of suctioning,

Discharge TimeSaver

Ensuring continued care for the patient with ALS

Review the following teaching topics, referrals, and follow-up appointments to make sure that your patient is adequately prepared for discharge.

Teaching topics
Make sure that the following topics have been covered and that your patient's learning has been evaluated:
□ explanation of amyotrophic lateral sclerosis (ALS) and its symptoms, treatment, and impact on life
□ medications, including possible adverse effects
□ need for rest periods and energy conservation techniques
□ activity and dietary guidelines
□ reinforcement of physical therapy program
□ alternative means of communication
□ techniques for nasogastric and gastrostomy tube feedings, if needed
□ measures to maintain independence and self-esteem
□ wheelchair operation
□ pulmonary care measures
□ modification of the home environment

□ sources of information and support.

Referrals
Make sure that the patient has been provided with appropriate referrals to:
□ social services, regarding equipment, medications, need for home health care services or placement in a long-term care facility
□ psychological counseling
□ physical therapist
□ occupational therapist
□ speech therapist
□ support groups for patient and family.

Follow-up appointments
Make sure that the necessary follow-up appointments have been scheduled and that the patient has been notified:
□ doctor or clinic.

teach the caregiver how and when to perform this procedure.
• As the patient's condition deteriorates, counsel the family on helping the patient through this difficult period and teach them how to perform comfort measures. (See *Ensuring continued care for the patient with ALS.*)
• Teach the patient and his family about a ventilator and tracheostomy and what to expect.
• Before discharge, refer the patient and his family to the social services

department. When warranted, help arrange for a home health care nurse to oversee the patient's status, to provide support, and to continue teaching the family about the illness.
• Help the patient and his family cope with the inevitable losses associated with terminal illness and assist them in the grieving process. Patients with ALS may benefit from a hospice program or the local chapter of an ALS support group.

When evaluating the patient's response to your nursing care, gather reassessment data and compare this information with the patient outcomes specified in your plan of care.

Teaching and counseling

Begin by determining the effectiveness of teaching and counseling. Consider the following questions:
• Has the patient demonstrated proper use of adaptive and assistive devices?
• Does he understand measures to promote effective communication?
• Does he participate in decisions about his care?
• Has he expressed feelings concerning terminal illness?
• Has he established goals for the remainder of his life?
• Has his caregiver requested needed support and respite?
• Have the patient and caregiver made use of resources to enhance coping, such as support groups?

Physical condition

A physical examination and diagnostic tests will also help evaluate the patient's response to therapy. Consider the following questions:
• Has the patient maintained maximal mobility within the limitations of the illness?
• Has he remained free of the complications of immobility?

Multiple sclerosis

A chronic degenerative disease that's a major cause of disability in adults ages 20 to 40, multiple sclerosis (MS) may progress rapidly, disabling the patient by early adulthood or causing death within months of onset. However, about 70% of patients experience prolonged remissions and lead active, productive lives. (See *Key points about MS*.)

MS results from progressive demyelination of the white matter of the brain and spinal cord. Patches of demyelination and lesions occur in various parts of the central nervous system (CNS), causing widespread neurologic dysfunction marked by periods of exacerbation and remission. (See *Understanding myelin breakdown,* page 244.)

Causes

The exact cause of MS is unknown. Theories point to a slow-acting viral infection, an autoimmune response of the nervous system, or genetic factors. Emotional stress, overwork, fatigue, pregnancy, and acute respiratory tract infections may precede the onset of illness.

Your findings will vary, depending on the part of the CNS that has been affected by demyelination. (See *Clinical findings in MS*, page 245.) Signs and symptoms may last for minutes, hours, or weeks and may vary from day to day with no predictable pattern. The patient may find it difficult, therefore, to describe her condition.

Health history

The patient may report initial visual problems, such as blurred vision or diplopia, and sensory impairment, such as numbness and tingling sensations (paresthesia). She also may complain of muscle stiffness and fatigue, especially involving the lower extremities.

After the initial episode, motor function may decline. The patient often reports a transient decrease in motor function after taking a hot bath or shower. Other findings may include dysphagia, sexual dysfunction, or urinary problems, such as incontinence or urine retention, frequency, urgency, or a history of urinary tract infections. The patient may report emotional lability—for example, mood swings, irritability, euphoria, and depression.

Obtain the patient's health history from a family member as well, especially concerning mental or emotional changes. A family member may report cognitive changes in the patient. For instance, she may be less attentive or more prone to poor judgment than usual.

Timesaving tip: While you obtain history data, save time by simultaneously assessing the patient's speech. Note scanning speech (the tendency to hesitate at the beginning of a word) or poorly articulated speech.

Also assess any known precipitating factors, such as stress or fatigue. Evaluate the patient's past coping skills and the effect of symptoms on her lifestyle. Find out if any other family members have ever been diagnosed with MS. Also probe for symptoms of MS that may have occurred in the past, even if the patient thinks it is unimportant. For instance, it is not unusual for a patient to report an episode of blurred vision that lasted a couple of days and occurred several years ago.

Physical examination

A mental status examination may reveal cognitive dysfunction, including changes in short-term memory, attention span, verbal fluency, and conceptual reasoning.

Assessment of motor function may reveal muscle weakness in the in-

FactFinder
Key points about MS

- *Incidence:* Multiple sclerosis (MS) is most prevalent in women and among people living in northern climates, in urban areas, and in higher socioeconomic groups.
- *Risk factors:* A family history of MS increases the risk of contracting MS, as does being white.
- *Prognosis:* Life expectancy following onset of symptoms averages 35 years.
- *Early signs and symptoms:* Sensory impairments, fatigue, visual symptoms, speech problems, and muscle weakness or spasticity all identify MS.
- *Complications:* MS may lead to injury from falls, urinary tract infections, joint contractures, pressure ulcers, and pneumonia.

volved area, such as an arm or leg. Other possible motor abnormalities include spasticity, hyperreflexia, intention tremor, and gait ataxia. In end-stage MS, paralysis of lower extremities may be evident.

Visual examination may reveal nystagmus, scotoma, optic neuritis, or ophthalmoplegia. Sensory examination may reveal impaired touch, pain, and temperature sensation.

Assess for Lhermitte's sign by having the patient flex her head forward. If the sign is present, she will feel an electric shock spread through her arms and legs.

Diagnostic test results

Because diagnosis is difficult, some patients undergo years of periodic

Understanding myelin breakdown

Myelin plays a key role in speeding electrical impulses to the brain for interpretation. A lipoprotein complex formed of glial cells or oligodendrocytes, the myelin sheath protects the neuron's long nerve fiber (the axon), much like the insulation on an electrical wire. Its high electrical resistance and low capacitance allow the myelin sheath to permit sufficient conduction of nerve impulses from one node of Ranvier to the next.

How demyelination occurs

In multiple sclerosis, patches of myelin in the long conduction pathways of the central nervous system degenerate for unknown reasons. In affected nerves, the myelin sheath becomes inflamed and the membrane layers break down into smaller components composed of well-circumscribed plaques filled with microglial elements, macroglia, and lymphocytes.

The damaged myelin sheath impairs normal conduction, causing partial loss or dispersion of the action potential and consequent neurologic dysfunction.

Abnormal neuron

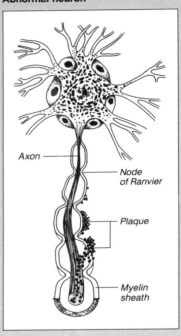

Axon

Node of Ranvier

Plaque

Myelin sheath

testing and close observation. Magnetic resonance imaging (MRI) is the most sensitive method of detecting MS lesions. More than 90% of patients with MS show multifocal white matter lesions when this test is performed. MRI is also used to evaluate disease progression and is the most important diagnostic tool for MS.

The following tests are also helpful in diagnosing the disease or confirming related problems of MS:
• EEG shows abnormalities in one-third of patients with MS.
• Cerebrospinal fluid analysis reveals elevated immunoglobulin G (IgG) levels but normal total protein levels. Such elevated IgG levels, which are significant only when serum gamma

globulin levels are normal, reflect hyperactivity of the immune system due to chronic demyelination. The white blood cell count may also be slightly increased.

• Evoked potential studies demonstrate slowed conduction of nerve impulses in 80% of patients with MS.

• Computed tomography may disclose lesions within the brain's white matter.

NURSING DIAGNOSIS

Common nursing diagnoses for the patient with MS include:

• Impaired physical mobility related to muscle weakness, gait disturbance, and intention tremor

• Sensory or perceptual alterations (visual, auditory, kinesthetic, and tactile) related to the demyelination process

• Sexual dysfunction related to impaired sensory or motor pathways or emotional or psychogenic disturbances

• Altered urinary elimination related to impaired sensory or motor pathways

• Ineffective individual coping related to impact of physical, mental, and emotional disabilities as well as the unpredictable course of illness

• Fatigue related to disease process.

PLANNING

Direct your plan of care toward helping the patient to maintain her mobility and independence for as long as possible and preventing complications.

Based on the nursing diagnosis *impaired physical mobility*, develop appropriate patient outcomes. For example, your patient will:

• maintain as much mobility as possible

Assessment TimeSaver
Clinical findings in MS

The list below provides a quick review of distinct signs and symptoms associated with the four types of multiple sclerosis (MS).

• *Cerebral type:* Intellectual and emotional changes, seizures, optic neuritis, hemiparesis, sensory loss, dysphagia

• *Cerebellar type:* Motor ataxia, hypotonia, asthenia

• *Brain-stem type:* Ocular disturbances, such as diplopia, blurred vision, and eye pain; dysarthria; vertigo; tinnitus; facial weakness

• *Spinal type:* Weakness of the lower extremities, spastic paraparesis, bowel and bladder disturbances, paresthesia

• remain free of complications related to immobility.

Based on the nursing diagnosis *sensory or perceptual alteration*s, develop appropriate patient outcomes. For example, your patient will:

• demonstrate successful strategies to compensate for sensory impairment

• remain free of injuries resulting from sensory impairment.

Based on the nursing diagnosis *sexual dysfunction*, develop appropriate patient outcomes. For example, your patient will:

• communicate sexual concerns

• maintain an intimate relationship with her partner.

Based on the nursing diagnosis *altered urinary elimination*, develop appropriate patient outcomes. For example, your patient will:

• remain continent for as long as possible

• remain free of urinary tract infections
• experience restful sleep uninterrupted by urinary problems.

Based on the nursing diagnosis *ineffective individual coping*, develop appropriate patient outcomes. For example, your patient will:
• express feelings about her illness
• identify effective coping mechanisms used in the past
• agree to use support services
• participate in care-related decisions
• express satisfaction with adjustments made to her lifestyle.

Based on the nursing diagnosis *fatigue*, develop appropriate patient outcomes. For example, your patient will:
• communicate an understanding that fatigue is a common symptom
• identify strategies to maximize energy level
• perform activities when energy level is high.

IMPLEMENTATION

Treatment seeks to shorten exacerbations and, if possible, relieve neurologic deficits, so that the patient can resume a normal lifestyle. (See *Medical care of the patient with MS*.)

Nursing interventions
• Provide emotional and psychological support for the patient and her family, and answer their questions honestly. Stay with them during crisis periods. Encourage the patient by suggesting ways to help her cope, based on coping mechanisms used effectively in the past. Refer the patient and her family to support groups and counseling, if appropriate.
• Increase patient comfort with massages and relaxing baths. Make sure that the water isn't too hot.

• Assist with active, resistive, and stretching exercises to maintain muscle tone and joint mobility, decrease spasticity, improve coordination, and boost morale. Provide rest periods between exercises because fatigue may contribute to exacerbations.
• Administer medications as ordered and watch for adverse reactions. For instance, dantrolene may cause muscle weakness and decreased muscle tone.
• If the patient is experiencing visual or other sensory alterations, modify the environment to help the patient perform daily activities more easily and to prevent injury.
• Suggest techniques to compensate for neurologic deficits. For example, if the patient's peripheral vision is affected, help her learn scanning techniques. Show the patient with diplopia how to use an eye patch or a frosted lens over one eye, alternating the patch or lens every 2 hours. If visual acuity is a problem, suggest large-print books or books on cassette.
• Advise the patient with a hearing deficit to always face the speaker. Refer her for lipreading instruction, unless she has visual difficulties.
• Help the patient establish a daily routine to maintain optimal functioning. Encourage daily physical exercise and regular rest periods to prevent fatigue.
• Suggest ways for the patient to enhance her emotional well-being. Encourage her to maintain contacts with family and friends.
• Refer the patient for vocational counseling, as needed.
• Contact the social services department to ensure discharge planning early in the course of the patient's hospitalization. Arrange for home health care equipment and services.

Treatments

Medical care of the patient with MS

Although drugs are the mainstay of therapy in multiple sclerosis (MS), supportive measures are also important.

Drug therapy
Corticotropin, prednisone, or dexamethasone is used to reduce the associated edema of the myelin sheath during exacerbations. Corticotropin and corticosteroids may relieve symptoms and hasten remission, but don't prevent future exacerbations.

Other drugs
• Chlordiazepoxide may be prescribed to mitigate mood swings.
• Baclofen or dantrolene may relieve spasticity.
• Bethanechol or oxybutynin are used to relieve urine retention and minimize urinary frequency and urgency.

• Antibiotics are prescribed to treat urinary tract infections, a common complication.
• Cyclophosphamide and azathioprine may be used for severe MS when it is progressive and there is no response to steroids.
• Interferon beta-1b (Betaseron) may be used for exacerbating-remitting MS.

Supportive measures
During acute exacerbations, supportive measures include:
• bed rest and other measures to lessen fatigue
• comfort measures, such as massages
• prevention of pressure ulcers
• bowel and bladder training, if necessary
• physical therapy
• counseling.

(See *Ensuring continued care for the patient with MS,* page 248.)
• Help family members plan ways to adapt their home for the patient, if needed. Discuss safety considerations and wheelchair access with them.

Patient teaching
Timesaving tip: Before you begin teaching, assess the patient's cognitive function, visual status, and auditory status. Adapt your teaching style according to your assessment findings to save valuable time. For example, if the patient has difficulty hearing, rely on illustrations and other visual teaching devices.

• Educate the patient and her family about the chronic nature of MS. Help them identify factors that precipitate exacerbations, such as trauma, menstruation, and pregnancy.
• Emphasize the need to avoid undue stress and discuss stress reduction techniques. Also emphasize the importance of avoiding exacerbating factors, including infections, temperature extremes, and fatigue.
• Teach the patient to maintain independence as long as possible by developing new ways of performing daily activities.
• Inform the patient about all prescribed medications, including signs of adverse reactions, particularly

Ensuring continued care for the patient with MS

Review the following teaching topics, referrals, and follow-up appointments to make sure that your patient is adequately prepared for discharge.

Teaching topics
Make sure that the following topics have been covered and that your patient's learning has been evaluated:
☐ explanation of multiple sclerosis (MS) and its symptoms, treatment, and impact on life
☐ medications, including possible adverse effects
☐ bowel and bladder programs
☐ need for rest periods and energy conservation techniques
☐ activity and dietary guidelines
☐ reinforcement of physical therapy program
☐ reinforcement of speech therapy program
☐ avoidance of precipitating factors
☐ measures to maintain independence and self-esteem
☐ sexual concerns
☐ safe use of wheelchairs
☐ safety in the home environment
☐ strategies for sensory deficits
☐ sources of information and support.

Referrals
Make sure that your patient has been provided with necessary referrals to:
☐ social services, regarding equipment, medications, need for home health care services, or placement in a long-term care facility
☐ psychological counseling
☐ physical therapist
☐ speech therapist
☐ vocational rehabilitation
☐ sexual counseling
☐ support groups for patient and his family.

Follow-up appointments
Make sure that the necessary follow-up appointments have been scheduled and that your patient has been notified:
☐ doctor or clinic.

those due to the effects of steroids, including mood swings and increased anxiety, insomnia, and appetite.
• Encourage the patient to exercise. Tell her that a walking exercise program may improve her gait. If her motor dysfunction causes coordination or balance problems, teach her to walk with a wide base of support. If she has trouble with proprioception, tell her to watch her feet.
• The patient may need a walker or a wheelchair to prevent falls during an exacerbation. Make certain that the patient and family members can demonstrate proper use of all assistive and adaptive equipment.
• Stress the importance of rest periods, preferably lying down. Also teach energy conservation techniques.
• If the patient has difficulty communicating, encourage her to perform phonetic exercises. Consult with the speech therapist and use a communi-

cation board and voice amplifiers, if necessary.

• Address the patient's sexual concerns. Explain that, although no cure exists for neurologically based sexual dysfunction, she and her partner can still maintain an intimate relationship.

• If the patient is experiencing bladder dysfunction, she should be evaluated by a urologist. The urologist will be able to determine the type of bladder dysfunction by urodynamic studies and to recommend the appropriate treatment.

• For urinary incontinence or retention, advise the patient to drink about 2 to 3 quarts (2 to 3 liters) of fluid daily but to restrict fluid intake about 2 hours before bedtime. If she is incontinent, teach her how to reestablish a normal pattern to spare her the embarrassment and frustration of incontinence. Tell the patient to record her fluid intake, including ice cream, gelatin, and pudding, noting excess fluid intake. Ask the patient to keep a diary of voiding times, both intentional urination and incontinent episodes. Review the diary with her to detect a pattern of incontinence. Then, instruct her to void at the most appropriate times—for example, after meals. Teach the patient to follow a voiding schedule, beginning with every 2 hours, increasing to every 3 hours, and progressing to every 4 hours. Suggest that she wear a wristwatch with a time signal or set an alarm clock to remind her to void. Advise the patient to wear incontinence briefs during bladder retraining to prevent embarrassment and to promote a sense of security. Caution the patient to avoid plastic or rubber bed sheets. They promote skin breakdown.

• Teach the patient to completely empty her bladder or perform intermittent catheterization to help prevent infection. Also suggest that she stimulate voiding by stroking her thighs and vulva (for the male patient, the glans penis), and by tapping the center of the abdomen below the navel up to 15 times or until urination occurs. Over time, the duration and intensity of tapping needed to produce bladder emptying will decrease.

• Credé's maneuver can also help empty the bladder. Direct the patient to tap her abdomen. A dull sound indicates a full bladder. Next, tell the patient to use the flat part of her fingertips to knead the bladder, progressively applying more pressure but not grinding her fingertips into her skin. Then, to ensure complete voiding, describe the hollow sound she'll hear when she taps her bladder.

• Discuss the importance of eating a well-balanced diet with sufficient roughage to prevent constipation. Recent research suggests that a low-fat diet may help prolong life and lessen neurologic complications.

• Suggest that the patient with constipation plan to have a bowel movement about 30 minutes after a meal (usually breakfast). Discuss using suppositories, as needed, before the scheduled time.

• Inform the patient that fecal incontinence usually results from illness, such as the flu, or from irritating substances, such as alcohol, spicy foods, or cigarettes, rather than from MS. Also advise her to avoid hot liquids.

• Counsel the patient that exacerbations are unpredictable, and that physical and emotional adjustments to her lifestyle will be necessary. Advise her to contact her doctor when she feels that an exacerbation is occurring or that symptoms are worsening.

• If the patient is planning a pregnancy, explain that there is a higher chance of an exacerbation occurring after delivery. During the pregnancy, the patient should be followed closely by a neurologist.

• If the patient's condition deteriorates, explain home health care measures and services available to the family, and discuss placement options, according to family needs. Contact the social services department for assistance.

Timesaving tip: Be sure to inform family members that most services and placement facilities have long waiting lists. To prevent needless and time-consuming delays, encourage them to plan at least 6 months ahead of time, based on the patient's pattern of illness.

• Refer the patient to the National Multiple Sclerosis Society.

EVALUATION

When evaluating a patient's response to your care, gather reassessment data and compare this with the outcomes specified in your plan of care.

Teaching and counseling

Begin by determining the effectiveness of teaching and counseling. Consider the following questions:

• Does the patient appear to understand MS and its treatment?
• Is she willing to comply with prescribed treatment?
• Has she discussed sexual concerns?
• Has she had success maintaining an intimate relationship?
• Has she demonstrated techniques to compensate for sensory impairment?
• Does she practice daily energy-conserving activities?
• Has she identified coping mechanisms used successfully in the past?
• Will she use support services?

• Does she participate in care-related decisions?
• Has she expressed satisfaction regarding an altered lifestyle?

Physical condition

Physical assessment and diagnostic tests also will help you evaluate the effectiveness of your plan of care. If your patient has complied with treatment, your ongoing assessment should indicate:

• maximum mobility (within physical limitations)
• absence of complications related to immobility
• urinary continence (for as long as possible)
• absence of urinary tract infections
• restful sleep uninterrupted by urinary problems
• absence of injuries resulting from sensory impairment.

CHAPTER 8

Caring for patients with CNS tumors

Brain tumors

Frightening for the patient and his family alike, brain tumors can occur at any age. Peak incidence occurs during early childhood and again between ages 50 and 80. In North America, brain tumors account for approximately 2% of all cancer deaths each year.

Tumors can develop within any area of the brain. *Primary* tumors originate within the brain, while *secondary* tumors originate most often in the lungs, breasts, GI tract, or kidneys and metastasize to the brain. Brain tumors may be further classified by the manner of cell growth (malignant or benign), location, cellular or histologic origin, or histologic features. (See *Classifying brain tumors,* opposite, and *Quick review of primary brain tumors,* pages 254 and 255.)

Causes

The exact cause of primary brain tumors isn't known; however, the processes that produce signs and symptoms are well understood. As the tumor develops, tissue destruction, distortion, and displacement compress blood vessels, obstruct the flow of cerebrospinal fluid (CSF), and increase intracranial pressure (ICP). These mechanisms result in focal neurologic deficits, cerebral edema, and tissue hypoxia. Ultimately, death may result from brain herniation.

ASSESSMENT

Signs and symptoms depend on tumor development and location. (See *Correlating sites and signs of brain tumors,* pages 256 to 258.) In most patients, symptoms result from increased ICP and focal neurologic impairment. Your assessment should include a complete health history and careful consideration of physical examination findings and diagnostic test results. In addition, expect to perform a psychosocial assessment.

Health history

Typically, the patient reports intermittent, moderate headaches that occur upon awakening. They may be generalized or localized in the frontal or occipital regions.

The patient may also complain of seizures, vomiting (occasionally, projectile vomiting), or changes in personality or behavior. When present, vomiting is most likely to occur in the morning and isn't related to eating a meal. If papilledema is present, the patient may report visual problems, such as diplopia or visual field deficits.

Family members may describe changes in the patient's behavior, personality, or mentation. They may report forgetfulness, depression, confusion, lethargy, loss of inhibition, or poor judgment.

Physical examination

Observation may reveal symptoms, indicating weakness or paralysis, cranial nerve abnormalities, gait disturbances, and changes in the patient's level of consciousness (LOC). Ophthalmoscopic examination may detect papilledema.

If ICP is severely increased, you may detect widened pulse pressure, bradycardia, and changes in the patient's respiratory pattern. If the patient has a pituitary tumor, endocrine dysfunction may result in Cushing's syndrome, gigantism, acromegaly, or hypopituitarism with accompanying changes in body function, such as

(Text continues on page 258.)

Classifying brain tumors

A brain tumor may be classified as primary or secondary and as malignant or benign. It may also be classified by location, cellular origin, or histologic features.

Primary or secondary

In primary brain tumors, cells in the central nervous system undergo rapid proliferation or abnormal growth. In secondary brain tumors, malignant cells from distant tumors metastasize to the brain.

Malignant or benign

Characteristics of malignant tumors include anaplasia, invasion, and metastasis. Prognosis is poor unless the tumor is diagnosed early and removed surgically.

Benign tumors, which are less virulent than malignant ones, aren't recurrent. Prognosis is generally more favorable, but possible complications include cerebral edema, focal neurologic deficits, and increased intracranial pressure. Benign tumors may also undergo histologic changes and become malignant.

Location

Supratentorial tumors are located within the cerebral hemispheres; infratentorial tumors are found within the brain stem and cerebellum.

Cellular origin

Astrocytomas originate in neuroglial cells called astrocytes; oligodendrogliomas, in oligodendroglial cells; and ependymomas, in ependymal cells.

Histologic features

Tissue structure may be used to classify brain tumors.

Intracerebral tumors

Intracerebral tumors include the following malignant gliomas: astrocytomas, glioblastoma multiforme, oligodendrogliomas, ependymomas, and medulloblastomas.

Tumors arising from supporting structures

Tumors may grow in supporting structures of the brain such as the meninges, cranial nerves, and the pituitary gland. Tumor types include meningiomas, neuromas (acoustic neuroma, schwannoma), and pituitary adenomas.

Developmental tumors

Dermoid and epidermoid cysts, teratoma, craniopharyngioma, and angioma are classified as developmental (congenital) tumors.

Others

This category of tumors contains unclassified tumors (mostly gliomas), sarcomas, and miscellaneous tumors (pinealoma, chordoma, granuloma).

Quick review of primary brain tumors

Type of tumor	Location and characteristics	Treatment and prognosis
Gliomas		
Astrocytoma Grades I (well differentiated) and II (moderately well differentiated) *Cellular origin:* astrocytes	• Usually in frontal, temporal, or parietal lobes of cerebral hemispheres • Slow-growing gliomas	• Surgery: complete removal rare, multiple excisions possible, partial removal may prolong life. Possible radiation therapy of residual tumor (grade II) • Prognosis: 6 to 7 years after surgery
Astrocytoma Grades III and IV (grossly undifferentiated); also called glioblastoma multiforme *Cellular origin:* mature astrocytes	• Frequently in white matter of anterior or frontal part of cerebral hemispheres • Malignant, rapidly growing tumor	• Surgery: resection and bulk removal to reduce intracranial pressure (ICP) and relieve cerebral compression • Prognosis: typically 12 to 18 months (only 10% of patients live beyond 24 months)
Oligodendroglioma *Cellular origin:* oligodendroglia cells	• In cerebral hemispheres, particularly frontal and temporal lobes • Slow-growing tumor; radiologic examination reveals calcification in 50% of all cases — seizure often first sign	• Surgery, radiation therapy, or both: used to remove bulk or destroy cells • Prognosis: 5 years or more
Ependymoma *Cellular origin:* ependymal cells	• In ventricles, particularly the fourth ventricle; may attach to roof or floor, or grow into cerebral hemisphere • Glioma arising from the ventricular lining	• Surgery: excision, if accessible; radiation therapy or chemotherapy possible; shunting often used • Prognosis: 1 month if malignant; 7 to 8 years if benign
Cranial nerve and spinal nerve and root		
Acoustic neuroma Also called a schwannoma or neurofibroma *Cellular origin:* Schwann cells	• In cranial nerve VIII, cerebellopontine angle • Benign, slow-growing tumors that arise from sheath of Schwann cells; often inaccessible; if large, may compress cranial nerves V, VII, IX, and X	• Surgery: may require microsurgery to remove tumor or diminish bulk to preserve cranial nerve function • Radiation therapy: may be alternative for older patients • Prognosis: generally good; excellent if tumor is small and surgically accessible
Pituitary		
Pituitary adenomas *Cellular origin:* pituitary cells	• Most common in anterior lobe of pituitary gland • Usually benign, slow-growing tumors; may cause visual disorders, headaches, and various endocrine disorders	• Surgery: may use microsurgery to remove smaller tumors; craniotomy for larger tumors • Radiation therapy: common after surgery; hormonal replacement therapy may be necessary • Prognosis: very good

Quick review of primary brain tumors *(continued)*

Type of tumor	Location and characteristics	Treatment and prognosis
Neural cell		
Medulloblastoma *Cellular origin:* embryonic cells	• Most often in cerebellar vermis, occupying fourth ventricle; may infiltrate floor • Rapidly growing childhood tumor; more common in males — vision disturbances frequently first sign	• Surgery: may be used to remove part of tumor • Tumor highly radiosensitive; radiation therapy typically involves head and spinal cord due to seeding via cerebrospinal fluid • Chemotherapy possible • May use shunting to reduce increased ICP • Prognosis: 5 years
Mesodermal tissue		
Meningioma *Cellular origin:* arachnoid cells; may be from fibroblasts	• Most common in areas proximal to venous sinuses: superior sagittal sinus, over convexities, or on the sphenoid ridge, anterior fossa floor, or posterior fossa • Firm, slow-growing, encapsulated tumor	• Surgery: complete or partial removal • Radiation therapy: to address residual tumor • Prognosis: excellent, especially with complete removal
Blood vessel		
Angioma *Cellular origin:* arises from congenitally malformed arteriovenous connections	• Predominantly in posterior cerebral hemispheres • Slow-growing tumor; may cause seizures, cerebral bleeding, and increased ICP	• Surgery: used to remove bulk • Prognosis: good
Hemangioblastoma *Cellular origin:* embryonic vascular tissue	• Most common in cerebellum as a single or multiple lesion; less frequent in medulla or cerebral hemispheres • Vascular, slow-growing tumor	• Surgery: complete removal possible • Radiation therapy: addresses recurrence • Prognosis: excellent, usually curable
Congenital		
Craniopharyngioma *Cellular origin:* arises from remnants of the hypophyseal stalk (Rathke's pouch)	• In or near the sella pituitary • Slow-growing, solid or cystic tumors; may compress the pituitary or sever the pituitary stalk; endocrine dysfunction common; congenital, more common in children	• Surgery: complete excision possible; however, most tumors recur • Radiation therapy: any remaining tumor highly radiosensitive after surgery • Prognosis: excellent if tumor removed

Assessment TimeSaver

Correlating sites and signs of brain tumors

Usually, signs and symptoms directly reflect a brain tumor's location. Recognizing them can help you plan nursing care and recognize potentially life-threatening complications, such as increased intracranial pressure (ICP) and brain herniation.

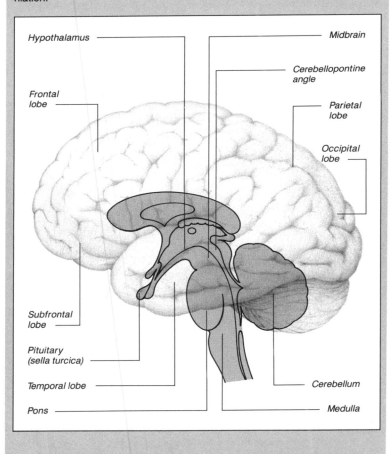

Assessment TimeSaver

Correlating sites and signs of brain tumors *(continued)*

Frontal lobe
• Expressive, or Broca's, aphasia (dominant hemisphere)
• Personality and behavior changes
• Headache
• Sensory and motor changes (unilateral if one lobe is affected; bilateral if both lobes are affected)
• Seizures

Subfrontal lobe
• Cranial nerve I (olfactory)
• Loss of smell

Pituitary
• Amenorrhea
• Cushingoid signs and symptoms
• Gigantism
• Acromegaly
• Headache
• Galactorrhea
• Impotence
• Visual field deficits
• Hypothalamic effects

Temporal lobe
• Changes in personality and mental status (for example, irritability, depression, poor judgment, or childish behavior)
• Auditory hallucinations
• Impaired memory (if tumor is bilateral)
• Psychomotor seizures
• Visual field deficits
• Receptive, or Wernicke's, aphasia (dominant hemisphere)
• Dysarthria

Pons
Cranial nerve V (trigeminal)
• Loss of ipsilateral facial or forehead sensation
• Loss of corneal reflex

Cranial nerve VI (abducens)
• Ipsilateral loss of ability to gaze outward

Cranial nerve VII (facial)
• Ipsilateral drooping of facial muscles

Medulla
Cranial nerve IX (glossopharyngeal)
• Difficulty swallowing

Cranial nerve X (vagus)
• Loss of gag and cough reflex
• Difficulty swallowing
• Hoarseness
• Projectile vomiting

Cranial nerve XI (spinal accessory)
• Inability to shrug shoulders or turn head toward side with tumor

Cranial nerve XII (hypoglossal)
• Protrusion of tongue, deviating toward side of tumor
• Changes in respiratory pattern

Cerebellum
• Disturbed gait
• Impaired balance
• Loss of coordination
• Signs of increased ICP (such as headache, vomiting)

Cerebellopontile angle
Cranial nerve VII (facial)
• Drooping of ipsilateral facial muscles

(continued)

Correlating sites and signs of brain tumors *(continued)*

Cerebellopontile angle *(continued)*
Cranial nerve VIII (acoustic)
• Tinnitus
• Hearing loss

Occipital lobe
• Contralateral homonymous hemianopia
• Visual hallucinations
• Possible seizure (generalized or focal)

Parietal lobe
• Hyperesthesia
• Paresthesia
• Loss of two-point discrimination
• Asterognosis (inability to recognize an object by feeling its size and shape)
• Autotopagnosia (inability to locate or recognize parts of the body)
• Finger agnosia (inability to identify or select specific fingers of the hands)
• Agraphia (loss of ability to write)
• Acalculia (difficulty in calculating numbers)
• Construction apraxia (loss of ability to draw a simple object)
• Homonymous hemianopia

Midbrain
• Ptosis
• Diplopia
• Dilated pupil
• Inability to gaze up, down, or inward (all ipsilateral)

Hypothalamus (possible pituitary tumor that extends upward)
• Diabetes insipidus
• Loss of temperature control
• Altered fat and carbohydrate metabolism
• Altered sleep pattern
• Pituitary effects

swelling of the breasts and menstrual changes in females.

Diagnostic test results
The following tests may help confirm a brain tumor:
• Computed tomography (CT) scan and magnetic resonance imaging help locate the tumor and determine its size and magnitude. A CT scan may help analyze the effects of increased ICP, such as shifts in midline structures and changes in cerebral ventricular size.
• Brain scan may reveal that isotope uptake increases within the tumor itself, which can help determine the tu-

mor's precise location and measurement.
• Cerebral angiography may delineate the deviation of blood vessels caused by highly vascular tumors. The pattern of vascularity may provide clues about the tumor's pathology.
• Positron emission tomography scan may identify vascular tumors, shifts in midline structures, and changes in cerebral ventricular size. It may also reveal sites of glucose metabolism, a common indicator of tumor activity in the brain.
• Open biopsy or stereotactic biopsy may identify the histologic type.

• Skull X-ray may reveal space-occupying lesions or the presence of intracranial calcifications.

• Ophthalmic examination may reveal visual field deficits, which help locate the lesion.

• EEG tracings may help pinpoint the tumor's location.

• Lumbar puncture may be used to determine whether CSF pressure has changed. Increased CSF pressure reflects elevated ICP and protein levels and reduced glucose levels. Lumbar puncture may also reveal tumor cells in CSF.

NURSING DIAGNOSIS

Common nursing diagnoses for a patient with a brain tumor include:

• Altered cerebral tissue perfusion related to increased ICP

• High risk for injury related to seizures, altered LOC, motor impairment or sensory impairment, or both

• Anticipatory grieving related to perceived losses, poor prognosis, or impending death

• Pain related to headache caused by increased ICP

• Knowledge deficit related to the disease process, methods of treatment, and support services.

PLANNING

Based on the nursing diagnosis *altered cerebral tissue perfusion,* develop appropriate patient outcomes. For example, your patient will:

• maintain normal ICP (15 mm Hg or less)

• remain free of signs and symptoms of increased ICP, such as deteriorating LOC, seizures, vomiting, papilledema, bradycardia, hypertension, worsening headache, increased weakness, or changes in behavior or respiratory pattern.

Based on the nursing diagnosis *high risk for injury,* develop appropriate patient outcomes. For example, your patient will:

• remain free of injury during hospitalization

• describe measures that will reduce his risk of injury when he returns home.

Based on the nursing diagnosis *anticipatory grieving,* develop appropriate patient outcomes. For example, your patient will:

• express his fears and feelings of loss

• show a willingness to grieve

• participate in care decisions

• identify measures to enhance coping with losses caused by illness

• develop achievable plans for the future.

Based on the nursing diagnosis *pain,* develop appropriate patient outcomes. For example, your patient will:

• identify factors that precipitate or intensify pain

• identify factors that alleviate pain

• communicate a reduction in pain.

Based on the nursing diagnosis *knowledge deficit,* develop appropriate patient outcomes. For example, your patient will:

• describe the nature of his brain tumor and related signs and symptoms

• express an understanding of treatment, including surgery, drug or radiation therapies, and supportive measures

• identify the risks and adverse reactions associated with treatment, and understand appropriate preventive measures

• describe measures to take for managing neurologic deficits and maintaining optimal quality of life at home

• identify five or more sources of support.

IMPLEMENTATION

The most common methods of treating brain tumors include surgery, radiation therapy, and chemotherapy. The specific regimen depends on the tumor's histologic type, radiosensitivity, and location. (See *Medical care of the patient with brain tumor,* pages 261 to 263.)

Nursing interventions

• Assess the patient's vital signs and neurologic status frequently. Watch for signs of worsening focal neurologic deficits and increasing ICP.

Timesaving tip: Establish priorities for your neurologic examinations — you may not always have time to thoroughly assess neurologic status. Your top priority is to frequently assess vital signs, pupils, and LOC. Keep in mind that changes in LOC, the first sign of rising ICP, may include short-term memory deficit and loss of orientation to time, then place, and then person.

• Initiate measures to reduce the patient's risk of increased ICP. Promote venous drainage by elevating the head of the bed 30 to 45 degrees (instructions will vary according to the doctor's preference). Keep the patient's head in neutral alignment to prevent flexion or rotation, and prevent hip flexion of more than 90 degrees.

• If the patient's status is deteriorating, watch for signs of herniation: fixed, dilated, unresponsive pupils; abnormal respiratory pattern; and Cushing's triad (increased systolic pressure, bradycardia, and widening pulse pressure).

• If the patient is at risk for seizure, pad the side rails of the bed and keep them elevated. Keep suction and airway equipment readily available. If you witness a seizure, carefully document the event, including its type and duration. Administer prescribed anticonvulsant drugs.

• Take steps to ensure the patient's safety. Place the call light and all the patient's important personal belongings within easy reach. Tell him to call for assistance before getting out of bed.

• Assess for pain. Administer prescribed analgesics and monitor their effectiveness. Intensifying pain may indicate increasing ICP.

• Carefully monitor temperature. Each 1.8°F (1°C) increase raises the brain's metabolic demand by 10%, which, in turn, can increase ICP. If fever occurs, give antipyretics. Use a hypothermia blanket if necessary.

• Monitor fluid and electrolyte status closely. Maintain precise intake and output records, and check for signs of dehydration and electrolyte depletion. Treatment for increased ICP often includes corticosteroids, osmotic diuretics (such as mannitol), and fluid restrictions to reduce cerebral edema. However, patients receiving radiation therapy or chemotherapy may become dehydrated due to vomiting, diarrhea, and inadequate intake. In these instances, *cautiously* replace fluids.

• Observe and report signs of ulcers, including abdominal distention, pain, vomiting, and tarry stools. Give prescribed antacids and histamine-receptor antagonists.

• If the patient has residual neurologic deficits that result in a physical or mental handicap, begin rehabilitation early.

Timesaving tip: To save nursing time, while also fostering the patient's self-esteem, consult with occupational and physical therapists for ways to promote independence in daily activities. As necessary, provide aids for self-care and mobilization

Medical care of the patient with brain tumor

The most common medical treatments for brain tumor are surgery, radiation therapy, and chemotherapy. Supportive therapy is also crucial.

Surgery
Surgery may be performed to remove a tumor or to reduce a nonresectable tumor. *Craniotomy* is the surgical opening of a flap of bone in the skull to provide access to the tumor, which is then removed by resection. Laser surgery may be an adjunct. This procedure is most often used for supratentorial tumors. *Craniectomy* is the excision of a portion of the skull to provide access to the tumor. It is used for infratentorial tumors or supratentorial tumors when intracranial expansion is suspected.

Radiation therapy
Radiation therapy may be used alone, after surgery, or with chemotherapy to destroy rapidly dividing cancer cells. Conventional radiation therapy employs a cobalt machine or a linear accelerator that rotates around the head.

Brachytherapy is an alternative method of delivering radiation to the tumor site. In brachytherapy, a flexible catheter is used to implant radioactive "seeds" at the site of the brain tumor.

Adverse effects
Possible adverse effects of radiation therapy include:
- nausea
- vomiting
- drowsiness
- anorexia
- itching
- scalp and ear discomfort
- dry mouth
- alopecia (hair grows back after treatment).

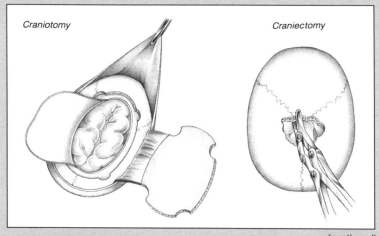

Craniotomy

Craniectomy

(continued)

Treatments

Medical care of the patient with brain tumor *(continued)*

Chemotherapy
Chemotherapy may be used alone or in conjunction with radiation therapy; however, it is most often used with surgery. Usually, the patient receives a combination of chemotherapeutic drugs, which may be administered orally, intravenously, intrathecally (by repeated lumbar punctures), or intraventricularly, depending on the drugs selected. Commonly used drugs include lomustine (CCNU), carmustine (BCNU), procarbazine hydrochloride, cisplatin, and etoposide (VP-16).

An Ommaya reservoir may be implanted under the patient's scalp to allow for intraventricular drug administration. This device consists of a self-sealing silicone injection dome (reservoir) and an attached catheter. A surgeon drills a burr hole in the patient's skull, inserts the catheter through the nondominant frontal lobe into the lateral ventricle, and places the dome over the burr hole, just under the scalp.

Chemotherapeutic drugs are injected into the Ommaya reservoir with a syringe. The reservoir permits consistent and predictable drug distribution throughout the subarachnoid space and central nervous system.

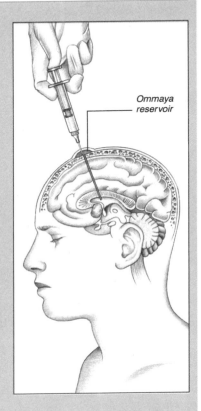

Ommaya reservoir

Adverse effects
Common adverse effects of chemotherapy include:
- nausea
- vomiting
- anorexia
- diarrhea
- stomatitis
- bone marrow depression
- alopecia.

Other possible complications include:
- hepatotoxicity
- nephrotoxicity
- burning at the I.V. injection site
- burning and hypopigmentation due to skin contact with the drug
- pulmonary infiltrate or fibrosis, or both (with prolonged use of BCNU).

Supportive therapy
Supportive therapy frequently includes measures to control intracranial pressure. Shunting may be performed to treat hydrocephalus, and corticosteroids may be administered to control cerebral edema. When therapy involves corticosteroids, antacids and a histamine-receptor antagonist, (such as cimetidine, ranitidine, or famotidine) may be administered to control gastric adverse effects. Anticonvulsants are used to prevent or treat seizures.

Because pain can be severe, many cancer centers now have a pain service responsible for determining and administering the appropriate form of pain relief. Pain relief may be provided through narcotic I.V. drips, patient-controlled analgesia, or nerve blocks.

(for example, bathroom rails for a patient in a wheelchair). If the patient is aphasic, arrange a consultation with a speech pathologist.
• Monitor the patient's nutritional status. Consult with the dietician and doctor to plan a program that considers the patient's emotional status, any residual neurologic deficits, and his response to radiation therapy or chemotherapy.
• Provide a clear, accurate explanation of all aspects of the patient's care. Encourage his participation in care decisions to promote feelings of independence.
• Help the patient and members of his family talk about feelings that may seem overwhelming, such as fear of death. Counsel them to focus on one day at a time.
• Describe the stages of grieving and help them identify sources of strength and support.
• Help the patient and family members cope with changes in their lifestyles. For example, the disease may cause changes in roles (for example, the patient may no longer be able to work) or self-image (for example, he may experience loss of function due to motor weakness).
• Refer the patient and members of his family to appropriate support services, such as the social service department, home health care agencies, hospice counseling, psychological counseling, and the American Cancer Society.
• Before surgery, help prepare the patient physically and emotionally by shampooing his hair, teaching him about coughing and deep breathing, preparing him for an alteration in his appearance following the operation, and advising him what to expect while recovering in the intensive care unit.

Postoperative care
• After craniotomy, monitor the patient's vital signs and neurologic status frequently. Watch for signs of increased ICP, including an elevated bone flap as well as typical neurologic changes. If an ICP monitoring device is inserted, report ICP elevations. Connect the patient to a cardiac monitor and observe for arrhythmias.

• Strictly enforce measures to reduce the risk of increased ICP. For example, restrict fluids to a maximum of 1,500 ml/24 hours, or as ordered.
• After supratentorial craniotomy, promote venous drainage and reduce cerebral edema by elevating the head of the bed about 30 degrees. (After infratentorial craniotomy, ask the doctor whether the patient should lie flat.) Position him on his side to encourage drainage of secretions and to prevent aspiration. Prevent excessive pressure on the surgical site, and reposition him every 2 hours.
• Instruct the patient to avoid actions that increase intrathoracic pressure, thereby raising ICP, such as Valsalva's maneuver and isometric muscle contractions (when moving or sitting up). Withhold oral fluids to reduce the risk of vomiting, which increases ICP.
• Give prescribed osmotic diuretics and corticosteroids, or loop diuretics (such as furosemide) to reduce cerebral edema.
• Perform passive range-of-motion exercises with all extremities three or more times each day. Apply antiembolism stockings.
• Check the dressing for excessive drainage (more than 50 ml in 8 hours). Keep the wound clean and check for signs of infection. Administer antibiotics, if prescribed.
• Closely monitor the patient's fluid and electrolyte status.
• Initiate measures to prevent respiratory complications. Hypoxia can contribute to increased ICP. However, keep in mind that aggressive postural drainage and chest percussion also can increase ICP.
• If mechanical ventilation is initiated to stimulate cerebral vasoconstriction, thereby preventing or treating increased ICP, anticipate maintaining partial pressure of arterial carbon dioxide at 25 to 30 mm Hg and partial pressure of arterial oxygen greater than 80 mm Hg.

Patient teaching
• Reinforce the doctor's explanation of the diagnosis and treatment. Describe all associated care.
• If surgery is ordered, explain the reason for surgery and describe the procedure. Also explain all preoperative, postoperative, and home care measures.
• Teach the patient about all prescribed medications, including their purposes, proper dosages, schedules of administration, and adverse reactions.
• Some antineoplastic drugs used as adjuncts to radiation therapy and surgery (carmustine, lomustine, and procarbazine, for example) can cause delayed bone marrow depression. Tell the patient to report immediately any sign of infection or bleeding that appears within 4 weeks after the start of chemotherapy.
• If the patient is receiving chemotherapy, radiation therapy, or both, explain all possible adverse reactions and steps to alleviate them. .
• Help the patient and members of his family prepare for home care. Explain safety measures, such as the use of grip bars, side rails, and shower chairs, and the proper use of medical equipment. Help them explore ways to maintain the patient's independence.
• Stress the importance of proper nutrition and regular exercise.
• Encourage the patient to maintain relationships with family and friends.
• Describe the early signs of tumor recurrence and stress the importance of complying with all aspects of treatment, including follow-up appointments. (See *Ensuring continued care for the patient with brain tumor.*)

Discharge TimeSaver

Ensuring continued care for the patient with brain tumor

Review the following teaching topics, referrals, and follow-up appointments to make sure that your patient is adequately prepared for discharge.

Teaching topics

Make sure that the following topics have been covered and that your patient's learning has been evaluated:
☐ disease process and management
☐ prescribed medications, including dosage, adverse reactions, and related precautions
☐ surgery and related care
☐ radiation therapy and related skin care
☐ warning signs and symptoms of complications
☐ safety measures
☐ guidelines for proper nutrition
☐ physical therapy
☐ coping with self-care deficits
☐ understanding the grieving process
☐ importance of follow-up care.

Referrals

Make sure that the patient has been provided with necessary referrals to:
☐ social services specializing in financial assistance

☐ home health care agency
☐ support services, such as the American Cancer Society
☐ medical equipment supplier
☐ rehabilitation facility for physical, speech, or occupational therapy, if needed
☐ pain control therapy
☐ psychological counseling service
☐ hospice center.

Follow-up appointments

Make sure that the necessary follow-up appointments have been scheduled and that the patient has been notified:
☐ neurologist
☐ neurosurgeon
☐ nutritionist
☐ laboratory for radiation therapy, if necessary
☐ laboratory for chemotherapy, if necessary
☐ diagnostic test center for reevaluation.

EVALUATION

When evaluating the patient's response to your nursing care, gather reassessment data and compare this information to the patient outcomes specified in your plan of care.

Teaching and counseling

Begin by determining the effectiveness of teaching and counseling. During the course of evaluation, observe the patient's actions and listen to him. Consider the following questions:
• Does the patient express an understanding of the nature of his illness?
• Is he willing to follow the treatment plan?
• Is he complying with the medication regimen?
• Are members of the family willing to discuss their feelings about the disease and necessary lifestyle changes?

• Are the patient and members of his family coping effectively with stress? Have they identified strategies to cope with loss?

• Do they know the signs and symptoms that require prompt medical attention, especially signs of increased ICP and seizure?

Mental status
As you evaluate your patient's mental status, consider the following questions:

• Is the patient oriented to person, place, and time?

• If surgery was performed, does he show any signs of presurgical (retrograde) or postsurgical (anterograde) memory loss?

Physical condition
Physical examination and diagnostic testing will also help you evaluate the effectiveness of your care. Consider the following questions:

• Does the patient maintain a normal ICP?

• Is he free of signs and symptoms of increased ICP, including deteriorating LOC, seizures, vomiting, papilledema, bradycardia, hypertension, worsening headache, increased weakness, or changes in behavior or respiratory pattern?

• Is he free of injuries?

• Does he report or demonstrate reduced pain?

Spinal cord tumors

Occurring anywhere along the spinal cord or its roots, spinal cord tumors account for less than 1% of cancers in North America. They affect men and women equally (except meningiomas, which occur more often in women) and are most likely to occur between ages 20 and 60.

Primary tumors originate from epidural vessels, spinal meninges, or glial elements of the spinal cord. Secondary tumors may be intraspinal extensions of tumors in the spinal column, but are more likely to metastasize from distant sites, such as the lungs or breast.

Most spinal cord tumors are benign. However, they can cause numerous complications, including motor weakness, paralysis, sensory deficits, loss of sphincter control, bladder and bowel dysfunction, and respiratory failure. In later stages, especially if paralysis occurs, the patient may experience complications of immobility, such as skin breakdown or pneumonia. If left untreated, spinal cord tumors can be fatal.

Causes
The cause of primary spinal cord tumors isn't known.

ASSESSMENT

Clinical findings depend on the tumor's location and growth rate and on the severity of cord compression. Include in your assessment an evaluation of the patient's psychosocial status and coping skills.

Health history
The patient may have a history of severe pain that originates in the area of the tumor and radiates around the trunk or along the limbs on the affected side. The pain is usually not alleviated by analgesics or bed rest and may be aggravated by straining or coughing.

If you suspect spinal cord tumor, ask about bladder difficulties or changes in the urinary stream, because the patient may dismiss or

Reviewing signs and symptoms of spinal cord tumors

The signs and symptoms of a spinal cord tumor depend on the location of the tumor along the spinal column.

Location	Possible signs and symptoms
Cervical levels C4 and above	• Respiratory distress (if bilateral) • Quadriparesis • Occipital headache • Stiff neck • Downbeat nystagmus (occurs when attempting to look down) • Cranial nerve involvement, such as dysphagia or deviated tongue (upper cervical region)
Cervical levels below C4	• Pain in shoulders, arms, and hands; then atrophy of muscle in these areas • Unilateral or bilateral Horner's syndrome
Thoracic levels T1 to T12	• Beevor's sign (when patient sits up or raises head while lying down, umbilicus displaces toward head) • Hyperesthesia (band in thoracic area) • Positive Babinski's sign • Paresis and plegia of lower extremities
Lumbosacral levels L1 to S5	• Lower back pain • Bowel and bladder changes • Sexual dysfunction (such as impotence) • Pain radiating to legs, then paresis and atrophy of muscles in lower extremities

overlook these signs. Note if the patient reports constipation or difficulty emptying his bladder. In advanced disease, spinal cord compression may cause urine retention. In a patient with a cauda equina tumor, bladder and bowel incontinence may result from flaccid paralysis.

The patient may report sensory disturbances such as paresthesias (caudal lesions invariably produce paresthesias in the nerve pathways of the involved roots), weakness, or clumsiness. He may also report sexual dysfunction.

Physical examination

Focus on sensory and motor impairment and any existing sphincter disturbances. (See *Reviewing signs and symptoms of spinal cord tumors.*)

Assessment of motor response may reveal symmetrical spastic weakness, decreased muscle tone, exaggerated reflexes, and a positive Babinski's sign. If the cauda equina is involved, you may note muscle flaccidity and decreased reflexes. In advanced disease, paraplegia or quadriplegia may be evident.

Sensory deficits vary according to the tumor's level on the spinal cord. Look for signs of diminished pain, temperature, and proprioception sen-

Understanding Brown-Séquard syndrome

In these illustrations, you'll see the characteristics of Brown-Séquard syndrome.

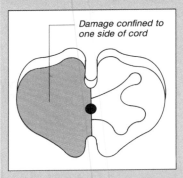

Damage confined to one side of cord

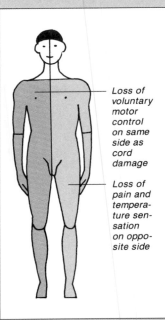

Loss of voluntary motor control on same side as cord damage

Loss of pain and temperature sensation on opposite side

sations. (The patient may be more aware of motor deficits than sensory deficits.) If lateral cord compression occurs, you may note Brown-Séquard syndrome. (See *Understanding Brown-Séquard syndrome.*)

If the tumor is located in the lumbosacral segment or cauda equina, sphincter control may be decreased or lost.

Diagnostic test results
The following tests can help confirm the diagnosis:
• X-ray may reveal distortions of the intervertebral foramina of sacrum, changes in the vertebrae or collapsed areas in the vertebral body, or localized enlargement of the spinal canal, indicative of an adjacent blockage.
• Lumbar puncture reveals clear yellow cerebrospinal fluid (CSF), resulting from increased protein levels related to completely and partially blocked CSF flow.
• Computed tomography scan and magnetic resonance imaging (MRI) may reveal cord compression and location of the tumor.
• Bone scan may indicate metastatic invasion of the vertebrae by revealing a characteristic increase in osteoblastic activity.
• Myelography identifies the tumor's level. If obstruction is partial, the myelogram outlines the tumor, showing its anatomic relationship to the cord and the dura. If obstruction is complete, the contrast media will be unable to flow past the tumor. This study can be dangerous if the patient has substantial cord compression because withdrawn or escaping CSF allows the tumor to exert greater pressure on the cord. Because of the popularity of the MRI, this test is no longer performed as frequently.
• Electromyography (EMG) aids differential diagnosis.

• Frozen section biopsy may identify the tissue type.

NURSING DIAGNOSIS

Common nursing diagnoses for a patient with a spinal tumor include:
• Altered urinary elimination related to spinal cord compression or damage
• Functional incontinence related to sensory or mobility deficits
• High risk for injury related to sensory or motor deficits
• Ineffective breathing pattern related to decreased energy or fatigue
• Impaired physical mobility related to spinal cord compression or damage
• Pain related to pressure on the spinal cord
• Powerlessness related to mobility and sensory impairment, altered body image, or poor prognosis
• Sexual dysfunction related to altered body structure or function.

PLANNING

Based on the nursing diagnosis *altered urinary elimination,* develop appropriate patient outcomes. For example, your patient will:
• recognize and report signs of changes in voiding
• remain free of signs of urinary tract infection, such as fever, cloudy or foul-smelling urine, or changes in intake or output
• demonstrate an absence of residual urine
• demonstrate competence in performing intermittent catheterization
• participate in a bladder training program.
Based on the nursing diagnosis *functional incontinence,* develop appropriate patient outcomes. For example, your patient will:

• void at specific times
• balance fluid intake with output
• demonstrate knowledge of managing incontinence.
Based on the nursing diagnosis *high risk for injury,* develop appropriate patient outcomes. For example, your patient will:
• express understanding of safety measures
• increase activities of daily living (ADLs) within limits
• remain free of injury.
Based on the nursing diagnosis *ineffective breathing pattern,* develop appropriate patient outcomes. For example, your patient will:
• maintain respiratory rate within established limits
• maintain arterial blood gas levels within established limits
• report feeling comfortable when breathing
• perform diaphragmatic pursed-lip breathing
• demonstrate ability to conserve energy while performing ADLs.
Based on the nursing diagnosis *impaired physical mobility,* develop appropriate patient outcomes. For example, your patient will:
• remain free of complications of impaired mobility, including contractures, skin breakdown, venous stasis, atelectasis, and pneumonia
• maintain the highest level of motor function possible.
Based on the nursing diagnosis *pain,* develop appropriate patient outcomes. For example, your patient will:
• identify pain characteristics
• describe pain on a scale of 1 to 10
• carry out appropriate interventions for pain relief
• report relief from pain.
Based on the nursing diagnosis *powerlessness,* develop appropriate

patient outcomes. For example, your patient will:
• express feelings of powerlessness
• identify and use effective coping mechanisms
• participate in care decisions
• perform care-related activities, if possible
• demonstrate increased acceptance of his disability and changes in lifestyle.

Based on the nursing diagnosis *sexual dysfunction,* develop appropriate patient outcomes. For example, your patient will:
• acknowledge a potential or real problem in sexual function
• express his feelings over changes in his sexual function
• explain the relationship between spinal cord tumor and sexual dysfunction
• express a willingness to obtain counseling, if appropriate
• communicate effectively with his partner.

IMPLEMENTATION

Whenever possible, surgery is used to excise spinal cord tumors. Radiation therapy and chemotherapy may be used adjunctively. (See *Medical care of the patient with spinal cord tumor.*)

Nursing interventions
• Using data from the initial neurologic evaluation, assess the patient's motor strength and sensory status frequently. Monitor for loss of proprioception and sense of temperature as well as any increase in pain.

Timesaving tip: Stay alert for early signs of acute cord compression, such as changes in the patient's temperature sensation, numbness, or tingling. If acute cord compression does occur, the patient's

status may deteriorate suddenly, so keep corticosteroids readily available, when prescribed, and anticipate immediate diagnostic testing and, possibly, surgery. Also, be prepared to treat cord edema.
• If the patient's mobility is impaired, perform passive range-of-motion exercises three to four times each day. Align his body properly and turn him frequently. Monitor for complications.
• Encourage the patient to express feelings of loss of control and other emotional responses to illness. Help him identify factors that contribute to his sense of helplessness and point out his strengths whenever possible. Continue to monitor his emotional state.
• Promote independent activity to the greatest extent possible. Provide the patient with choices about his care. Making decisions may help him regain a sense of control.
• If the patient experiences urine retention, initiate an intermittent catheterization program.
• Monitor intake and output as needed. Encourage the patient to drink sufficient fluids during the day, and caution him against taking fluids before bedtime.
• If appropriate, develop a bowel-training program. Encourage the patient to consume sufficient fiber and fluids. If prescribed, administer stool softeners and suppositories.
• Help the patient manage pain. If pain is not intense, suggest nonpharmacologic interventions such as distraction and relaxation techniques. Administer prescribed analgesics, as needed. To avoid aggravating pain, move the patient slowly and make sure his body is aligned properly when providing care. If pain is intense, consult with the doctor about

Medical care of the patient with spinal cord tumor

Surgery is the preferred treatment for spinal cord tumors. In addition, radiation therapy, chemotherapy, or both may be warranted.

Surgery
If the surgeon removes the tumor before the cord degenerates from compression, signs and symptoms are likely to subside and function may be restored. If the patient has experienced the rapid onset of incomplete paraplegia, emergency surgical decompression may save cord function. In a patient with a nonresectable malignant tumor, laminectomy may be performed to relieve acute cord compression.

Drug therapy
Corticosteroids, such as dexamethasone, control spinal cord edema. Antacids and a histamine-receptor antagonist, such as cimetidine or ranitidine, may be given to minimize or prevent adverse GI effects associated with corticosteroids. Analgesics, such as acetaminophen, morphine, or meperidine, may help to relieve pain.

Radiation therapy and chemotherapy
Radiation therapy may be used when only partial removal can be accomplished by surgery. Chemotherapy, however, isn't usually preferred for spinal cord tumors; it's commonly reserved for treatment of metastasis. The following list identifies different types of spinal cord tumors and the recommended treatment combinations:
• Extradural tumors: decompression by laminectomy may be followed by radiation therapy for malignant tumors. When the tumor is benign, laminectomy alone is used.
• Intradural extramedullary tumors: decompression by laminectomy may be followed by radiation therapy. When the tumor is benign, radiation may not be used.
• Intradural intramedullary tumors: decompression by laminectomy may be followed by radiation therapy for tumors only partially removed by surgery. Complete surgical removal is rare.

Additional treatments
Transcutaneous electrical nerve stimulation (TENS) may relieve radicular pain from spinal cord tumors and provides a useful alternative to opioid analgesics. TENS works by applying an electrical charge to the skin, thereby stimulating large-diameter nerve fibers and inhibiting the transmission of pain impulses along nerve fibers. The doctor may also prescribe a physical rehabilitation program. The specific regimen will depend on the patient's needs and prognosis.

using transcutaneous electrical nerve stimulation. Monitor the patient to determine the effectiveness of pain management.

• If the patient has sensory or motor deficits, institute safety precautions. Keep the side rails of the bed elevated if the patient is on strict bed rest. If he's ambulatory, encourage him to wear flat, comfortable shoes when walking. Remind family members to remove scatter rugs and clutter at home to prevent falls.

• If the patient has respiratory problems, plan rest periods between activities. If oxygen is prescribed, help him into a position that allows maximal chest expansion.

• After laminectomy, perform neurologic checks frequently and monitor the patient for signs of infection. Use logrolling techniques to change his position and provide assistance when he begins to walk again.

• After radiation therapy, administer prescribed corticosteroids for spinal cord edema. Monitor for sensory or motor dysfunction, which indicates the need for increased steroid therapy. Administer prescribed antacids and histamine-receptor antagonists.

• If the patient had radiation therapy 6 to 18 months prior to your care, be alert for signs of radiation myelopathy, including pain, motor dysfunction, changes in temperature sensation, spastic paraplegia, loss of sensation, Brown-Séquard syndrome, and bowel or bladder incontinence.

• If the patient has vertebral body involvement, enforce bed rest until the doctor determines he can walk safely. Body weight alone can cause vertebral column collapse and cord laceration from bone fragments.

• Roll and position the patient on his side every 2 hours to prevent pressure ulcers and other complications of immobility.

• If the patient requires a back brace, make sure he wears it whenever he gets out of bed. Make sure the brace is put on *before* he gets out of bed.

• Help the patient and his family understand and cope with the diagnosis, treatment, and necessary changes in lifestyle. Refer them for additional counseling as needed.

• If the patient develops sexual dysfunction, be aware that he may be uncomfortable discussing his concerns. If appropriate, refer the patient to a sex therapist, clinical nurse specialist, psychologist, marriage counselor, or member of the clergy. Afterward, be willing to discuss the patient's reaction to counseling sessions.

Patient teaching
• Reinforce the doctor's explanation of the diagnosis and all treatment measures.

• If the patient is scheduled for surgery, explain all preoperative and postoperative measures and discuss home care.

• If the patient is to receive radiation therapy or chemotherapy, explain these therapies fully. Discuss possible adverse reactions and ways to minimize or prevent them.

• Teach the patient and his primary care provider about the prescribed medications. Include a discussion of proper dose, schedule, administration, and possible adverse effects for each of them.

• Provide the patient and his family members with instruction about the care he requires at home. For example, explain how to maintain skin integrity, prevent infection, and reduce pain and discomfort.

• Encourage the patient to participate in a physical therapy program as soon as his condition permits.

Discharge TimeSaver

Ensuring continued care for the patient with spinal cord tumor

Review the following teaching topics, referrals, and follow-up appointments to make sure that your patient is adequately prepared for discharge.

Teaching topics
Make sure that the following topics have been covered and that your patient's learning has been evaluated:
☐ nature and progression of spinal cord tumor and its management
☐ drug therapy, including adverse reactions and related precautions
☐ surgery and related care
☐ radiation therapy and related safety measures
☐ physical therapy
☐ guidelines for proper nutrition
☐ possible complications and preventive measures
☐ pain relief
☐ bowel- and bladder-training program
☐ support services
☐ importance of follow-up care.

Referrals
Make sure that the patient has been provided with necessary referrals to:
☐ social services specializing in financial assistance
☐ home health care agency
☐ medical equipment supplier
☐ physical therapist
☐ pain control therapy
☐ psychological counseling.

Follow-up appointments
Make sure that the necessary follow-up appointments have been scheduled and that the patient has been notified:
☐ neurologist
☐ neurosurgeon
☐ rehabilitation program
☐ laboratory for radiation therapy
☐ laboratory for chemotherapy.

Timesaving tip: When providing patient teaching, gather all people involved for a group session. For example, when discussing the physical therapy program, ask the patient, his care provider, and his physical therapist to attend. Doing so saves you time, prevents needless repetition, and minimizes the chance of a misunderstanding.
• Teach the patient and family members how to implement a bowel- or bladder-program and assess their ability to perform intermittent catheterization.
• Describe necessary safety measures. Explain that the patient may

need to make some adaptations to his home, such as the installation of grab rails in the bathroom or a ramp at an entrance. Be sure that he and his family understand the proper use of all prescribed devices and equipment.
• Explain the importance of attending all follow-up appointments.
• As needed, provide the patient, family members, and close friends with referrals to support groups, the social service department, and home health care agencies. (See *Ensuring continued care for the patient with spinal cord tumor.*)

EVALUATION

When evaluating the patient's response to nursing care, gather reassessment data and compare this information to the patient outcomes specified in your plan of care.

Teaching and counseling

Begin by determining the effectiveness of teaching and counseling. Consider the following questions:

• Does the patient understand the nature of his spinal cord tumor?

• Does he fully understand the treatment plan?

• Is he willing to cooperate with the treatment plan?

• If the patient is participating in a bladder program, can he or his care provider perform intermittent catheterization?

• Is he using effective coping mechanisms?

• Does he participate in decisions and activities related to his care?

• Is he able to perform diaphragmatic pursed-lip breathing?

• Does he take steps to conserve energy while performing ADLs?

• Has he expressed feelings of fear or powerlessness?

• What steps has he taken to adapt to his disability?

• Has he expressed feelings regarding changes in his sexual function?

• Can he explain the relationship between the disorder and sexual dysfunction?

• Has he expressed a willingness to obtain counseling, if appropriate?

• Do the patient and members of his family know the signs and symptoms of tumor recurrence?

• Have they identified resources to assist with care following discharge?

• Have they developed a strategy to maintain safety at home?

Physical condition

Physical examination and diagnostic testing will also help you evaluate the effectiveness of your care. Note whether the patient:

• remains free of urinary tract infection

• voids at specific times

• demonstrates a residual urine level of 50 ml or less

• remains free of complications, such as contractures, skin breakdown, venous stasis, atelectasis, or pneumonia

• reports feeling comfortable when breathing

• maintains respiratory rate within established limits

• maintains arterial blood gas levels within established limits

• maintains the highest level of mobility possible

• maintains muscle and joint function

• reports pain relief

• reports feeling rested each day.

Caring for patients with paroxysmal disorders

Headache

A common and frequently recurrent disorder, headache can seriously disrupt a patient's functioning. Its pain may be generalized or localized and may range from mild to severe. Common types include migraine, cluster, tension, and combined tension-vascular headaches. (See *Classifying headaches*.)

Causes

Primary headaches may result from tension, menstruation, loud noises, menopause, or alcohol ingestion. Postural changes, prolonged coughing, sneezing, or exposure to sunlight may also be contributing factors. Occasionally, a headache may be symptomatic of a serious underlying condition, such as intracranial bleeding, head trauma, cerebral hypoxia, inflamed meninges, or a tumor.

ASSESSMENT

Although a headache doesn't usually signal a serious underlying disorder, expect to take a detailed history to determine the need for further investigation.

Health history

Obtain information about the patient's headache pattern. Ask about age of onset, changes in headache pattern, and a family history of headaches. Also ask about recent physical, social, or work-related changes in the patient's life. Then have the patient describe headache episodes. (See *Helping the patient describe his headache,* page 279.)

The patient with a tension headache may report a dull, persistent ache; tender spots on the head and neck; and a feeling of tightness around the head, beginning in the forehead, the temple, or the back of the neck (a "hatband" distribution of pain). The patient with a migraine headache may report unilateral, pulsating pain that gradually becomes more generalized and lasts 4 to 72 hours. (See *Key points about tension and migraine headaches*, page 280.)

The patient with a headache from intracranial bleeding may report sudden, severe occipital pain. The patient with a headache from a tumor may report that his pain is most severe upon awakening but diminishes when he lifts his head to an upright position.

Medication history

Determine if the patient uses any over-the-counter drugs to relieve headache pain. To remain functional despite pain, the patient may require frequent use of analgesics, such as aspirin or acetaminophen. If so, he may be vulnerable to *analgesic rebound headache,* which stems from analgesic overuse. He may report a chronic daily headache, which may wax and wane during the day.

Determine whether the patient uses any drugs or other substances that can cause a headache, such as vasodilators (nitrates and alcohol), vasopressors (caffeine, ergotamine, and adrenergic drugs), or indomethacin. Withdrawal from vasopressors may cause throbbing pain. Indomethacin produces morning headache in about half of all patients who take it.

Physical examination

Palpation may reveal some local tenderness on the scalp or tightness of the head and neck muscles. Note whether the patient has a fever, a common cause of headache, and ob-

Classifying headaches

The following system, developed by the International Headache Society, groups headaches into 13 classifications.

Migraine

This group includes migraine with and without an aura, ophthalmoplegic migraine, and retinal migraine. It also encompasses childhood periodic syndromes that may be precursors to or associated with migraine (benign paroxysmal vertigo, alternating hemiplegia) and complications of migraine, such as status migrainosus and migrainous infarction.

Tension-type headache

This group includes episodic and chronic tension-type headaches, which may or may not be associated with a disorder of the pericranial muscles.

Cluster headache and chronic paroxysmal hemicrania

This group of headaches covers episodic and chronic cluster headaches as well as chronic paroxysmal hemicrania.

Miscellaneous headaches unassociated with structural lesions

In this group, idiopathic stabbing headache is listed along with external compression and cold stimulus headaches, benign cough and benign exertional headaches, and headache that is associated with sexual activity.

Headache associated with head trauma

This group includes acute and chronic posttraumatic headaches.

Headache associated with vascular disorders

This group covers headache brought on by acute ischemic cerebrovascular disease, intracranial hematoma, subarachnoid hemorrhage, unruptured vascular malformation, arteritis, carotid or vertebral artery pain, venous thrombosis, arterial hypertension, and other vascular disorders.

Headache associated with nonvascular intracranial disorders

This group includes headache resulting from high or low cerebrospinal fluid pressure, intracranial infection, intracranial sarcoidosis and other noninfectious inflammatory diseases, intrathecal injections, intracranial neoplasm, and other intracranial disorders.

Headache associated with substances or their withdrawal

This group covers headache induced by acute use of or exposure to nitrates or nitrites, monosodium glutamate, carbon monoxide, alcohol, or other substances; chronic use of or exposure to ergotamine, analgesics, or other substances; withdrawal from acute use of alcohol or other substances; withdrawal from chronic use of ergotamine, caffeine, narcot-

(continued)

Classifying headaches *(continued)*

ics, or other substances; and use of oral contraceptives or estrogens.

Headache associated with noncephalic infection
Headache-inducing viral, bacterial, and other infections make up this group.

Headache associated with metabolic disorders
This group includes headache resulting from hypoxia, hypercapnia, mixed hypoxia and hypercapnia, hypoglycemia, dialysis, or other metabolic abnormalities.

Headache or facial pain associated with disorders of the head and neck
This group includes headache resulting from disorders of the cranium, neck, eyes, ears, nose, sinuses, teeth, mouth or other facial or cranial

structures. Examples include retropharyngeal tendinitis, acute glaucoma, heterophoria or heterotropia, acute sinus headache, and temporomandibular joint disease.

Cranial neuralgias, nerve trunk pain, and deafferentation pain
This group includes persistent (in contrast to ticlike) pain of cranial nerve origin, trigeminal neuralgia, glossopharyngeal neuralgia, nervus intermedius neuralgia, superior laryngeal neuralgia, occipital neuralgia, central causes of head and facial pain other than tic douloureux, and other miscellaneous types of facial pain.

Unclassifiable headache
This group includes headaches that don't fall into the preceding 12 categories because of unknown or obscure etiology.

serve the character of the patient's respirations.

If the patient has a history of head trauma, examine his head for evidence of bruising, bleeding, swelling, or obvious bone abnormalities. Also check for neck stiffness, otorrhea, rhinorrhea, raccoon's eyes, or Battle's sign.

Assess the patient's level of consciousness (LOC), and check his pupils for equality, size, and reaction to light. Note photophobia if present. The patient may exhibit dilated pupils, suggesting an adverse drug reaction. Ophthalmoscopic evaluation

may also reveal signs of intracranial hemorrhaging or papilledema.

Measure the patient's blood pressure to determine if hypertension may be causing the headache. Auscultation may detect bruits, indicating an aneurysm, another possible cause of headaches.

Check for cranial nerve involvement by having the patient raise his eyebrows, smile (tests cranial nerve VII), and clench his teeth (tests cranial nerve V).

If the patient complains of an acute, severe headache, assess for a serious problem, such as meningitis.

Assessment TimeSaver

Helping the patient describe his headache

To help your patient describe his headache, ask the following questions:
• At what age did your first attack occur?
• Can you recall particular circumstances that occur at the time of your attacks, such as a hard day at work, a disagreement with a friend or family member, a traffic jam or — more seriously — the onset of menses, pregnancy, menopause, marriage or divorce, the death of a loved one, or an illness?
• Has there been any change in your headache pattern?
• Does anyone in your family have a history of headaches?
• Do you have a headache now? If you do, how severe is it? Did the pain begin gradually and then worsen? Or did it begin suddenly?

• Is the pain dull or achy, throbbing, sharp, or stabbing? Does it feel like a tight band of pressure?
• How often do you get headaches?
• Is the pain unilateral or bilateral?
• Does it usually occur in the same location? Or does the location vary with each attack?
• Do your headaches interfere with your daily activities?
• Are your headaches accompanied by nausea, weakness, facial pain, or areas of partial or complete blindness?
• How long does the pain usually last with medication? Without medication?
• Do you feel well rested?
• Is your sleep sound or fitful and easily disturbed?
• Do you awaken early without an obvious cause?

If you suspect meningeal irritation, test for Kernig's and Brudzinski's signs.

Diagnostic test results
The following tests may help identify the type of headache or reveal its underlying cause:
• Magnetic resonance imaging (MRI) may help determine if intracranial bleeding has occurred or if occlusive disease is present.
• Computed tomography scan can rule out lesions and other abnormalities and, like MRI, will show cerebrospinal fluid flow in the ventricles.
• Lumbar puncture can rule out infection, subarachnoid hemorrhage, or abnormal intracranial pressure. This test may be ordered if scans are negative, but intracranial bleeding is still suspected.
• Transcranial Doppler studies may be performed if auscultation reveals bruits.

NURSING DIAGNOSIS

Common nursing diagnoses for a patient with headache include:
• Pain related to severe headache
• Sleep pattern disturbance related to insomnia caused by headache
• Altered role performance related to headache.

FactFinder

Key points about tension and migraine headaches

Tension headache
• *Pain characteristics:* Frequently occurs in occipital and upper cervical areas and radiates over the top of the head. Pain develops gradually and may be unilateral or bilateral. It may be accompanied by feelings of tightness or pressure, dizziness, tinnitus, lacrimation, nausea, and vomiting. Exposure to cold may precipitate or aggravate the pain.
• *Causes:* Usually results from muscle contraction. Other causes or contributing factors include stress, fatigue, and noise; certain disorders, such as glaucoma, inflammation of the eyes or nasal passages, and muscle spasms; and use of certain drugs, such as nitrates.
• *Incidence:* Tension headaches from muscle contraction are the most common type of headache. Women experience this type of headache more often than men; incidence is higher in adults ages 20 to 40.

Migraine headache
• *Pain characteristics:* Paroxysmal, throbbing, unilateral head pain possibly accompanied by nausea and vomiting. The patient may experience a visual, auditory, or other sensory aura. Unlike tension headaches, migraines usually appear after a period of stress has ended.
• *Causes:* Although the exact cause is unknown, migraine headaches are believed to result from a serotonin imbalance in the brain combined with subsequent constriction and dilation of intracranial and extracranial arteries. Other biochemical abnormalities are thought to occur during an attack, including local leakage of a vasodilating polypeptide through the dilated arteries.
• *Incidence:* Migraines are more common in women than men and tend to run in families. They usually appear initially in childhood or adolescence and recur throughout adulthood.

PLANNING

Based on the nursing diagnosis *pain,* develop appropriate patient outcomes. For example, your patient will:
• report pain relief within a reasonable time after taking prescribed drugs
• help develop a plan to control pain
• adjust his lifestyle to alleviate or minimize factors that contribute to headache

• express satisfaction with his pain management regimen.

Based on the nursing diagnosis *sleep pattern disturbance,* develop appropriate patient outcomes. For example, your patient will:
• sleep a specified number of hours nightly
• show no signs of sleep deprivation
• perform relaxation exercises at bedtime.

Based on the nursing diagnosis *altered role performance,* develop ap-

Treatments

Medical care of the patient with headaches

For many patients, analgesics — ranging from aspirin or ibuprofen to codeine or meperidine — may provide relief. An antianxiety agent, such as diazepam, may help during acute attacks. Low-dose antidepressants, such as imipramine or amitriptyline, may be used to relieve stress-related headaches. Patients who experience chronic tension headaches may benefit from muscle relaxants.

Other measures include identification and elimination of causative factors, including headache-triggering foods. Psychotherapy may benefit patients whose headaches appear to be related to emotional stress.

Treating migraine headaches
Treatment of migraines includes administering prescribed drugs at the onset of pain, administering fluids to avoid dehydration, and eliminating causative factors. Despite the severity of pain that they inflict, migraines rarely require hospitalization, unless vomiting is severe enough to induce dehydration or shock.

Drug therapy
Ergotamine preparations, taken alone or with caffeine, are the most effective treatment for migraines. Other drugs may include analgesics, antiemetics, metoclopramide, propranolol, verapamil, and naproxen. These drugs work best when taken early in the course of an attack. If nausea and vomiting make oral administration problematic, drugs may be administered rectally or given by injection.

Supportive measures
Patients who are prone to headaches may benefit from supportive measures, such as:
• regular exercise (30 minutes, three times a week)
• biofeedback if stress is a major cause
• physical therapy, especially if headaches are chronic and associated with stiff and sore muscles of the neck, shoulders, and back. Therapy should include exercises that the patient can perform at home.

propriate patient outcomes. For example, your patient will:
• express his feelings about his diminished capacity to carry out his usual roles
• make decisions regarding the course of treatment
• continue to function in his usual roles as much as possible.

IMPLEMENTATION

Treatment hinges on the type of headache. Stress the importance of following the prescribed regimen and avoiding over-the-counter drugs. For pain stemming from environmental stimuli such as stress, emphasize supportive measures such as relaxation therapy. (See *Medical care of the patient with headaches*.)

Nursing interventions

• Establish and document the patient's baseline neurologic status, including mentation, LOC, judgment, insight, orientation, and sensation. Monitor his neurologic status periodically throughout his hospitalization.

• Obtain baseline vital signs; reassess them if the patient complains of a headache.

• Administer prescribed drugs.

• Adjust the patient's head position to avoid a rigid posture that may aggravate a tension headache.

• Keep his room dark and quiet. Place ice packs on his forehead or a cold cloth over his eyes to decrease the severity of pain.

• Provide a warm bath and take other steps to promote relaxation.

• Encourage the patient to discuss problems with family, friends, and members of the health care team.

• Promote adequate exercise and rest.

• If the patient reports that his headache is stress related, discuss ways to improve coping.

Patient teaching

• Provide information on the patient's type of headache and its treatment.

• Using the health history as a guide, help the patient understand which factors precipitate his headaches so that he can avoid them.

• Provide information on relaxation techniques, and explain that these may help change his responses to stress and thus decrease headache frequency.

• Explain the importance of regular exercise in promoting relaxation.

• Advise him to prevent dehydration by drinking plenty of fluids, to avoid long intervals between meals, and to awaken at the same time every day.

• Warn him to avoid headache-triggering foods and beverages, such as alcohol (particularly red wines), aged cheeses, peanuts, chocolate, foods with a high preservative content, and artificial sweeteners. (See *Headache prevention diet.*)

• Stress the importance of avoiding over-the-counter drugs.

Timesaving tip: When discussing headache-relieving drugs, assemble patients with common complaints and provide group teaching. Your job will be easier, you'll save time, and the patients will benefit from group interaction.

• Refer the patient who experiences migraine headaches to the National Headache Foundation for a list of doctors and clinics in the United States that specialize in migraines.

• If the patient's headache results from analgesic overuse, stress that analgesic use must be tapered slowly and as recommended by the doctor. Warn that headache symptoms will worsen before improvement is noticeable. (See *Ensuring continued care for the patient with headaches,* page 285.)

EVALUATION

When evaluating the patient's response to nursing care, gather reassessment data and compare this information with the patient outcomes specified in your plan of care.

Teaching and counseling

Begin by determining the effectiveness of your teaching. Consider the following questions:

• Is the patient willing to take all prescribed drugs at the headache's onset?

• Does he use relaxation techniques to reduce stress?

Headache prevention diet

Guiding and monitoring a patient's diet can help prevent migraine headaches. Be sure to tell your patient:
- to avoid fasting or skipping meals
- to eat three or more small meals a day
- to eat at the same times each day
- to carefully read all snack food labels
- to eat all foods in moderation.

Provide the patient with a list of foods that he can eat safely as well as those that he should avoid.

Permitted foods
- all fruits and vegetables except those listed under *Fruits and vegetables to avoid*
- beef
- most breads, such as white, whole wheat, rye, French, Italian, English muffins, melba toast, crackers, and bagels
- broth, homemade
- butter or margarine
- cake and cookies made without chocolate or yeast
- cereals, hot and cold, such as farina, oatmeal, corn flakes, puffed wheat and rice, and bran cereal
- cottage, cream, farmer's, processed, and ricotta cheeses
- chicken
- cooking oil
- cream, whipped
- fish, fresh or frozen
- hard candy
- honey
- ice milk
- jam, jellies
- lamb
- lemon juice, natural

- pasta
- pork
- potato, white or sweet
- rice
- soups, cream (made from permitted foods)
- sugar
- tuna
- turkey, fresh or frozen
- veal
- vinegar, white

Permitted beverages
- beer, nonalcoholic
- coffee, decaffeinated
- milk
- natural fruit juice
- club soda
- noncola soda

Foods and beverages permitted in limited amounts
- coffee, tea, cola, and other caffeinated drinks (two cups per day)
- eggs (three a week)
- citrus fruit (½ cup per day)
- commercial salad dressing
- salt

Foods to avoid
- all foods containing monosodium glutamate (including but not limited to restaurant-prepared Oriental foods)
- all foods containing nitrites, nitrates, or amines
- any pickled, preserved, or marinated foods
- bacon
- bologna
- bouillon cubes
- hot, fresh homemade yeast bread

(continued)

Headache prevention diet *(continued)*

Foods to avoid *(continued)*
- bread or crackers containing cheese
- bread, sourdough
- buttermilk
- cheeses (blue, brick, Camembert, cheddar, Swiss, Gouda, Roquefort, Stilton, mozzarella, Parmesan, provolone, and romano)
- cheese sauce
- chocolate, including chocolate syrup and any ice cream, pudding, cookies, or cake containing chocolate
- sour cream
- doughnuts
- fish, salted and dried
- game, aged
- gelatin
- herring, pickled
- hot dogs
- chicken liver
- meat (aged, canned, cured or processed)
- meat tenderizer
- milk, chocolate
- mincemeat pie
- mixed dishes (such as lasagna, macaroni and cheese, beef Stroganoff, and cheese blintzes)
- nuts and seeds
- pizza
- salt, seasoned
- sausage, fermented (such as salami or pepperoni)
- soup base with yeast or monosodium glutamate
- soup, canned
- soup cubes
- soy sauce
- TV dinners
- yeast, yeast extract, brewer's yeast; any fresh product baked with yeast

Beverages to avoid
- alcohol
- cocoa

Fruits and vegetables to avoid
- apples, applesauce
- apricots
- avocados
- beans (lima, pole, broad, Italian, fava, navy, pinto, and garbanzo)
- carob
- cherries
- figs
- fruit cocktail
- lentils
- olives
- onions (except for flavoring)
- papaya
- passion fruit
- peaches
- pears
- pickles
- raisins
- snow peas
- pea pods
- red plums
- sauerkraut

- Does he understand that environmental stimuli and certain foods may trigger headaches?

- Does he express his feelings and concerns openly?
- Has he taken steps to improve his coping skills?

Discharge TimeSaver

Ensuring continued care for the patient with headaches

Review the following teaching topics, referrals, and follow-up appointments to make sure that your patient is adequately prepared for discharge.

Teaching topics
Make sure that the following topics have been covered and that your patient's learning has been evaluated:
□ explanation of headache, including its causes, management, and prevention
□ activity and rest guidelines
□ prescribed drugs
□ warning signs of headache
□ sources of information and support.

Referrals
Make sure that the patient has been provided with necessary referrals to:
□ dietitian
□ psychological counseling
□ support group.

Follow-up appointments
Make sure that the necessary follow-up appointments have been scheduled and that the patient has been notified:
□ doctor
□ diagnostic tests for reevaluation.

Physical condition

Consider the following questions:
• Have the patient's headaches been alleviated?
• Does he sleep a specified number of hours nightly?
• Are signs of sleep deprivation absent?
• Has he resumed his usual activities?

Epilepsy

A recurrent paroxysmal disorder of cerebral function, epilepsy is characterized by sudden, brief attacks of altered level of consciousness (LOC), motor activity, or sensory phenomena. The term "epilepsy" applies to patients with recurrent seizures; a single, isolated seizure doesn't constitute epilepsy.

Epilepsy occurs most commonly in patients under age 20. Although about 80% of them achieve good seizure control with strict adherence to the treatment regimen, many continue to have seizures despite compliance. (See *Classifying seizures,* pages 286 and 287.)

Causes

Epilepsy may result from cerebral, biochemical, posttraumatic, or idiopathic causes. Genetic predisposition plays a dominant role in about 20% of patients. In about 50% of patients, the cause is unknown. (See *Causes of epilepsy,* page 288.)

ASSESSMENT

If the patient is experiencing repetitive seizures without recovery (status epilepticus), you'll need to provide

Classifying seizures

Caused by abnormal electrical discharges of neurons in the brain, seizures produce skeletal muscle convulsions and disturbances in consciousness and behavior. Recurring seizures can be classified as *partial* or *generalized*. Some patients may be affected by more than one type.

Partial seizures
Arising from a localized area in the brain, partial seizures cause specific symptoms. In some patients, seizure activity may spread to the entire brain, causing a generalized seizure. Partial seizures include simple partial (jacksonian motor type and sensory type), complex partial (psychomotor or temporal lobe), and secondary generalized partial seizures.

Simple partial seizures
This type of seizure begins as a localized motor seizure that is characterized by a spread of abnormal activity to adjacent areas of the brain. Typically, the patient experiences a stiffening or jerking in one extremity, accompanied by a tingling sensation in the same area. The patient seldom loses consciousness, although the seizure may progress to a generalized tonic-clonic seizure.
Perception is distorted in this type of seizure. Symptoms can include hallucinations, paresthesia, a foul odor, vertigo, or déjà vu.

Complex partial seizures
Symptoms vary but usually include purposeless behavior. The patient may experience an aura and exhibit overt signs, including a glassy stare, picking at his clothes, aimless wandering, lip-smacking or chewing motions, and unintelligible speech. A sei-

zure may last for a few seconds or as long as 20 minutes. Afterward, confusion may last for several minutes. As a result, an observer may mistakenly suspect psychosis or drug or alcohol intoxication. The patient has no memory of his actions during the seizure.

Secondary generalized partial seizures
This type of seizure can be simple or complex and can progress to generalized seizures. An aura may precede the progression. Loss of consciousness occurs immediately or within 2 minutes of onset.

Generalized seizures
As the term suggests, these seizures cause a generalized electrical abnormality within the brain. They include several distinct types.

Absence seizures
Formerly known as petit mal seizures, absence seizures occur most often in children, although they may affect adults as well. They usually begin with a brief change in level of consciousness, indicated by a blinking or rolling of the eyes, a blank stare, and slight mouth movements. The patient retains his posture and continues preseizure activity without difficulty. Typically, this type of seizure lasts from 1 to 10 seconds. The impairment is so

Classifying seizures *(continued)*

brief that the patient is sometimes unaware of it. If not properly treated, these seizures can recur as often as 100 times a day.

Myoclonic seizures
Also called bilateral massive epileptic myoclonus, this seizure type is marked by brief, involuntary muscular jerks of the body or extremities which may occur in a rhythmic manner, and a brief loss of consciousness.

Generalized tonic-clonic seizures
Formerly known as grand mal seizures, these seizures typically begin with a loud cry precipitated by air rushing from the lungs through the vocal cords. The patient falls to the ground, losing consciousness. The body stiffens (tonic phase) and then alternates between episodes of muscle spasm (tonic phase) and relaxation (clonic phase). Tongue biting, incontinence, labored breathing, apnea, and subsequent cyanosis may also occur. The seizure typically ends in 2 to 5 minutes, when abnormal electrical conduction of the neurons is completed. The patient then regains consciousness but is somewhat confused and may have difficulty talking. If he can talk, he may complain of drowsiness, fatigue, headache, muscle soreness, and arm or leg weakness. He may fall into a deep sleep after the seizure.

Akinetic seizures
Characterized by a general loss of postural tone and a temporary loss of consciousness, this type occurs in young children. It's also known as a drop attack because it causes the child to fall.

---

emergency treatment. (See *Understanding status epilepticus,* page 289.)

If the patient is stable, proceed with the health history (including a medication history), a physical examination, and a review of diagnostic test results. You may need to ask a family member to describe the patient's reactions during a seizure.

Health history
If the cause of the patient's epilepsy is known, his history and physical examination may reveal identifiable signs and symptoms. However, some causes of epilepsy, such as a brain tumor, may produce no signs other than the seizure itself.

Try to determine what precipitates the patient's seizures. Find out if they usually take place at a particular time — for example, during sleep. Seizures can be triggered by such factors as fatigue, lack of sleep, stress, electric shock, alcohol or excessive water consumption, constipation, menstruation, flashing lights, hyperventilation, loud noises, particular odors, heavy musical beats, video games, and television. In many patients, seizures occur unpredictably.

Determine if the patient experiences an aura, commonly a visual

Causes of epilepsy

Epilepsy may be associated with cerebral, biochemical, posttraumatic, or idiopathic causes.

Cerebral causes
Cerebral lesions, a major cause of seizures, may result from:
• birth injuries, such as trauma and anoxia, jaundice, and maternal infections or drug use
• infectious disorders, such as meningitis, encephalitis, and abscesses, or high fever
• cerebral circulatory disturbances, such as subarachnoid hemorrhage, cerebrovascular accident, hypertensive encephalopathy, vasospasms, and vascular anomalies
• cerebral trauma, such as hematoma or laceration
• brain tumors.

Biochemical causes
Biochemical disturbances that may produce seizures include:
• alcohol ingestion
• drug overdose

• seizure-inducing drug use
• electrolyte imbalance (such as hyponatremia)
• vitamin deficiency
• diabetes mellitus and other metabolic disorders
• endocrine disorders caused by pregnancy and menstruation.

Posttraumatic causes
Common causes include craniocerebral trauma and cerebral infections. Seizures can occur at any time following a head injury but usually occur 6 months to 2 years after the injury. Few patients develop seizures less than 2 months or more than 5 years after trauma.

Idiopathic causes
Idiopathic epilepsy has no identifiable cause. It probably results from a biochemical imbalance.

disturbance (such as a flashing light), a few seconds or minutes before the seizure. Other possible auras include a pungent smell, GI distress (nausea or indigestion), a rising or sinking feeling in the stomach, a dreamy feeling, or an unusual taste.

Ask the patient how seizures affect his daily activities. Note if he has experienced status epilepticus.

Medication history
Take a thorough drug history. Toxic blood levels of aminophylline, the-ophylline, or lidocaine, or excessive doses of meperidine, penicillin, or cimetidine may cause generalized seizures. Contrast agents used in radiologic tests may also cause generalized seizures. In patients with preexisting epilepsy, certain drugs — including phenothiazines, tricyclic antidepressants, alprostadil, and amphetamines — may trigger seizures. Some drugs, such as isoniazid and vincristine, actually lower the seizure threshold.

In alcohol-dependent patients, seizures and status epilepticus may occur 7 to 48 hours after sudden withdrawal. Barbiturate withdrawal after chronic use may produce generalized seizures and, possibly, status epilepticus 2 to 4 days after the last dose.

Physical examination

Assess the patient's mental status (including LOC), pupillary constriction, bowel and bladder control, and sensorimotor function (weakness and paralysis, for example). Also check for photophobia, meningeal irritation, and hypertension.

In idiopathic epilepsy, your assessment findings may reveal nothing if the patient is examined while his condition is stable.

Diagnostic test results

The following tests may reveal predisposing factors and help identify causes of epilepsy:

• EEG can help to classify the disorder. Because paroxysmal abnormalities can occur intermittently, a negative EEG doesn't rule out epilepsy.

• Computed tomography scan provides density readings of the brain and may indicate abnormalities in internal structures.

• Magnetic resonance imaging may help identify the seizure's cause by providing images of cerebral regions where bone normally hampers visualization.

• Serum chemistry studies can detect hypoglycemia, hypocalcemia, and other electrolyte imbalances, increased blood urea nitrogen levels, elevated alcohol levels, and elevated liver enzyme levels.

NURSING DIAGNOSIS

Common nursing diagnoses for a patient with epilepsy include:

FactFinder

Understanding status epilepticus

Marked by continuous seizure activity with no return to baseline, status epilepticus can occur in any epilepsy patient. Its most life-threatening form is *generalized tonic-clonic status epilepticus,* a continuous generalized tonic-clonic seizure that is accompanied by respiratory distress and that should always be considered an emergency.

Causes

Status epilepticus can result from:

• abrupt withdrawal of anticonvulsant drugs

• hypoxic or metabolic encephalopathy

• acute head trauma

• septicemia from encephalitis or meningitis.

Treatment

Emergency treatment usually consists of:

• breaking the continuous seizure activity by administering diazepam or lorazepam

• using anticonvulsants, such as phenytoin, phenobarbital, or carbamazepine, once the seizure activity has been interrupted, to prevent the return of seizure activity

• administering dextrose 50% in water I.V. (when seizures result from hypoglycemia)

• administering thiamine I.V. (if seizures are associated with chronic alcoholism or drug withdrawal).

• Fear related to seizures or loss of bodily control
• High risk for injury related to seizures
• Ineffective individual coping related to inability to use adaptive behaviors
• Knowledge deficit related to epilepsy and the skills needed to manage the disorder
• Social isolation related to fear of experiencing a seizure in public.

PLANNING

Based on the nursing diagnosis *fear,* develop appropriate patient outcomes. For example, your patient will:
• report feeling more control over his condition
• communicate an understanding of how drug therapy reduces seizure risk
• recognize the physical and emotional signs of anxiety.

Based on the nursing diagnosis *high risk for injury,* develop appropriate patient outcomes. For example, your patient will:
• adjust his behavior and activities to adapt to his disorder
• provide the safest possible environment for himself
• teach family, friends, and coworkers how to protect him from injury during a seizure
• wear a medical identification necklace or bracelet to identify his disorder.

Based on the nursing diagnosis *ineffective individual coping,* develop appropriate patient outcomes. For example, your patient will:
• demonstrate a willingness to adapt to demands or changes imposed by his disorder
• comply with his prescribed drug regimen

• comply with his prescribed activity, exercise, and rest regimen.

Based on the nursing diagnosis *knowledge deficit,* develop appropriate patient outcomes. For example, your patient will:
• express an understanding of his disorder, drug and activity regimens, and their implications for his lifestyle.

Based on the nursing diagnosis *social isolation,* develop appropriate patient outcomes. For example, your patient will:
• express feelings of loneliness
• make an effort to increase social contacts
• identify organizations and support groups available to help him adapt to the demands of his disorder and altered lifestyle.

IMPLEMENTATION

Epilepsy can usually be controlled with drug therapy. For many patients, though, the fear of an uncontrolled seizure overshadows everyday life. Such patients need psychosocial support to deal with their concerns about the social and emotional hardships associated with epilepsy. (See *Medical care of the patient with epilepsy.*)

Nursing interventions
• Provide a safe, protected environment for the patient in the hospital.
• Administer all prescribed drugs.
• Establish baseline neurologic status upon the patient's admission to the hospital. Perform neurologic examinations periodically and document deteriorations or improvements.
• Observe and document any seizure activity.

Timesaving tip: Remember to document any seizure activity as soon as possible after the event. This will save time when trying to recall the event, ensure the accuracy of

Treatments

Medical care of the patient with epilepsy

Treatment typically consists of drug therapy for the specific seizure type. More severe cases may require surgery.

Drug therapy

First, an antianxiety agent, such as diazepam or lorazepam, is prescribed to break the seizure activity. Then an anticonvulsant may be given to prevent the return of seizures. Commonly prescribed anticonvulsants include:

• phenobarbital — for all seizure types; may be used in combination with other drugs
• primidone — for tonic-clonic seizures; may be the drug of choice for complex partial and other partial seizures
• diazepam — for status epilepticus
• clonazepam — for myoclonic, akinetic, absence, and complex partial seizures

• phenytoin — for tonic-clonic seizures, complex partial and other partial seizures, and psychomotor seizures
• carbamazepine — for tonic-clonic seizures, complex partial and other partial seizures, and psychomotor seizures
• ethosuximide — for absence seizures
• trimethadione — for refractory absence seizures
• valproic acid — for absence seizures.

Surgery

If drug therapy fails, treatment may include surgical removal of a demonstrated focal lesion in an attempt to end seizures. Surgery is also performed when epilepsy results from an underlying problem, such as intracranial tumors, brain abscess or cysts, and vascular abnormalities.

your documentation, help the doctor determine the best treatment, and possibly shorten the patient's hospital stay.
• If the patient is taking anticonvulsants, monitor for signs and symptoms of toxicity, such as slurred speech, ataxia, lethargy, dizziness, drowsiness, nystagmus, irritability, nausea, and vomiting.
• Because reduced glucose and sodium levels may exacerbate or precipitate seizures, monitor serum chemistry findings and correlate them with the patient's progress in gaining control over his disorder.

• Prepare the patient for surgery if necessary.
• During emergency treatment, ensure the patient's safety. Be aware that you may have to teach emergency techniques to the patient's family. (See *Responding to seizures,* pages 292 and 293.)

Patient teaching
• Teach the patient and his family about his disorder and its management. When possible, teach patients with epilepsy in a group setting.
• Answer any questions the patient may have about his condition. Assure

Responding to seizures

The following guidelines describe steps for preventing a seizure, providing care during and after a seizure, and documenting a seizure.

Seizure precautions
• Administer the precise doses of anticonvulsant drugs on time.
• Be sure to use a rectal thermometer, not an oral one, with the seizure-prone patient.
• Pad the bed's side rails and headboard to protect the patient from injury.
• Keep the padded side rails in place if the patient has frequent or generalized seizures or severe muscle contractions.
• If the patient has an oral endotracheal tube in place, insert an airway to prevent him from occluding or biting the tube during seizure activity and to allow for suctioning.
• Keep suction equipment handy if the patient's airway becomes clogged with oral secretions.
• Monitor the patient's cardiovascular and respiratory status closely to detect hypoxia, which may lead to seizures.
• Accompany the seizure-prone patient when he takes a walk.

Care during a seizure
• Stay with the patient and call for assistance.
• Have the patient lie flat on a bed or on the floor. Don't lift him onto a bed during a seizure.
• Turn him on his side to allow his tongue to fall away from his airway and permit drainage of saliva.

• Don't force open the patient's clenched teeth or put anything in his mouth.
• Loosen tight clothing, such as a collar or belt.
• Move objects out of the way to protect his head and limbs from injury.
• Don't restrain him, but try to guide his movements.
• Provide privacy if possible.

Care after a seizure
• Place the patient in bed.
• Turn him on his side to permit continued drainage. Check his level of consciousness. If it's depressed, insert an oral airway. Suction as needed.
• If this is the patient's first seizure, notify the doctor immediately. If the patient has had seizures before, notify the doctor only if the seizure activity is prolonged or if the patient fails to regain consciousness.
• Check for injuries.
• Reorient and reassure the patient as necessary.
• When the patient is comfortable and safe, document what happened during the seizure.

Documenting a seizure
• *Onset:* Was it sudden or preceded by an aura? If preceded by an aura, have the patient describe what he experienced.
• *Duration:* When did the seizure begin and end?

Responding to seizures *(continued)*

- *Frequency and number:* Did the patient have one seizure or several?
- *Level of consciousness:* Was the patient unconscious? If so, for how long? Could you wake him? Note any changes in consciousness.
- *Motor activity:* Where did the movements begin? What parts of his body were involved? Was there a pattern of progression to the activity? Describe the patient's movements.
- *Eyes:* Did they deviate to one side? Did the pupils change in size, shape, equality, or reaction to light?
- *Teeth:* Were they clenched or open?

- *Respirations:* What was the patient's respiratory rate and quality? Was he cyanotic?
- *Body functions:* Did he become incontinent, vomit, salivate, or bleed from his mouth?
- *Drug response:* If any drugs were administered during the seizure, how did the patient respond? Did the seizure cease? Did it worsen?
- *Seizure awareness:* Is the patient aware of what happened? Did he fall into a deep sleep following the seizure? Was he upset? Did he seem ashamed?

him that epilepsy is usually controllable if he follows the prescribed drug regimen, and that most patients maintain a normal lifestyle.

- Arrange for appropriate health care professionals (pharmacist, physical therapist, dietitian) to instruct the patient in their areas of expertise.
- Explain diagnostic tests as necessary, including what to expect before, during, and after each procedure.
- Explain the uses and actions of each prescribed drug.
- Assure the patient that anticonvulsants are safe when taken as prescribed. Provide written dosage instructions. Teach the patient methods to help him remember when to take his medications. For example, if a drug is to be taken three times a day, suggest that the patient take one dose at each meal. If the drug is to be taken once a day, he could take it at night before going to bed. Schedule doses

around the patient's routine. Stress that skipping or doubling doses can cause a seizure. Caution him to monitor the amount of medication he has left so that he doesn't run out.

- Teach the patient and his family about the possible adverse effects of anticonvulsants: drowsiness, lethargy, hyperactivity, confusion, and visual and sleep disturbances. Inform them that these effects indicate the need for dosage adjustment. Instruct them to report adverse reactions immediately.
- Explain the importance of having anticonvulsant blood levels checked regularly even if seizures are under control.
- Instruct the patient to avoid alcohol.
- Teach him to eat balanced, regular meals. Low blood glucose levels and vitamin deficiencies can lead to seizures.

Discharge TimeSaver

Ensuring continued care for the patient with epilepsy

Review the following teaching topics, referrals, and follow-up appointments to make sure that your patient is adequately prepared for discharge.

Teaching topics
Make sure that the following topics have been covered and that your patient's learning has been evaluated:
☐ explanation of epilepsy, including its causes and treatments
☐ warning signs and symptoms
☐ emergency care during seizures
☐ activity and rest guidelines
☐ medication therapy, including adverse effects, precautions, and need for compliance with therapy
☐ need for high-calorie, well-balanced diet
☐ prescriptions and medication teaching cards
☐ need for follow-up care and testing.

Referrals
Make sure that the patient has been provided with necessary referrals to:
☐ social service agencies
☐ public health nurse or visiting nurse association
☐ Alcoholics Anonymous, or other support groups, if appropriate
☐ sources of information and support, such as the Epilepsy Foundation of America.

Follow-up appointments
Make sure that the necessary follow-up appointments have been scheduled and that the patient has been notified:
☐ neurologist
☐ diagnostic tests for reevaluation.

• Instruct him to check with his doctor before dieting.
• Encourage him to get sufficient sleep; excessive fatigue can precipitate a seizure.
• Stress the need to treat fever early during an illness. If the patient can't reduce a fever, he should notify the doctor.
• Teach the patient how to control stress. If appropriate, suggest learning relaxation techniques, such as deep-breathing exercises.
• Emphasize the importance of avoiding factors that may trigger a seizure, such as loud rhythmic music, video games, and television.

• Refer the patient to sources of information and support, such as the Epilepsy Foundation of America.
• Meet with family members to establish their roles in patient care.
• Advise family members about positive reinforcement techniques and about procedures to be followed during and after a seizure. Such instruction is especially important if the patient experiences generalized tonic-clonic seizures.
• Instruct the family to allow the patient to lie quietly as he recovers from a seizure.
• Tell them to reassure the patient after the seizure, to orient him to time

Assessing failure to respond to anticonvulsant therapy

If your patient fails to respond to anticonvulsant therapy, this checklist can help you evaluate the possible reasons. Consult with the patient, his family, and members of the health care team. The doctor will evaluate drug therapy if necessary.

Factors interfering with compliance

☐ Unclear instructions
☐ Failure to provide written instructions
☐ Inadequate patient teaching
☐ Memory deficits
☐ Inability to afford medication
☐ Inability to tolerate adverse effects of medication
☐ Inconvenient dosage form

Factors interfering with treatment effectiveness

☐ Insufficient drug dosage
☐ Metabolic factors, such as genetic predisposition to rapid drug metabolism
☐ Alcohol withdrawal syndrome
☐ Barbiturate withdrawal
☐ Inappropriate drug combinations
☐ Toxic blood levels of certain drugs, including aminophylline, theophylline, lidocaine, meperidine, penicillins, or cimetidine

☐ Use of drugs that may increase the risk of seizures in patients with epilepsy, including phenothiazines, tricyclic antidepressants, alprostadil, amphetamines, isoniazid, and vincristine
☐ Daily alcohol consumption exceeding 1 oz (28 g)
☐ Decreased serum albumin levels

Seizure-triggering disorders

☐ Vascular anomalies or lesions, including emboli, cerebrovascular accident, and hemorrhages
☐ Brain abscesses, tumors, or hematomas
☐ Craniocerebral trauma
☐ Acute cerebral edema
☐ Infections, such as encephalitis
☐ Degenerative disorders
☐ Cerebral anoxia
☐ Renal insufficiency causing uremia
☐ Ingestion of toxins, such as lead
☐ Electrolyte imbalances
☐ Febrile state

and place, and to inform him that he has had a seizure.
• Train the family to keep a precise written record of the seizure's onset and duration, the patient's recovery, and any memories the patient may have of feelings before, during, and after the seizure.
• If the patient has an injury, such as a bleeding tongue, instruct the family

to seek medical care immediately. (See *Ensuring continued care for the patient with epilepsy.*)

EVALUATION

When evaluating a patient's response to your nursing care, gather reassessment data and compare this information with the patient outcomes specified in your plan of care. (See *Assessing failure to respond to anticonvulsant therapy,* page 295.)

Teaching and counseling
Begin by determining the effectiveness of your teaching and counseling. Listen for statements from the patient indicating:
• an understanding of his disorder, its management, and its effects upon his lifestyle
• an understanding of the importance of drug therapy
• a willingness to adjust his behavior and activities to adapt to his condition
• an acknowledgment of his feelings of loneliness and a willingness to increase contact with others.

Also note whether or not the patient:
• complies with the prescribed medication regimen
• follows prescribed activity, exercise, and rest regimens
• wears his medical identification necklace or bracelet.

Physical condition
Physical assessment and diagnostic tests will also help to evaluate the effectiveness of care. If the treatment has been successful, your ongoing assessment should indicate that the patient:
• displays fewer physical and emotional signs of anxiety and fear, as evidenced by decreased heart and respiratory rates, blood pressure, diaphoresis, voice and limb trembling, insomnia, restlessness, irritability, impatience, angry outbursts, crying, and withdrawal
• maintains or returns to optimal neurologic status, as evidenced by adequate mentation, LOC, judgment, insight, orientation, and sensation

• remains free of injury during seizure activity.

CHAPTER 10

Caring for patients with cranial nerve disorders

Trigeminal neuralgia

Also known as tic douloureux, trigeminal neuralgia is a painful disorder of one or more branches of cranial nerve V, the trigeminal nerve. (See *Three branches of the trigeminal nerve.*) This nerve affects chewing movements and sensations of the face, scalp, and teeth. When a tender area or trigger zone is stimulated, the patient experiences paroxysmal attacks of excruciating facial pain, probably produced by an interaction or short-circuiting of the sensory fibers that relay sensations of touch and pain. Unlike other cranial nerve disorders, trigeminal neuralgia produces no motor or sensory deficits. (See *Key points about trigeminal neuralgia,* page 300.)

Causes
Although its ultimate cause remains unknown, trigeminal neuralgia may be associated with one of the following:
• an afferent reflex phenomenon located centrally in the brain stem or more peripherally in the sensory root of the trigeminal nerve
• middle fossa tumors or vascular lesions that compress the nerve root
• tortuous arteries adjacent to the nerve
• myelin deterioration
• unstable electrolyte transfer across the nerve membrane
• multiple sclerosis or herpes zoster.

ASSESSMENT

Trigeminal neuralgia may produce many symptoms, often involving eating and sleeping. Assess the patient's lifestyle and environment for factors that may trigger pain.

Health history
The patient may report searing, electrifying jolts of pain on one side of the head over the scalp, eye, cheek, or teeth. (The pain is localized in an area innervated by one or more branches of the trigeminal nerve.) Typically, she reports that the pain occurs in lightning-like jabs lasting 1 to 2 minutes. However, the pain can last for as little as a few seconds or as long as 15 minutes. At times, the severity of the pain may make talking, chewing, and swallowing very difficult. The pain may even cause difficulty sleeping.

Although attacks can occur at any time, the patient may report that they are precipitated by eating, smiling, talking, blinking, drinking hot or cold beverages, or exposure to a draft of hot or cold air. A light touch to a hypersensitive area, such as the scalp, eyebrow, eyelid, cheek, nose, or gum on the affected side, can also cause pain.

Between attacks, most patients report that they are free of pain, but some may complain of a constant, dull ache.

Usually, the patient begins to feel facial pain during her twenties and thirties. She may have developed various techniques to cope with the pain, such as favoring the affected area (splinting) and avoiding activities. (See *Complications of trigeminal neuralgia,* page 301.)

Timesaving tip: Rather than asking the patient multiple questions about her problem, which can be time-consuming, simply have her describe the characteristics of her pain.

Medication history
Determine if the patient has ever taken phenytoin, carbamazepine, or analgesics to control neuralgic pain. If she has, note how often she takes the

Three branches of the trigeminal nerve

The trigeminal nerve (cranial nerve V) innervates the face through the ophthalmic, maxillary, and mandibular branches.

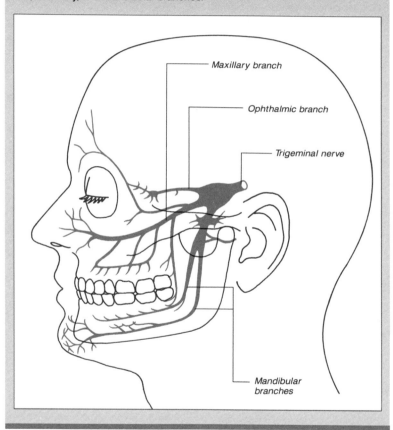

Maxillary branch

Ophthalmic branch

Trigeminal nerve

Mandibular branches

drug, the dosages, and the effects. Note how long she has been taking phenytoin or carbamazepine because their effectiveness wanes over time. If the patient has stopped taking the medication, ask why.

Physical examination
You should notice no loss of sensory or motor function. (See *Testing for pain and sensory dysfunction,* page 302.) If a sensory abnormality is found, it suggests a disorder other than trigeminal neuralgia. The pa-

Key points about trigeminal neuralgia

- *Incidence:* Idiopathic trigeminal neuralgia affects approximately 15,000 adults per year. It strikes mostly those over age 40 (about 25% more women than men), and it develops in the right side of the face more often than in the left side.
- *Patterns and prognosis:* Symptoms may worsen during the spring and fall. The frequency of attacks varies greatly, from almost continual pain to attacks occurring several times a month or year. The attacks can subside spontaneously, with remissions lasting from several months to years. The patient may fear her next attack and limit her activities to prevent pain. As she ages, the attacks may last longer and become more severe.

tient may have a neoplasm or other lesion impinging on cranial nerves other than cranial nerve V.

On inspection, you may observe splinting. If you witness a painful attack, you may notice that the patient holds her face immobile, abruptly stops talking, or attempts to shield her face with her hand to ward off the attack. She may also quickly draw away from the jablike pain, suggesting a tic. The affected side of the face may be unwashed and, in male patients, unshaven. When asked where the pain occurs, the patient typically points to — but avoids touching — the affected area.

Timesaving tip: Perform two tasks at once by inspecting the patient for facial abnormalities while eliciting her history.

Diagnostic test results

The diagnosis primarily hinges on the patient's history and clinical signs. A computed tomography scan and magnetic resonance imaging may be performed to rule out sinus or tooth infections and space-occupying lesions.

NURSING DIAGNOSIS

Common nursing diagnoses for a patient with trigeminal neuralgia include:
- Pain related to stimulation of a trigger zone
- Fear related to recurring attacks of pain
- Powerlessness related to inability to control attacks.

PLANNING

Based on the nursing diagnosis *pain,* develop appropriate patient outcomes. For example, your patient will:
- learn how to avoid stimulation of trigger zones
- express relief after taking prescribed pain medication
- express long-term relief from pain following alcohol injection or other procedure.

Based on the nursing diagnosis *fear,* develop appropriate patient outcomes. For example, your patient will:
- communicate feelings of fear
- join a support group to help reduce fear
- show no physical signs of fear.

Based on the nursing diagnosis *powerlessness,* develop appropriate

patient outcomes. For example, your patient will:
• describe feelings of powerlessness
• identify measures that can relieve attacks, such as taking medications and avoiding stimulation of trigger zones
• make decisions about her course of treatment.

IMPLEMENTATION

Nursing interventions include helping the patient cope effectively with pain. If medications are prescribed, watch for efficacy and possible adverse reactions. Help the patient maintain a balanced diet and achieve emotional well-being through self-care and an active lifestyle. (See *Medical care of the patient with trigeminal neuralgia,* pages 303 and 304.)

Nursing interventions
• Provide emotional support. Help the patient communicate her pain clearly, and provide feedback to indicate that you understand.
• Promote independence through self-care and physical activity.
• Encourage the patient to stay active and to allow time for rest. Explain that this will improve her sense of well-being and help her cope with the pain.
• Establish and document a baseline neurologic status.
• Monitor neurologic status, including mentation, level of consciousness, judgment, orientation, and sensation.
• Explore therapy choices with the patient, and note her responses to treatment.
• Observe and record the characteristics of each attack, including the patient's protective mechanisms.
• If brushing the teeth is painful, suggest trying a water-powered dental

---

Complications of trigeminal neuralgia

The pain associated with trigeminal neuralgia may be so incapacitating that the patient fails to care for herself properly, leading to the following complications:
• excessive weight loss
• poor hygiene
• depression
• physical inactivity
• social isolation.

Postoperative complications
A patient who undergoes surgery for trigeminal neuralgia may experience damage to cranial nerve V or VII during the procedure, which may lead to paresthesia or paralysis in portions of the face or jaw or loss of feeling or tearing in the affected eye. Such a patient may experience corneal or buccal lacerations or dental caries without being aware of it.

---

device, which will reduce jaw movement.
• Encourage the patient to wash her face without a washcloth, or to wash using soft touches and straight motions instead of tension-causing circular motions.
• Suggest tub baths if the patient can't tolerate showers.
• Provide adequate nutrition in small, frequent meals served at room temperature.
• If poor appetite due to pain is causing the patient to lose weight, help her plan a balanced diet that requires minimal chewing. Suggest that she puree foods and eat soft or liquid

Assessment TimeSaver

Testing for pain and sensory dysfunction

Use the following techniques when assessing the location and degree of the patient's trigeminal neuralgia.

Pain test
Have the patient open and clench her jaw and perform chewing and swallowing motions. These motions may cause pain and reveal the pattern of facial pain, thereby enabling you to better identify the involved branch of the trigeminal nerve.

Sensory tests
Perform sensory tests by lightly touching a wisp of cotton to the cornea or by touching or pricking the eyelids, forehead, nose, teeth, tongue, and facial skin. Sensation should be intact in true trigeminal neuralgia. If the patient wears contact lenses, her cornea may be less sensitive to touch.

To assess temperature sensation of the facial skin, fill one test tube with hot water and one with ice and then lightly touch each to the patient's face bilaterally. The patient should be able to discriminate between hot and cold sensations on both sides of the face.

If testing causes pain, allow the patient to rest before proceeding.

procedure and postoperative treatment. Counsel her to review her options with the doctor and to ask about potential complications, such as facial numbness and paralysis.

• Provide postoperative care, including fluid, respiratory, pain, and neurologic management.

• After any neurosurgical procedure, check neurologic and vital signs frequently.

• After any neurosurgical procedure that may cause facial paralysis or paresthesia, check the buccal cavity for cuts and use mouth rinses if necessary. Inspect the eyes for redness and conjunctival erythema, which should be reported to the doctor.

Patient teaching
• Teach the patient about trigeminal neuralgia's symptoms and its usual progression. Discuss the procedures and treatments as they occur, as well as any possible complications.

• Show the patient how to ward off neuralgic attacks. For example, remind her to protect trigger zones from wind and cold by wearing a scarf or turning up her coat collar.

• Teach the patient about her medications. Be sure that she understands the desired effects and knows which adverse effects to report.

• Following surgery, teach the patient appropriate eye care.

• Instruct the patient to comply with ongoing outpatient therapy, doctor visits, and routine visits to the dentist. (See *Ensuring continued care for the patient with trigeminal neuralgia,* page 305.)

foods, such as soups, custards, and stews. If necessary, consult a nutritionist.

• Monitor for adverse reactions to drug therapy.

• If the patient plans to undergo a craniotomy, carefully explain the

EVALUATION

When evaluating a patient's response to your nursing care, gather reassessment data and compare this information with the patient outcomes speci-

Treatments

Medical care of the patient with trigeminal neuralgia

Treatment of trigeminal neuralgia may include drug therapy, nerve blocking, and surgery.

Drug therapy
Oral administration of carbamazepine or phenytoin may temporarily relieve pain by reducing the transmission of nerve impulses at affected nerve terminals. Although these drugs benefit some patients, their adverse effects are numerous and serious. Narcotic analgesics may also be helpful.

Nerve blocking
When medications fail or attacks become increasingly frequent or severe, nerve blocks (avulsions) are performed. This procedure involves blocking one or more of the branches of the trigeminal nerve or blocking the gasserian ganglion by injecting a nerve-blocking anesthetic. This results in loss of sensation in some portions of the face. Either procedure may provide long-lasting relief.

Alcohol injection
Alcohol injection into the nerve branches through the infraorbital foramen located near to the junction of the nose and cheek, and through the supraorbital notch located in the eyebrow, has been very successful. The procedure is performed under local anesthesia so that the patient may assist in identifying the affected branches. Alcohol injections may provide relief for 8 to 16 months, but the nerve eventually regenerates, so the injections may need to be repeated.

Complications include regeneration of pain impulses and, with recurrent injections, scar tissue formation and more pain.

Blocking the gasserian ganglion may provide more permanent relief from pain. Complications include extraocular palsies, keratitis, blindness, and masticatory paralysis.

Glycerol injection
In this procedure, small amounts of glycerol are injected percutaneously into the subarachnoid spaces surrounding the gasserian ganglion. Glycerol injection provides some relief of trigeminal neuralgia with fewer adverse effects.

Surgery
Surgical alternatives include open surgical retrogasserian rhizotomy, decompression of the sensory root, vascular decompression of the trigeminal nerve, and electrocoagulation.

Open surgical retrogasserian rhizotomy
In this surgical procedure, a craniotomy is performed and part of the sensory root of the trigeminal nerve is severed. Complications include paresthesia, anesthesia dolorosa, facial paralysis, corneal ulceration, keratitis, extraocular palsies, hemiparesis, and aphasia.

Decompression of the sensory root
Cutting the dural sheath and root surrounding the gasserian ganglion produces decompression of the intact

(continued)

Treatments

Medical care of the patient with trigeminal neuralgia *(continued)*

nerve. This results in the relief of pain without loss of feeling or sensation. Complications include recurrent pain and injury to the facial nerve or temporal lobe.

Vascular decompression of the trigeminal nerve
If vascular compression of the trigeminal nerve is believed to be the cause of pain, a small craniotomy in which the artery is resected away from the trigeminal nerve is performed. This microsurgical procedure requires the same extensive postoperative management as any craniotomy. The advantage of this procedure is that normal sensation in the face may be preserved. Complications include headache, persistent facial pain, and postsurgical deficits.

Electrocoagulation
Performed under local anesthesia (small doses of I.V. diazepam and fentanyl), percutaneous electrocoagulation of nerve rootlets and percutaneous radio frequency rhizotomy cause partial root destruction, which relieves pain but doesn't compromise the sense of touch or motor function. One to three treatments are usually necessary. These procedures cause partial numbness of the face and the patient may be unable to wear contact lenses or sense food between the cheek and gums. The major complication is anesthesia dolorosa.

fied in your plan of care. Consider the level and frequency of the patient's pain and how the pain affects the patient's emotional well-being and diet.

Teaching and counseling
Talk to the patient to determine the effectiveness of teaching and counseling. Consider the following questions:
• Does the patient report any pain relief?
• Can she describe treatment alternatives and list their advantages and disadvantages?
• Can she explain the medications prescribed and identify the adverse effects that necessitate calling the doctor?

• Does she use support systems and stress reduction techniques to manage anxiety?
• Does she function at optimal self-care and activity levels?
• Does she know what triggers painful attacks, and can she help ward them off and respond constructively if they do occur?
• Does she take steps to maintain health and hygiene, including washing her face, performing water-powered dental cleansing, eating small frequent meals, and protecting trigger zones?
• Does she express a reduction in, and display fewer signs of, fear?

Discharge TimeSaver

Ensuring continued care for the patient with trigeminal neuralgia

Review the following teaching topics, referrals, and follow-up appointments to make sure that your patient is adequately prepared for discharge.

Teaching topics
Make sure that the following topics have been covered and that your patient's learning has been evaluated:
☐ explanation of trigeminal neuralgia, including its cause, management, and treatment
☐ prescribed medications, including possible adverse effects, precautions, and the need for compliance with therapy
☐ activity and rest guidelines
☐ need for a well-balanced diet
☐ sources of information and support.

Referrals
Make sure that the patient has been provided with necessary referrals to:

☐ nutritionist
☐ social worker
☐ home health care nurse or visiting nurse association
☐ support groups for people with chronic pain or depression.

Follow-up appointments
Make sure that the necessary follow-up appointments have been scheduled and that the patient has been notified:
☐ doctor
☐ neurosurgeon
☐ complete blood count and liver function tests for patients receiving drug therapy.

Physical condition
Evaluate the patient's adherence to treatment and medical regimens, and consider the following questions:
• Does the patient maintain stable vital signs and neurologic status?
• Does she maintain a stable nutritional status and adequate hydration?
• Is she within 5 lb (2.3 kg) of her baseline weight?

Bell's palsy

In this idiopathic facial paralysis, impulses from cranial nerve VII — the nerve responsible for motor innervation of the facial muscles — are blocked. This blockage causes unilateral facial weakness or paralysis. (See *Facial paralysis in Bell's palsy,* page 306.) The blockage apparently results from inflammation around the nerve (usually at the internal auditory meatus). In most instances, the condition isn't permanent — spontaneous recovery usually occurs within several weeks.

Causes
The causes of Bell's palsy aren't known. Ischemia, viral diseases such as herpes simplex or herpes zoster, local traumatic injury, or an autoimmune disease may be involved. (See *Key points about Bell's palsy,* page 307.)

Facial paralysis in Bell's palsy

Unilateral facial paralysis characterizes Bell's palsy. The paralysis distorts the patient's appearance, and he may be unable to wrinkle his forehead, close his eyelid, show his teeth, or puff out his cheek.

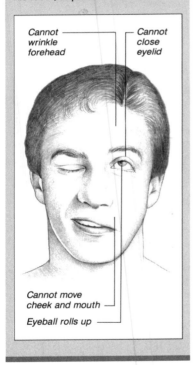

Cannot wrinkle forehead

Cannot close eyelid

Cannot move cheek and mouth

Eyeball rolls up

ASSESSMENT

Note carefully the patient's descriptions of the onset of his symptoms, which can begin up to several days before facial weakness. Be aware that other conditions, such as upper motor neuron lesions, have similar, but not identical, symptoms.

Health history

The patient may have pain on the affected side around his jaw or behind the ear for a few hours or days before the onset of weakness. Initially, he may feel a pulling sensation of the skin on the affected side and then numbness as the paralysis develops. Relaxation of the facial muscles may cause difficulty eating, and taste perception may be distorted over the affected anterior two-thirds of the tongue. Some patients report an aching pain behind the affected eye.

Involuntary contractions of the facial muscles — for example, wincing in response to pain — may be normal, whereas voluntary contractions, such as retracting the corner of the mouth, may be weak or absent.

Timesaving tip: To quickly test cranial nerve VII, ask the patient to smile, wrinkle his forehead, puff out his cheeks, and close his eyes. The patient with Bell's palsy may be unable to perform these tasks. In patients with upper motor neuron lesions, such as tumors, abscesses, or depressed skull fractures, upper motor neuron paralysis is usually incomplete. The patient can raise both eyebrows and wrinkle his forehead.

If the patient reports a visual field deficit — the loss of vision in a portion of each eye's field of view — suspect cerebrovascular disease rather than Bell's palsy. Also suspect cerebrovascular disease if the patient has a history of hypertension. A history of other neurologic symptoms that may relate to a brain tumor or a past history of cancer suggests the presence of lesions that mimic symptoms.

Medication history

Determine if the patient has ever had an anaphylactic reaction to any drug or if he has a history of cocaine or crack use. Both may be responsible for causing an ischemic event. Also ask if he's currently taking an antihypertensive medication. To avoid adverse drug interactions with any new medications, note the amounts of any medications the patient may be taking as well as how often he takes them.

Physical examination

The affected side of the patient's face is masklike and sags. His mouth may droop on the affected side, allowing saliva to drool from the corner. He may not be able to smile, whistle, or grimace. His eye doesn't close, tears constantly, and rolls upward (Bell's phenomenon) with any attempt to close it. (Bell's phenomenon is actually a normal occurrence but isn't usually noticed because of complete lid closure.) The patient may have difficulty speaking clearly because of facial muscle relaxation, and his sense of taste may be affected.

Diagnostic test results

• Electromyography 10 days after the onset of symptoms can indicate denervation and imply a prolonged, possibly incomplete recovery.
• Magnetic resonance imaging or a computed tomography scan may rule out compression of the nerve by a lesion, tumor, or other agent.

NURSING DIAGNOSIS

Common nursing diagnoses for a patient with Bell's palsy include:
• Body image disturbance related to unilateral facial paralysis
• High risk for injury related to inability to close affected eyelid

FactFinder
Key points about Bell's palsy

• *Incidence:* Bell's palsy strikes both sexes almost equally and all age-groups, but mostly those between ages 20 and 60. Its onset is rapid. Any or all of the three branches of cranial nerve VII may be affected, resulting in bilateral facial paralysis or the more common unilateral paralysis.
• *Complications:* The patient is at risk for corneal ulceration and blindness (because his eye won't close), impaired nutrition secondary to paralysis of the lower face, long-term psychosocial problems secondary to his altered body image, and permanent facial paralysis.
• *Prognosis and recovery:* In 80% to 90% of patients, the disorder subsides spontaneously and completely in 1 to 8 weeks, although maximum recovery may not occur until 1 year after the episode. Older patients may take longer to recover. The disorder may recur on the same or the opposite side of the face. If recovery is partial, contractures may develop on the paralyzed side of the face.

• Altered nutrition: Less than body requirements, related to eating difficulties caused by facial muscle paralysis.

PLANNING

Direct your nursing care toward managing drug therapy, encouraging the patient to experience and express positive feelings about himself, providing teaching on proper eye care and how to avoid injury, and ensuring that the patient doesn't suffer weight loss.

Based on the nursing diagnosis *body image disturbance,* develop appropriate patient outcomes. For example, your patient will:
• discuss concerns about facial appearance
• demonstrate the ability to practice two new coping behaviors
• express positive feelings about himself.

Based on the nursing diagnosis *high risk for injury,* develop appropriate patient outcomes. For example, your patient will:
• understand and comply with the prescribed eye care regimen
• protect the affected eye from injury.

Based on the nursing diagnosis *altered nutrition: less than body requirements,* develop appropriate patient outcomes. For example, your patient will:
• maintain body weight within 5 lb (2.3 kg) of baseline
• show no signs or symptoms of malnutrition
• maintain a daily balanced diet.

IMPLEMENTATION

Nursing interventions include helping the patient manage with his temporary impairment and cope with his changed body image. (See *Medical care of the patient with Bell's palsy.*)

Nursing interventions
• Work with the patient to develop a consistent vocabulary that describes his pain.
• Establish and document a baseline neurologic status.
• Monitor neurologic status, including mentation, level of consciousness, judgment, insight, orientation, and sensation.

• Document variations from the baseline neurologic status.
• Assess eyes for muscle paralysis, dryness, or excessive tearing to determine the degree of eye impairment.
• Determine the patient's ability to chew and swallow to assess the extent of facial paralysis.
• Provide psychological support for the patient, reassuring him that he has not had a stroke.
• To help relieve his anxiety about his appearance, inform him that spontaneous recovery usually occurs within 8 weeks.
• During treatment with prednisone, watch for adverse reactions, especially GI distress and fluid retention. An antacid given concomitantly usually provides relief from GI distress. Cimetidine or ranitidine may also be prescribed. Prednisone is used cautiously in patients with diabetes mellitus; monitor their serum glucose levels frequently.
• Apply moist heat to the patient's face to reduce pain, being careful not to burn him.
• Administer pain medications as prescribed.
• Use prescribed eye lubricants every 1 to 2 hours to prevent corneal damage.
• Massage the patient's face with a gentle upward motion two to three times daily for 5 to 10 minutes to help maintain muscle tone and alleviate pain.
• As muscle tone returns, encourage facial exercises, such as wrinkling the brow, tightly shutting the eyes, whistling, and puffing out the cheeks several times daily for 5 to 10 minutes.
• Apply a facial sling to support the sagging face, as ordered.
• Provide a soft, balanced diet, eliminating hot foods and fluids. Consult a nutritionist if necessary.

- Arrange for privacy at mealtimes to reduce embarrassment.
- If surgery is necessary (usually only when Bell's palsy is associated with other disorders), provide the patient with complete preoperative and postoperative care.

Patient teaching
- Teach the patient about the symptoms of Bell's palsy and treatment plans and goals.
- Advise the patient to cover his affected eye with an eye patch, especially when outdoors, and to avoid rubbing it. Tell him to keep warm and avoid exposure to dust and wind.
- Teach him how to inspect the cornea for irritation.
- Explain to the patient that applying moist heat to his face will help to reduce the pain. Warn him to be careful not to burn himself.
- Instruct the patient to massage his face with a gentle upward motion two to three times daily for 5 to 10 minutes.
- When the patient is ready to exercise the facial muscles, teach him to grimace in front of a mirror, wrinkle his forehead, tightly close his eyes and keep them closed, whistle, and puff out his cheeks.
- Help the patient cope with eating and drinking difficulties.
- Instruct him to chew on the unaffected side of his mouth and to eat semisolid foods.
- Instruct the patient to perform complete mouth care, taking special care to remove residual food that collects between the cheek and gums.
- Give the patient complete information about his medications. (See *Ensuring continued care for the patient with Bell's palsy*, page 310.)

Treatments
Medical care of the patient with Bell's palsy

Medical treatment for the patient with Bell's palsy includes drug therapy, supportive care and, in rare cases, surgery.

Drug therapy
Prednisone, an oral corticosteroid, reduces facial nerve edema and improves nerve conduction and blood flow. Prednisone treatment is especially helpful when begun in the first week after the disorder's onset. After 14 days of prednisone therapy, electrotherapy may help prevent facial muscle atrophy.

Supportive therapy
Analgesics, such as salicylates or codeine, control facial pain and discomfort. Moist heat on the affected side may provide comfort. Eye lubricants or salves can protect and lubricate the affected eye.

Surgery
If the patient fails to recover from facial paralysis and a lesion can be demonstrated through diagnostic tests, decompression surgery or exploratory surgery of the facial nerve may be necessary.

EVALUATION

When evaluating a patient's response to your nursing care, gather reassessment data and compare this information with the patient outcomes specified in your plan of care. Consider the level and frequency of the patient's pain and how the pain affects his

Discharge TimeSaver

Ensuring continued care for the patient with Bell's palsy

Review the following teaching topics, referrals, and follow-up appointments to ensure that your patient is adequately prepared for discharge.

Teaching topics
Make sure that the following topics have been covered and that your patient's learning has been evaluated:
□ explanation of Bell's palsy and its causes, management, and treatment
□ prescribed medications, including possible adverse effects, precautions, and the need for compliance
□ activity and rest guidelines
□ need for continuing eye and mouth care
□ importance and methods of facial exercises, heat applications, facial sling, and massage
□ sources of information and support.

Referrals
Make sure that the patient has been provided with necessary referrals to:
□ dietitian
□ otolaryngologist
□ support group
□ speech therapist, if necessary.

Follow-up appointments
Make sure that the necessary follow-up appointments have been scheduled and that the patient has been notified:
□ doctor
□ additional diagnostic tests (if condition persists).

emotional well-being and diet. Also be aware of the patient's self-image.

Teaching and counseling
Talk to the patient to determine the effectiveness of teaching and counseling. Consider the following questions:
• Does the patient comply with treatment measures, such as using a facial sling, heat, massage, and facial exercises?
• Can he provide adequate self-care to his affected eye, gums, and teeth?
• Does he chew food on the unaffected side of his mouth?
• Can he accurately describe his disorder, medications, and treatments?

Physical condition
Evaluate the patient's adherence to treatment and medical regimens, and consider the following questions:
• Does the patient report adequate pain relief with medication?
• Does he display minimal signs and symptoms of discomfort?
• Does he maintain or return to optimal neurologic status, including mentation, level of consciousness, judgment, insight, orientation, and sensation?
• Does he maintain his body weight within 5 lb (2.3 kg) of baseline?
• Does he maintain adequate hydration as determined by tissue turgor and moisture of mucous membranes?

Appendices and index

Quick reference to neurologic treatments

Carotid endarterectomy

In this procedure, a surgeon removes atherosclerotic plaque from the internal or external carotid arteries or the common carotid artery. Accumulation of plaque can reduce cerebral blood flow, thereby causing transient ischemic attacks or a cerebrovascular accident.

First, the surgeon heparinizes the artery, and clamps it above and below the obstruction. Then he makes a small incision to open the artery and remove the plaque. Depending on the artery's condition, the surgeon will suture it closed or patch it with an autologous vein or Gore-tex graft. Next, he removes the clamps, sutures the neck incision, and applies a sterile dressing.

Indications
• Transient ischemic attacks
• Asymptomatic carotid bruit (controversial)

Complications
• Hypotension or hypertension
• Airway obstruction
• Infection
• Cerebral infarction
• Cardiac arrhythmias
• Damage to cranial nerves VII, X, XI, and XII
• Vocal cord paralysis

Cerebrospinal fluid drainage

Cerebrospinal fluid (CSF) drainage is used to manage increased intracranial pressure (ICP) and to promote spinal or cerebral dural healing after a traumatic injury or surgery. The drain may withdraw fluid from the lateral ventricle (ventriculostomy) or the lumbar subarachnoid space.

A catheter drains CSF into a sterile, closed collection system. Placement of a *ventricular drain* may take place at the bedside with the patient under local anesthesia or in the operating room with the patient under general anesthesia. The doctor inserts a ventricular catheter through a burr hole in the patient's skull and dural lining and into the ventricle. Its distal end is connected to a closed drainage system.

To place a *lumbar subarachnoid drain,* the doctor may administer a local spinal anesthetic at the bedside or in the operating room before suturing the drain in place or taping it externally. He places the catheter beneath the dura into the L3-L4 interspace and connects its distal end to a closed drainage system.

Indications
• ICP monitoring
• Instillation of drugs or contrast media directly into the subarachnoid space (done only by a doctor)
• Aspiration of CSF for laboratory analysis; the specimen is usually taken from the catheter or collection bag.

Complications
• Excessive CSF drainage
• Clots in the catheter or ventriculostomy tube
• Increased ICP
• Infection

Craniotomy

In this procedure, a neurosurgeon makes an incision into the skull, thereby exposing the brain before performing brain surgery.

After the patient receives a general anesthetic, the surgeon marks an incision line and cuts through the scalp to the cranium, forming a scalp flap that he turns to one side. Then he bores two or more holes through the skull in the corners of the cranial incision, using an air-driven or electric drill, and cuts out a bone flap with a small saw. After pulling aside or removing the bone flap, he incises and retracts the dura, exposing the brain.

The surgeon may insert a Jackson-Pratt drain to remove or prevent any fluid accumulation under the scalp. Then, he reverses the incision procedure, covers the site with a sterile dressing, and wraps the patient's head with a turban-style dressing.

Indications
• Ventricular shunting
• Excision of a tumor, abscess, hematoma, or aspiration
• Aneurysm clipping
• Excision of an arteriovenous malformation
• Treatment of hydrocephalus
• Repair of cerebral injury

Complications
These depend largely on the patient's condition and complexity of surgery.
• Infection
• Hemorrhage
• Respiratory compromise
• Increased ICP
• Meningitis
• Diabetes insipidus
• Seizures
• Vasospasm
• Syndrome of inappropriate secretion of antidiuretic hormone
• Hydrocephalus
• Cerebral infarction

Halo device

This device provides skeletal immobilization for treatment of cervical injuries. It allows the patient some mobility, with minimal risk of disturbing his spinal alignment during position changes. To apply a halo device, the doctor places an adjustable stainless steel hoop around the patient's head and secures it to his skull with two occipital and two temporal screws. Steel bars anchor the brace on the patient's shoulders, which are protected by a padded, sheepskin-lined vest, ensuring that

alignment and traction can be maintained without ropes or weights.

Halo devices are generally made of graphite so that the patient may undergo MRI.

Indications
• Cervical injury

Complications
• Infection
• Osteoporosis

Laminectomy

In this procedure, the surgeon removes one or more of the bony laminae that cover the vertebrae. Laminectomy may be performed in the cervical, lumbar, or thoracic areas.

During laminectomy, the patient is placed in a prone, side-lying, or knee-to-chest position and is given general anesthesia. The surgeon makes a midline incision and then retracts the paravertebral muscles. Next, he removes portions of one or two laminae and their attached ligamentum flavum.

Indications
• Trauma to the spine that causes spinal cord compression
• Removal of spinal cord tumors or abscess
• Intolerable pain
• Removal of herniated intervertebral disks
• Progressive loss of motor and sensory function

Complications
• Infection
• Cerebrospinal fistula
• Urine retention and paralytic ileus (after a lumbar laminectomy)
• Nerve root damage (may cause paralysis of upper or lower extremities)
• Hematoma at the operative site
• Vocal cord paralysis and respiratory depression (after an anterior cervical diskectomy)

Ommaya reservoir

This mushroom-shaped device is used to administer medications directly into the CSF, to measure ICP, or to sample CSF. It consists of a catheter inserted through a burr hole into the lateral ventricle of the brain and a self-sealing silicone injection dome (reservoir) that rests over the burr hole, just under the scalp, and causes a small bulge.

The Ommaya reservoir is inserted in the operating room. After the surgeon evaluates ventricular size using a computed tomography (CT) scan, he makes an incision in the patient's right frontal region. Then he tunnels a subgaleal pocket and places the reservoir in it. Next, he drills a burr hole just anterior to the coronal suture, cauterizes the dura mater, and opens it to allow catheter insertion. Then he cauterizes the pia mater, opens the cortex, and introduces the catheter with its stylet into the nondominant frontal horn. He positions the catheter at the foramen of Monro and confirms its position by X-ray. Finally, he connects the catheter to the reservoir, sutures the system to the edge of the burr hole, and closes the wound.

A pressure dressing remains in place for 24 hours, then a gauze dressing for 1 or 2 days. The reservoir can usually be used by the third postoperative day.

Indications
- Measurement of ICP
- Tumor or cyst drainage
- Administration of medications directly into the CSF
- CSF sampling

Complications
- Infection
- Catheter migration or blockage
- Inadvertent injection of local anesthetic into the CSF (can cause spinal block)

Plasmapheresis

This treatment removes plasma from withdrawn blood and reinfuses formed blood elements, thereby helping to clean the blood of harmful substances and disease mediators, such as immune complexes and autoantibodies.

During plasmapheresis, a double-lumen catheter is inserted for the duration of treatment. In patients requiring long-term, frequent plasmapheresis, such as those with myasthenia gravis, an anteriovenous shunt may be used. Blood is removed from the patient through two large intravenous needles, usually in the antecubital veins, and flows into a cell separator (where it's divided into plasma and formed elements) at a rate of 40 to 60 ml/minute. The plasma is collected in a container for disposal, while the formed elements are mixed with a plasma replacement solution and returned to the patient through a vein. In a newer method of plasmapheresis, the plasma is separated out, filtered to remove a specific disease mediator, and then returned to the patient.

Both methods may be performed on an inpatient or outpatient basis. Plasmapheresis requires a doctor's supervision. A specially trained technician or nurse operates the cell separator and a primary nurse monitors the patient and provides supportive care.

Indications
- Guillain-Barré syndrome
- Multiple sclerosis
- Myasthenia gravis

Complications
- Hypersensitivity to replacement solution
- Hypocalcemia (from excessive binding of circulating calcium to the citrate solution used as an anticoagulant in the replacement solution)
- Hypomagnesemia
- Hypotension
- Hypokalemia
- Prolonged bleeding

- Air embolism
- Anemia
- Infection

Radiation therapy

This therapy delivers high-speed electrons, which are converted into X-rays, to neoplastic cells. It aims to alter the membranes of rapidly dividing cancer cells and destroy them, while minimizing damage to normal cells.

Radiation can be delivered externally via X-rays or internally. Internal radiation is delivered locally into the tissues surrounding the tumor or into the tumor itself (using the interstitial approach) or is systemically delivered into a hollow body cavity (using the intracavitary approach).

Indications
- Inoperable brain or spinal cord tumor
- Preoperatively to shrink a tumor
- Postoperatively to eradicate neoplastic cells undetected during surgery

Complications
These usually reflect the radiation dosage, the number of treatments, and the type of tissue and area treated.
- Headache
- Mucositis
- Pharyngitis
- Decreased salivation and taste sensation
- Erythema
- Desquamation
- Epilation
- Cranial nerve damage

Skull tongs

Skull tongs immobilize the spine and maintain vertebral alignment, preventing spinal cord damage from unstable bone fragments or misaligned vertebrae. When placing tongs, the doctor first shaves the patient's hair above the ears, cleans the area, and administers a local anesthetic. He then gently advances spring-loaded pins attached to the tongs into the patient's skull. After tightening the tongs to secure the apparatus, he creates traction by extending a rope with weights attached at one end from the center of the tongs over a pulley. Traction is usually attached to a Roto Rest bed or Stryker frame.

Graphite tongs are generally used so magnetic resonance imaging (MRI) may be performed without complications. Gardner-Wells (metal) tongs are not compatible with MRI because the metal is drawn to the MRI magnet.

When caring for a patient with skull tongs, provide meticulous care of the pin sites. Check the traction apparatus often to make sure it's working properly. If the tongs become loosened or dislodged, immobilize the patient's head with sandbags on each side and notify a doctor.

Indications
- Stabilization of the cervical spine after a fracture or dislocation, invasion by tumor or infection, or surgery

Complications
- Infection
- Excessive traction force
- Osteoporosis
Note: All of these complications can cause skull pins to slip or pull out.

Stereotactic surgery

This surgery is usually performed to facilitate biopsy or to place a catheter for delivering radiation seeds in tumor bed radiation. It allows the neurosurgeon to determine the precise location of a lesion that's thought to be inoperable.

The surgeon first attaches a stereotactic frame, with well-defined reference points, to the patient's head. He then performs a CT scan to locate the lesion; a computer calculates the exact location of the lesion with respect to the reference points. The surgeon then marks this point on the patient's scalp. After administration of a local anesthetic and, if appropriate, a sedative, the surgeon drills a burr hole in the patient's skull to expose the dura.

Indications
- Brain tumor biopsy
- Radiotherapeutic device insertion

Complications
- Bleeding into brain or above dura that results in increased ICP
- Infection
- Hemorrhage
- Meningitis

Transcutaneous electrical nerve stimulation

In this procedure, a mild electrical current is used to stimulate nerve fibers to block the transmission of pain impulses to the brain. The transcutaneous electrical nerve stimulation (TENS) unit consists of a portable, battery-powered generator that sends the current through electrodes placed relative to the pain loci.

Indications
- Pain management

Complications
- Pruritus
- Electrical burns (caused by improper electrode placement)

Ventricular shunting

During this procedure, the surgeon inserts a catheter into the patient's ventricular system to drain CSF into the peritoneal sac or another body space for absorption. The shunt extends from one of the cerebral ventricles to the scalp, where it's tunneled under the skin to the appropriate cavity. By draining excessive CSF or relieving blockage, shunting can lower ICP and prevent brain damage caused by persistently elevated ICP.

To implant a ventricular shunt, the surgeon must perform a craniotomy. To implant a *ventriculoperitoneal shunt,*

he performs the craniotomy, then inserts a catheter into the ventricular system through a lateral ventricle. He tunnels the distal end of the catheter through subcutaneous tissue to a point below the diaphragm and inserts it into the peritoneal sac for CSF drainage.

For a *ventriculoatrial* shunt, he runs the catheter from the ventricle through the jugular vein to the right atrium. In a *third ventriculostomy,* he elevates the frontal lobe to expose the third ventricle for catheter insertion. Then he passes the other end of the catheter into the cisterna chiasmatis of the subarachnoid space.

The *ventriculocisternal* shunt doesn't require a craniotomy; the surgeon drills a small burr hole in the occipital region. He then inserts a catheter into a lateral ventricle and passes it under the dura and into the cisterna magna.

Indications
- Communicating hydrocephalus (excessive accumulation of CSF in the subarachnoid space)
- Noncommunicating hydrocephalus (blockage of normal CSF flow from the lateral ventricles to the subarachnoid space)

Complications
- Infection
- Ventricular collapse
- Blocked, kinked, or displaced shunt, which may cause an increased ICP from excess CSF accumulation

Quick reference to neurologic drugs

amantadine hydrochloride

General
Brand names: Symadine, Symmetrel
Pharmacologic classification: synthetic cyclic primary amine
Therapeutic classification: antiviral, antiparkinsonian agent

Indications and dosage
• Drug-induced extrapyramidal reactions. *Adults:* 100 mg P.O. b.i.d., up to 300 mg daily in divided doses. Patient may benefit from as much as 400 mg daily, but dosages over 200 mg must be closely supervised.
• Idiopathic parkinsonism; parkinsonian syndrome. *Adults:* 100 mg P.O. b.i.d.; in patients who are seriously ill or receiving other antiparkinsonian agents, 100 mg daily for at least 1 week, then 100 mg b.i.d., p.r.n.

Adverse reactions
CNS: depression, fatigue, confusion, dizziness, psychosis, hallucinations, anxiety, *irritability,* ataxia, *insomnia,* weakness, headache, light-headedness, difficulty concentrating
CV: peripheral edema, orthostatic hypotension, *CHF*
GI: anorexia, nausea, constipation, vomiting, dry mouth
GU: urine retention
Skin: *livedo reticularis* (with long use)

ambenonium chloride

General
Brand name: Mytelase
Pharmacologic classification: cholinesterase inhibitor
Therapeutic classification: antimyasthenic

Indications and dosage
• Symptomatic treatment of myasthenia gravis in patients who can't take neostigmine bromide or pyridostigmine bromide. *Adults:* Dosage usually ranges from 5 to 25 mg P.O. t.i.d. to q.i.d. Starting dose usually is 5 mg t.i.d. to q.i.d. Increase gradually and adjust at 1- to 2-day intervals to avoid drug accumulation and overdosage. Usual range is 15 to 100 mg daily, but some patients may require as much as 75 mg b.i.d. to q.i.d.

Adverse reactions
CNS: headache, dizziness, muscle weakness, incoordination, confusion, jitters, sweating
CV: bradycardia, hypotension
EENT: miosis, blurred vision
GI: *nausea, vomiting, diarrhea, abdominal cramps,* increased salivation
GU: urinary frequency, incontinence
Other: ***bronchospasm,*** *muscle cramps,* ***bronchoconstriction,*** increased bronchial secretions, ***respiratory paralysis***

aspirin
(acetylsalicylic acid)

General
Brand names: Bayer Aspirin, Ecotrin
Pharmacologic classification: salicylate
Therapeutic classification: antiplatelet agent, nonnarcotic analgesic, anti-inflammatory agent

Indications and dosage
• Reduction of the risk of transient ischemic attacks (TIAs) and cerebrovascular accident (CVA) in patients with TIAs. *Adults:* 325 mg P.O. q.i.d. or 650 mg b.i.d.

Adverse reactions
Blood: *prolonged bleeding time*

Common adverse reactions in *italics;* life-threatening, in ***bold italics.***

EENT: *tinnitus and hearing loss*
GI: *nausea, vomiting, GI distress, occult bleeding*
GU: albuminuria, decreased glomerular filtration rate (GFR), analgesic nephropathy
Hepatic: abnormal liver function studies, hepatitis
Skin: *rash,* bruising
Other: *hypersensitivity manifested by anaphylaxis or asthma*

---

baclofen

General
Brand names: Lioresal, Lioresal DS
Pharmacologic classification: chlorophenyl derivative
Therapeutic classification: skeletal muscle relaxant

Indications and dosage
• Spasticity in multiple sclerosis, spinal cord injury. *Adults:* initially, 5 mg P.O. t.i.d. for 3 days, 10 mg t.i.d. for 3 days, 15 mg t.i.d. for 3 days, 20 mg t.i.d. for 3 days. Increase according to response up to maximum of 80 mg daily. *Note:* Not available in I.V. form.
Intrathecal use — 1,200 to 1,500 mcg daily as a continuous infusion using an implanted pump.

Adverse reactions
CNS: *drowsiness, dizziness,* headache, *weakness, fatigue,* confusion, insomnia, dysarthria, *seizures;* with intrathecal use—*coma, CNS depression,* dizziness, hypotonia
CV: hypotension
EENT: nasal congestion, blurred vision
GI: *nausea,* constipation; with intrathecal use—nausea, vomiting
GU: urinary frequency
Hepatic: increased aspartate aminotransferase and alkaline phosphatase
Metabolic: hyperglycemia
Skin: rash, pruritus
Other: ankle edema, excessive perspiration, weight gain, seizures and emotional or psychiatric crises possible with withdrawal

---

benztropine mesylate

General
Brand names: Apo-Benztropine, Cogentin, PMS Benztropine
Pharmacologic classification: anticholinergic
Therapeutic classification: antiparkinsonian agent

Indications and dosage
• Acute dystonic reaction. *Adults:* 1 to 2 mg I.V. or I.M., followed by 1 to 2 mg P.O. b.i.d. to prevent recurrence.
• Parkinsonism. *Adults:* 0.5 to 6 mg P.O. daily. Initial dose is 0.5 mg to 1 mg. Increase 0.5 mg q 5 to 6 days. Adjust dosage to meet individual requirements. Usual dose is 1 to 2 mg daily.

Adverse reactions
Some adverse reactions may be due to pending atropinelike toxicity and are dose related.
CNS: disorientation, restlessness, irritability, incoherence, hallucinations, headache, sedation, weakness
CV: palpitations, tachycardia, paradoxical bradycardia
EENT: dilated pupils, blurred vision, photophobia, difficulty swallowing
GI: *constipation, dry mouth,* nausea, vomiting, epigastric distress
GU: urinary hesitancy, urine retention
Skin: warming, dryness, flushing

---

biperiden hydrochloride
biperiden lactate

General
Brand names: Akineton, Akineton Lactate
Pharmacologic classification: anticholinergic
Therapeutic classification: antiparkinsonian agent

Indications and dosage
• Extrapyramidal disorders. *Adults:* 2 to 6 mg P.O. daily, b.i.d., or t.i.d., depending on severity; usual dose is 2 mg daily. Or 2 mg I.M. or I.V. q 30 min-

---

utes, not to exceed four doses or 8 mg total daily.
• Parkinsonism. *Adults:* 2 mg P.O. t.i.d. to q.i.d. Some patients may require as much as 16 mg daily.

Adverse reactions
Adverse reactions are dose related and may resemble atropine toxicity.
CNS: disorientation, euphoria, restlessness, irritability, incoherence, dizziness, increased tremor
CV: transient postural hypotension (with parenteral use)
EENT: blurred vision
GI: *constipation, dry mouth,* nausea, vomiting, epigastric distress
GU: urinary hesitancy, urine retention

bromocriptine mesylate

General
Brand name: Parlodel
Pharmacologic classification: dopamine-receptor agonist
Therapeutic classification: semisynthetic ergot alkaloid; dopaminergic agonist; antiparkinsonian agent

Indications and dosage
• Parkinson's disease. *Adults:* 1.25 mg P.O. b.i.d. with meals. Dosage may be increased q 14 to 28 days, up to 100 mg daily.

Adverse reactions
CNS: confusion, hallucinations, uncontrolled body movements, *dizziness, headache,* fatigue, mania, delusions, nervousness, insomnia, depression, *nightmares,* parkinsonian symptoms may appear and disappear intermittently
CV: *hypotension,* syncope
EENT: nasal congestion, tinnitus, blurred vision
GI: *nausea,* vomiting, *abdominal cramps,* constipation, diarrhea
GU: urine retention, urinary frequency
Other: *pulmonary infiltration and pleural effusion,* coolness and pallor of fingers and toes

carbamazepine

General
Brand names: Apo-Carbamazepine, Epitol, Mazepine, Tegretol
Pharmacologic classification: iminostilbene derivative; chemically related to tricyclic antidepressants
Therapeutic classification: anticonvulsant, analgesic

Indications and dosage
• Generalized tonic-clonic and complex-partial seizures, mixed seizure patterns. *Adults:* initially, 200 mg P.O. b.i.d. May increase by 200 mg P.O. daily, in divided doses at 6- to 8-hour intervals. Adjust to minimum effective level when control achieved. Maintain serum levels between 4 and 12 mcg/ml.
• Trigeminal neuralgia. *Adults:* initially, 100 mg P.O. b.i.d. with meals. Increase by 100 mg q 12 hours until pain is relieved. Don't exceed 1.2 g daily. Usual maintenance dose is 200 to 400 mg P.O. b.i.d.

Adverse reactions
Blood: *aplastic anemia, agranulocytosis,* eosinophilia, leukocytosis, *thrombocytopenia*
CNS: dizziness, *vertigo, drowsiness,* fatigue, *ataxia, worsening of seizures*
CV: *CHF,* hypertension, hypotension, aggravation of coronary artery disease
EENT: conjunctivitis, blurred vision, diplopia, nystagmus
GI: dry mouth and pharynx, *nausea,* vomiting, abdominal pain, diarrhea, anorexia, *stomatitis,* glossitis
GU: urinary frequency, urine retention, impotence, albuminuria, glycosuria, elevated blood urea nitrogen
Hepatic: abnormal liver function tests, *hepatitis*
Metabolic: water intoxication
Skin: *rash,* urticaria, erythema multiforme, *Stevens-Johnson syndrome*
Other: diaphoresis, fever, chills, pulmonary hypersensitivity

---

Common adverse reactions in *italics;* life-threatening, in ***bold italics.***

carmustine

General
Brand name: BiCNU
Pharmacologic classification: alkylating agent, nitrosourea (cell cycle–nonspecific phase)
Therapeutic classification: antineoplastic

Indications and dosage
• Brain cancer. *Adults:* 75 to 100 mg/m^2 I.V. by slow infusion daily for 2 days; repeat q 6 weeks if platelet count is above 100,000/mm^3 and WBC count is above 4,000/mm^3. Dosage is reduced by 30% when WBC count is 2,000 to 3,000/mm^3 and platelet count is 25,000 to 75,000/mm^3. Dosage is reduced by 50% when WBC count is below 2,000/mm^3 and platelet count is below 25,000/mm^3.
Alternative therapy — 200 mg/m^2 I.V. by slow infusion as a single dose, repeated q 6 to 8 weeks; or 40 mg/m^2 I.V. by slow infusion for 5 consecutive days, repeated q 6 weeks.

Adverse reactions
Blood: *cumulative bone marrow depression, delayed 4 to 6 weeks, lasting 1 to 2 weeks; leukopenia; thrombocytopenia*
CNS: ataxia, drowsiness
GI: *nausea, which begins in 2 to 6 hours (can be severe); vomiting*
GU: nephrotoxicity
Hepatic: *hepatotoxicity*
Metabolic: possible hyperuricemia in lymphoma patients when rapid cell lysis occurs
Skin: facial flushing
Local: *intense pain at infusion site from venous spasm*
Other: *pulmonary fibrosis*

ceftriaxone sodium

General
Brand name: Rocephin
Pharmacologic classification: third-generation cephalosporin

Therapeutic classification: antibacterial

Indications and dosage
• Meningitis. *Adults:* 100 mg/kg given in divided doses q 12 hours. May administer a loading dose of 75 mg/kg. Total daily dose depends on susceptibility of organism and severity of infection, but should not exceed 4 g.

Adverse reactions
Blood: eosinophilia; thrombocytosis, leukopenia
CNS: headache, dizziness
GI: pseudomembranous enterocolitis, nausea, vomiting, diarrhea, dysgeusia, abdominal cramps
GU: genital pruritus and moniliasis
Hepatic: transient elevation in liver enzymes, biliary sludge
Skin: maculopapular and erythematous rashes, urticaria, bleeding
Local: at injection site — pain, induration, sterile abscesses, tissue sloughing; phlebitis and thrombophlebitis with I.V. injection
Other: *hypersensitivity,* dyspnea, elevated temperature

clonazepam

General
Brand names: Klonopin, Rivotril
Controlled substance schedule: IV
Pharmacologic classification: benzodiazepine
Therapeutic classification: anticonvulsant

Indications and dosage
• Lennox-Gastaut syndrome and atypical absence seizures; akinetic and myoclonic seizures. *Adults:* initial dosage should not exceed 1.5 mg P.O. daily in three divided doses. May be increased by 0.5 to 1 mg q 3 days until seizures are controlled. If given in unequal doses, the largest dose should be given h.s. Maximum recommended daily dosage is 20 mg.

Common adverse reactions in *italics;* life-threatening, in ***bold italics.***

- Status epilepticus (where parenteral form is available). *Adults:* 1 mg by slow I.V. infusion.

Adverse reactions
Blood: *leukopenia,* thrombocytopenia, eosinophilia
CNS: *drowsiness, ataxia, behavioral disturbances (especially in children),* slurred speech, tremor, confusion
EENT: *increased salivation,* diplopia, nystagmus, abnormal eye movements
GI: constipation, gastritis, change in appetite, nausea, abnormal thirst, sore gums
GU: dysuria, enuresis, nocturia, urine retention
Skin: rash
Other: *respiratory depression*

clorazepate dipotassium

General
Brand names: Novoclopate, Tranxene, Tranxene-SD
Controlled substance schedule: IV
Pharmacologic classification: benzodiazepine
Therapeutic classification: antianxiety agent, anticonvulsant, sedative-hypnotic

Indications and dosage
- Adjunct in seizure disorder. *Adults:* Maximum recommended initial dosage is 7.5 mg P.O. t.i.d. Dosage increases should be no greater than 7.5 mg/week. Maximum daily dosage should not exceed 90 mg daily.

Adverse reactions
CNS: *drowsiness, lethargy, hangover,* fainting
CV: transient hypotension
GI: nausea, vomiting, abdominal discomfort
Respiratory: *respiratory depression*

codeine phosphate

General
Brand name: Paveral

Controlled substance schedule: II
Pharmacologic classification: opioid
Therapeutic classification: analgesic

Indications and dosage
- Mild to moderate pain. *Adults:* 15 to 60 mg P.O. or 15 to 60 mg S.C. or I.M. q 4 hours, p.r.n. or around the clock.

Adverse reactions
CNS: *sedation, clouded sensorium, euphoria,* dizziness, seizures with large doses
CV: hypotension, bradycardia
GI: *nausea, vomiting, constipation, dry mouth,* ileus
GU: *urine retention*
Skin: pruritus, flushing
Other: *respiratory depression,* physical dependence, drowsiness

corticotropin (adrenocorticotropic hormone)

General
Brand names: ACTH, Acthar, ACTH Gel, H.P. Acthar Gel
Pharmacologic classification: anterior pituitary hormone
Therapeutic classification: multiple sclerosis treatment

Indications and dosage
- Therapeutic use. *Adults:* 80 to 120 units daily in four divided doses (aqueous) or 40 units q 24 to 72 hours S.C. or I.M. (gel or repository form) for 2 to 3 weeks.
- Multiple sclerosis. *Adults:* 100 units I.V. daily over 8 hours for 10 days.

Adverse reactions
CNS: *seizures, dizziness,* papilledema, headache, *euphoria, insomnia,* mood swings, personality changes, depression, psychosis
EENT: cataracts, glaucoma
GI: peptic ulcer with perforation and hemorrhage, pancreatitis, abdominal distention, ulcerative esophagitis, nausea, vomiting

---

Common adverse reactions in *italics;* life-threatening, in ***bold italics.***

GU: menstrual irregularities
Metabolic: *sodium and fluid retention,* calcium and potassium loss, hypokalemic alkalosis, negative nitrogen balance
Skin: impaired wound healing, thin fragile skin, petechiae, ecchymoses, facial erythema, increased sweating, acne, hyperpigmentation, allergic skin reactions, hirsutism
Other: muscle weakness, steroid myopathy, loss of muscle mass, osteoporosis, vertebral compression fractures, cushingoid state, suppression of growth in children, activation of latent diabetes mellitus, progressive increase in antibodies, loss of ACTH stimulatory effect, *hypersensitivity*

---

cytarabine (ARA-C, cytosine arabinoside)

General
Brand names: Cytosar-U, Tarabine PFS
Pharmacologic classification: antimetabolite (cell cycle–specific phase, S phase)
Therapeutic classification: antineoplastic

Indications and dosage
• Meningeal leukemias and meningeal neoplasms. *Adults:* 10 to 30 mg/m^2 or 5 to 75 mg/m^2 intrathecally once q 4 days.

Adverse reactions
Blood: *leukopenia, WBC nadir 7 to 9 days after drug stopped;* anemia, reticulocytopenia; *thrombocytopenia,* platelet nadir occurring on day 10; *megaloblastosis*
CNS: neurotoxicity with high doses
EENT: *keratitis*
GI: *nausea, vomiting,* diarrhea, dysphagia; reddened area at juncture of lips, then sore mouth, oral ulcers in 5 to 10 days; high dose given via rapid I.V. may cause projectile vomiting

Hepatic: hepatotoxicity (usually mild and reversible)
Metabolic: hyperuricemia
Skin: rash
Other: flulike syndrome

---

dantrolene sodium

General
Brand names: Dantrium, Dantrium I.V.
Pharmacologic classification: hydantoin derivative
Therapeutic classification: skeletal muscle relaxant

Indications and dosage
• Spasticity and sequelae secondary to severe chronic disorders (multiple sclerosis, cerebral palsy, spinal cord injury, stroke). *Adults:* 25 mg P.O. daily. Increase gradually in increments of 25 mg at 4- to 7-day intervals, up to 100 mg b.i.d. to q.i.d., to maximum of 400 mg daily.

Adverse reactions
CNS: *muscle weakness, drowsiness,* dizziness, light-headedness, malaise, headache, confusion, nervousness, insomnia, *precipitation of seizures*
CV: tachycardia, blood pressure changes
EENT: excessive tearing, visual disturbances
GI: anorexia, constipation, cramping, dysphagia, metallic taste, severe diarrhea
GU: urinary frequency, incontinence, nocturia, dysuria, crystalluria, difficulty achieving erection
Hepatic: hepatitis
Skin: eczematous eruption, pruritus, urticaria, photosensitivity
Other: abnormal hair growth, drooling, sweating, pleural effusion, myalgia, chills, fever

---

Common adverse reactions in *italics;* life-threatening, in ***bold italics.***

dexamethasone
dexamethasone sodium phosphate

General
Brand names: Ak-Dex, Dalalone, Decadron, Hexadrol
Pharmacologic classification: glucocorticoid
Therapeutic classification: anti-inflammatory, immunosuppressant

Indications and dosage
• Cerebral edema. *Adults:* initially, 10 mg (phosphate) I.V., then 4 to 6 mg I.M. or I.V. q 6 hours for 2 to 4 days, then tapered over 5 to 7 days.
• Inflammatory conditions, neoplasias. *Adults:* 0.25 to 4 mg P.O. b.i.d., t.i.d., or q.i.d.

Adverse reactions
Most adverse reactions of corticosteroids are dose or duration dependent.
CNS: *euphoria, insomnia,* psychotic behavior, pseudotumor cerebri
CV: *CHF,* hypertension, edema
EENT: cataracts, glaucoma
GI: *peptic ulcer,* GI irritation, increased appetite
Metabolic: possible hypokalemia, *hyperglycemia* and carbohydrate intolerance, growth suppression in children
Skin: delayed wound healing, acne, various skin eruptions
Local: atrophy at I.M. injection sites
Other: muscle weakness, pancreatitis, hirsutism, susceptibility to infections.
Acute adrenal insufficiency may follow increased stress (infection, surgery, or trauma) or abrupt withdrawal after long-term therapy.
Withdrawal symptoms: rebound inflammation, fatigue, weakness, arthralgia, fever, dizziness, lethargy, depression, fainting, orthostatic hypotension, dyspnea, anorexia, hypoglycemia. ***Sudden withdrawal may be fatal.***

diazepam

General
Brand names: Apo-Diazepam, Diazemuls, Q-Pam, Rival, Valium
Controlled substance schedule: IV
Pharmacologic classification: benzodiazepine
Therapeutic classification: anticonvulsant, antianxiety agent, sedative-hypnotic

Indications and dosage
• Adjunct in seizure disorders or skeletal muscle spasm. *Adults:* 2 to 10 mg P.O. t.i.d. or q.i.d. Or, 15 to 30 mg (extended-release capsule) once daily.
• Seizures. *Adults:* 5 to 10 mg I.V. initially, up to 30 mg in 1 hour.
• Status epilepticus. *Adults:* 5 to 20 mg slow I.V. push at a rate of 2 to 5 mg/minute; may repeat q 5 to 10 minutes up to a maximum total dose of 60 mg. Use 2 to 5 mg in older or debilitated patients. May repeat therapy in 20 to 30 minutes with caution if seizures recur.

Adverse reactions
CNS: *drowsiness, lethargy, hangover,* fainting
CV: transient hypotension
EENT: diplopia, blurred vision, nystagmus
GI: nausea, vomiting, abdominal discomfort
Skin: rash, urticaria
Local: *pain, phlebitis at injection site*
Other: respiratory depression

dihydroergotamine mesylate

General
Brand name: D.H.E. 45
Pharmacologic classification: ergot alkaloid
Therapeutic classification: vasoconstrictor

Indications and dosage
• Vascular or migraine headache. *Adults:* 1 mg I.M. or I.V. May repeat q 1 to 2 hours, p.r.n., up to total of 2 mg I.V.

or 3 mg I.M. per attack. Maximum weekly dosage is 6 mg.

Adverse reactions
CV: numbness and tingling in fingers and toes, transient tachycardia or bradycardia, precordial distress and pain, increased arterial pressure
GI: nausea, vomiting
Skin: itching
Other: weakness in legs, muscle pains in extremities, localized edema

---

edrophonium chloride

General
Brand names: Enlon, Reversol, Tensilon
Pharmacologic classification: cholinesterase inhibitor
Therapeutic classification: cholinergic agonist, diagnostic agent

Indications and dosage
• Diagnostic aid in myasthenia gravis (Tensilon test). *Adults:* 1 to 2 mg I.V. within 15 to 30 seconds, then 8 mg if no response (increase in muscular strength); or 10 mg I.M. If cholinergic reaction occurs, give 2 mg I.M. 30 minutes later to rule out false-negative response. If Tensilon exacerbates cholinergic crisis, give 0.5 to 1.0 mg I.V. of atropine to counteract cholinergic effects.
• Differentiation of myasthenic crisis from cholinergic crisis. *Adults:* 1 mg I.V. If no response in 1 minute, repeat dose once. Increased muscular strength confirms myasthenic crisis; no increase or exaggerated weakness confirms cholinergic crisis.

Adverse reactions
CNS: *seizures,* weakness, dysarthria, dysphagia, sweating
CV: hypotension, bradycardia, AV block
EENT: excessive lacrimation, diplopia, miosis, conjunctival hyperemia
GI: nausea, vomiting, *diarrhea, abdominal cramps,* excessive salivation
GU: urinary frequency, incontinence

Respiratory: *respiratory paralysis, bronchospasm, laryngospasm,* increased bronchial secretions
Other: muscle cramps, muscle fasciculation

---

ergotamine tartrate

General
Brand names: Ergomar, Ergostat, Gynergen, Medihaler-Ergotamine
Pharmacologic classification: ergot alkaloid
Therapeutic classification: vasoconstrictor

Indications and dosage
• Vascular or migraine headache.
Adults: Initially, 2 mg P.O. or S.L., then 1 to 2 mg P.O. q hour or S.L. q 30 minutes, to a maximum of 6 mg daily and 10 mg weekly. Or use aerosol inhaler: 1 spray (360 mcg) initially, repeated q 5 minutes p.r.n. to a maximum of 6 sprays (2.16 mg) per 24 hours or 15 sprays (5.4 mg) per week.
Patient may also use rectal suppositories. Initially, 2 mg rectally at onset of attack, repeated in 1 hour p.r.n. Maximum dosage is 2 suppositories per attack or 5 suppositories per week.

Adverse reactions
CV: numbness and tingling in fingers and toes, transient tachycardia or bradycardia, precordial distress and pain, increased arterial pressure, *angina pectoris*
GI: nausea, vomiting, diarrhea, abdominal cramps
Skin: itching
Other: weakness in legs, muscle pains in extremities, localized edema

---

heparin sodium

General
Brand name: Liquaemin Sodium
Pharmacologic classification: anticoagulant
Therapeutic classification: antithrombotic

Indications and dosage
• Acute cardioembolic stroke. *Adults:* 50 to 100 units/kg by I.V. bolus, followed by 10 to 15 units/kg/hour adjusted to achieve a partial thromboplastin time of 1½ to 2 times control values.

Adverse reactions
Blood: hemorrhage from any site with excessive dosage, overly prolonged clotting time, ***thrombocytopenia***
Hepatic: elevated liver function tests
Local: irritation, hematoma, ulceration, cutaneous or subcutaneous necrosis, mild pain and burning on injection
Other: *"white clot" syndrome,* hypersensitivity reactions including chills, fever, pruritus, rhinitis, burning of the feet, conjunctivitis, lacrimation, arthralgia, urticaria

interferon beta-1b

General
Brand name: Betaseron
Pharmacologic classification: natural protein
Therapeutic classification: immunomodulator

Indications and dosage
• Multiple sclerosis. *Adults:* 1.6 million IU S.C. every other day.

Adverse reactions
Blood: neutropenia, *lymphopenia, leukopenia*
Other: *fever, chills, alopecia, myalgia,* flulike syndrome, sweating, injection site reactions

levodopa

General
Brand names: Dopar, Larodopa
Pharmacologic classification: precursor of dopamine
Therapeutic classification: antiparkinsonian agent

Indications and dosage
• Treatment of idiopathic parkinsonism, postencephalitic parkinsonism, and symptomatic parkinsonism after carbon monoxide or manganese intoxication; or in association with cerebral arteriosclerosis. *Adults:* initially, 0.5 to 1 g P.O. daily, given b.i.d., t.i.d., or q.i.d. with food; increase by no more than 0.75 g daily q 3 to 7 days, until usual maximum of 8 g is reached. Carefully adjust dosage to individual requirements, tolerance, and response. Higher dosage requires close supervision.

Adverse reactions
Blood: *hemolytic anemia,* leukopenia
CNS: *aggressive behavior; choreiform, dystonic, and dyskinetic movements; involuntary grimacing; head movements; myoclonic body jerks; ataxia; tremor; muscle twitching; bradykinetic episode; psychiatric disturbances; memory loss; mood changes; nervousness; anxiety; disturbing dreams; euphoria; malaise; fatigue; severe depression; **suicidal tendencies;** dementia; delirium; hallucinations (may necessitate reduction or withdrawal of drug); parkinsonian symptoms may appear and disappear intermittently*
CV: orthostatic hypotension, cardiac irregularities, flushing, hypertension, phlebitis
EENT: blepharospasm, blurred vision, diplopia, mydriasis or miosis, widening of palpebral fissures, activation of latent Horner's syndrome, oculogyric crises, nasal discharge
GI: nausea, vomiting, anorexia, weight loss perhaps occurring at start of therapy, constipation, flatulence, diarrhea, epigastric pain, hiccups, sialorrhea, dry mouth, bitter taste
GU: urinary frequency or incontinence, urine retention, darkened urine, excessive and inappropriate sexual behavior, priapism
Hepatic: hepatotoxicity
Other: dark perspiration, hyperventilation

levodopa-carbidopa

General
Brand names: Sinemet, Sinemet CR
Pharmacologic classification: decarboxylase inhibitor–dopamine precursor combination
Therapeutic classification: antiparkinsonian agent

Indications and dosage
• Treatment of idiopathic Parkinson's disease, postencephalitic parkinsonism, and symptomatic parkinsonism resulting from carbon monoxide or manganese intoxication. *Adults:* 3 to 6 tablets of 25 mg carbidopa/250 mg levodopa daily given in divided doses. Do not exceed 8 tablets of 25 mg carbidopa/250 mg levodopa daily. Optimum daily dosage must be determined by careful titration for each patient.

Adverse reactions
Blood: *hemolytic anemia*
CNS: *choreiform, dystonic, dyskinetic movements; involuntary grimacing, head movements, myoclonic body jerks, ataxia,* tremor, muscle twitching; bradykinetic episodes; psychiatric disturbances, memory loss, nervousness, anxiety, disturbing dreams, euphoria, malaise, fatigue; severe depression, *suicidal tendencies,* dementia, delirium, hallucinations (may necessitate reduction or withdrawal of drug)
CV: *orthostatic hypotension, cardiac irregularities,* flushing, hypertension, phlebitis
EENT: blepharospasm, blurred vision, diplopia, mydriasis or miosis, widening of palpebral fissures, activation of latent Horner's syndrome, oculogyric crises, nasal discharge
GI: *nausea, vomiting, anorexia,* weight loss perhaps occurring at start of therapy; constipation; flatulence; diarrhea; *epigastric pain;* hiccups; sialorrhea; *dry mouth;* bitter taste
GU: urinary frequency, urine retention, urinary incontinence, darkened urine, excessive and inappropriate sexual behavior, priapism
Hepatic: hepatotoxicity
Other: dark perspiration, hyperventilation

lomustine (CCNU)

General
Brand name: CeeNU
Pharmacologic classification: alkylating agent, nitrosourea
Therapeutic classification: antineoplastic

Indications and dosage
• Primary and metastatic brain tumors. *Adults:* 130 mg/m^2 P.O. as a single dose q 6 weeks. Reduce further doses of mannitol by 30% if nadir WBC count is below 3,000/mm^3 or platelet count is below 75,000/mm^3 and by 50% if nadir WBC count is below 2,000/mm^3 or platelet count is below 25,000/mm^3.

Adverse reactions
Blood: *leukopenia (delayed and up to 6 weeks after dose),* thrombocytopenia, anemia
GI: *nausea, vomiting,* stomatitis
Hepatic: *hepatitis*
Other: pulmonary infiltrates, *pulmonary fibrosis*

lorazepam

General
Brand name: Ativan
Pharmacologic classification: antianxiety agent
Therapeutic classification: anticonvulsant

Indications and dosage
• Status epilepticus. *Adults:* 0.05 to 0.15 mg/kg at a rate of 2 mg/minute repeated every 10 to 15 minutes p.r.n.

Adverse reactions
CNS: *drowsiness, lethargy, hangover,* fainting
CV: transient hypotension
GI: dry mouth, abdominal discomfort

mannitol

General
Brand name: Osmitrol
Pharmacologic classification: osmotic diuretic
Therapeutic classification: reduction of intracranial pressure

Indications and dosage
• Reduction of intracranial pressure.
Adults: 1.5 to 2 g/kg as a 15% to 25% solution I.V. over 30 to 60 minutes.

Adverse reactions
CNS: rebound increase in intracranial pressure 8 to 12 hours after diuresis; headache; confusion
CV: transient expansion of plasma volume during infusion, causing circulatory overload and *pulmonary edema,* tachycardia, angina-like chest pain
EENT: blurred vision, rhinitis
GI: thirst, nausea, vomiting
GU: urine retention
Metabolic: fluid and electrolyte imbalance, water intoxication, cellular dehydration

meperidine hydrochloride (pethidine hydrochloride)

General
Brand name: Demerol
Controlled substance schedule: II
Pharmacologic classification: opioid
Therapeutic classification: analgesic

Indications and dosage
• Moderate to severe pain. *Adults:* 50 to 150 mg P.O., I.M., or S.C. q 3 to 4 hours, p.r.n. or around the clock; or 15 to 35 mg/hour continuous I.V. infusion.

Adverse reactions
CNS: *sedation, somnolence, clouded sensorium, euphoria,* paradoxical excitement, tremor, dizziness, *seizures with large doses*
CV: *hypotension,* bradycardia, tachycardia

GI: *nausea, vomiting, constipation,* ileus
GU: *urine retention*
Local: pain at injection site, local tissue irritation and induration after S.C. injection; phlebitis after I.V. use
Other: *respiratory depression,* physical dependence, muscle twitching

mephobarbital

General
Brand name: Mebaral
Controlled substance schedule: IV
Pharmacologic classification: barbiturate
Therapeutic classification: anticonvulsant, nonspecific CNS depressant

Indications and dosage
• Generalized tonic-clonic or absence seizures. *Adults:* 400 to 600 mg P.O. daily or in divided doses.

Adverse reactions
Blood: megaloblastic anemia, *agranulocytosis,* thrombocytopenia
CNS: *dizziness,* headache, *hangover,* confusion, paradoxical excitation, exacerbation of existing pain, drowsiness
CV: hypotension, bradycardia
GI: nausea, vomiting, epigastric pain
Skin: urticaria, morbilliform rash, blisters, purpura, *erythema multiforme*
Other: allergic reactions (facial edema)

methocarbamol

General
Brand names: Marbaxin-750, Robaxin, Robomol-500, Robomol-750
Pharmacologic classification: carbonate derivative of guaifenesin
Therapeutic classification: skeletal muscle relaxant

Indications and dosage
• As an adjunct in acute, painful musculoskeletal conditions. *Adults:* 1.5 g P.O. q.i.d. for 2 to 3 days, then 1 g P.O. q.i.d. Alternatively, give no more than 500 mg (5 ml) I.M. into each gluteal re-

---

Common adverse reactions in *italics;* life-threatening, in ***bold italics.***

gion. May repeat q 8 hours. Or 1 to 3 g daily (10 to 30 ml) I.V. directly into vein at 3 ml/minute, or 10 ml may be added to no more than 250 ml of D₅W or 0.9% sodium chloride solution. Maximum dosage is 3 g daily.

Adverse reactions
Blood: hemolysis, decreased hemoglobin (I.V. only)
CNS: drowsiness, dizziness, lightheadedness, headache, syncope, mild muscular incoordination (I.M. or I.V. only), *seizures* (I.V. only)
CV: hypotension, bradycardia (I.M. or I.V. only)
GI: nausea, anorexia, GI upset, metallic taste
GU: hematuria (I.V. only), discoloration of urine
Skin: urticaria, pruritus, rash
Local: thrombophlebitis, extravasation (I.V. only)
Other: fever, flushing, *anaphylactic reactions* (I.M. or I.V. only)

---

methotrexate
methotrexate sodium

General
Brand names: Folex, Mexate, Rheumatrex
Pharmacologic classification: antimetabolite (cell cycle–specific phase, S phase)
Therapeutic classification: antineoplastic

Indications and dosage
• Meningeal leukemia. *Adults:* 10 to 15 mg/m² intrathecally q 2 to 5 days until CSF is normal. Use only 20-, 50-, or 100-mg vials of powder with no preservatives; dilute using 0.9% sodium chloride injection *without* preservatives. Use only new vials of drug and diluent. Use immediately.

Adverse reactions
Blood: WBC and platelet nadir occurring on day 7; *anemia, leukopenia, thrombocytopenia* (all dose related)

CNS: *arachnoiditis within hours of intrathecal use;* subacute neurotoxicity, which may begin a few weeks later; *necrotizing demyelinating leukoencephalopathy* a few years later
EENT: pharyngitis
GI: gingivitis, *stomatitis, diarrhea leading to hemorrhagic enteritis and intestinal perforation, nausea, vomiting*
GU: nephropathy, *tubular necrosis*
Hepatic: acute toxicity (elevated transaminases), *chronic toxicity* (cirrhosis, *hepatic fibrosis*)
Metabolic: hyperuricemia
Respiratory: *pulmonary fibrosis,* pneumonitis
Skin: *urticaria;* pruritus; hyperpigmentation; alopecia; exposure to sun may aggravate psoriatic lesions, rash, photosensitivity
Other: *pulmonary interstitial infiltrates;* long-term use in children may cause osteoporosis

---

methylprednisolone sodium succinate

General
Brand names: A-Metha-pred, Solu-Medrol
Pharmacologic classification: glucocorticoid
Therapeutic classification: antiinflammatory, immunosuppressant

Indications and dosage
• Decrease of residual damage after spinal cord trauma. *Adults:* 30 mg/kg I.V. as a bolus injection over 15 minutes, then wait 45 minutes before starting continuous infusion for 23-hour period.

Adverse reactions
Most adverse reactions of corticosteroids are dose or duration dependent.
CNS: *euphoria, insomnia,* psychotic behavior, pseudotumor cerebri
CV: *CHF,* hypertension, edema
EENT: cataracts, glaucoma
GI: *peptic ulcer,* GI irritation, increased appetite

Common adverse reactions in *italics;* life-threatening, in *bold italics.*

Metabolic: possible hypokalemia, *hyperglycemia* and carbohydrate intolerance, growth suppression in children
Skin: delayed wound healing, acne, various skin eruptions
Other: muscle weakness, pancreatitis, hirsutism, susceptibility to infections. Acute adrenal insufficiency may occur with increased stress (infection, surgery, or trauma) or abrupt withdrawal after long-term therapy.
Withdrawal symptoms: rebound inflammation, fatigue, weakness, arthralgia, fever, dizziness, lethargy, depression, fainting, orthostatic hypotension, dyspnea, anorexia, hypoglycemia. *Sudden withdrawal may be fatal.*

methysergide maleate

General
Brand name: Sansert
Pharmacologic classification: ergot alkaloid
Therapeutic classification: vasoconstrictor

Indications and dosage
• Prevention of frequent, severe, uncontrollable, or disabling migraine or vascular headache. *Adults:* 4 to 8 mg P.O. daily in divided doses with meals.

Adverse reactions
Blood: neutropenia, eosinophilia
CNS: insomnia, drowsiness, *euphoria, vertigo,* ataxia, *light-headedness,* hyperesthesia, weakness, hallucinations or feelings of dissociation
CV: *fibrotic thickening of cardiac valves and aorta, inferior vena cava, and common iliac branches (retroperitoneal fibrosis);* vasoconstriction, causing chest pain, abdominal pain, vascular insufficiency of lower limbs; cold, numb, painful extremities with or without paresthesia and diminished or absent pulses; postural hypotension; tachycardia; peripheral edema; murmurs; bruits
EENT: nasal stuffiness
GI: nausea, vomiting, diarrhea, constipation, epigastric pain

Skin: hair loss, dermatitis, sweating, flushing, rash
Other: *pulmonary fibrosis,* causing dyspnea, tightness and pain in chest, pleural friction rubs and effusion, arthralgia, myalgia

morphine hydrochloride
morphine sulfate

General
Brand names: Atramorph, Duramorph PF, Epimorph, MS Contin, M.O.S., Oramorph, RMS Uniserts
Controlled substance schedule: II
Pharmacologic classification: opioid
Therapeutic classification: narcotic analgesic

Indications and dosage
• Severe pain. *Adults:* 4 to 15 mg S.C. or I.M. (sulfate); or 30 to 60 mg P.O. or rectally q 4 hours, p.r.n. or around the clock. May be injected slow I.V. (over 4 to 5 minutes) diluted in 4 to 5 ml water for injection. May also administer controlled-release tablets q 8 to 12 hours. As an epidural injection, 5 mg via an epidural catheter by bolus or continuous infusion q 24 hours.
  Sometimes, morphine may be administered by continuous I.V. infusion or by intraspinal and intrathecal injection.

Adverse reactions
CNS: *sedation, somnolence, clouded sensorium, euphoria,* seizures with large doses, dizziness, *nightmares*
CV: *hypotension,* bradycardia
GI: *nausea, vomiting, constipation,* ileus
GU: *urine retention*
Other: respiratory depression, physical dependence, pruritus, skin flushing

neostigmine bromide
neostigmine methylsulfate

General
Brand name: Prostigmin Bromide
Pharmacologic classification: cholinesterase inhibitor

Common adverse reactions in *italics;* life-threatening, in ***bold italics.***

Therapeutic classification: muscle stimulant

Indications and dosage
• Myasthenia gravis. *Adults:* initially, 15 to 30 mg P.O. t.i.d. Increase q 1 to 2 days to a maximum of 375 mg daily. Or 0.5 to 2.5 mg S.C., I.M., or I.V. q 1 to 3 hours. Dosage must be individualized, depending on response. Large doses should be accompanied by 0.6 to 1.2 mg of atropine. Therapy may be required day and night.

Adverse reactions
CNS: dizziness, muscle weakness, mental confusion, jitters, sweating
CV: bradycardia, hypotension
EENT: blurred vision, lacrimation, miosis
GI: *nausea, vomiting, diarrhea, abdominal cramps,* excessive salivation
GU: urinary frequency
Respiratory: *depression, bronchospasm, bronchoconstriction*
Skin: rash (bromide)
Other: *muscle cramps,* muscle fasciculations

---

nimodipine

General
Brand name: Nimotop
Pharmacologic classification: calcium channel blocker
Therapeutic classification: cerebral vasodilator

Indications and dosage
• Improvement of neurologic deficits after subarachnoid hemorrhage from ruptured congenital aneurysms. *Adults:* 60 mg P.O. q 4 hours for 21 days. Therapy should begin within 96 hours after subarachnoid hemorrhage.

Adverse reactions
CNS: headaches
CV: decreased blood pressure, flushing, edema

---

penicillin G potassium (benzylpenicillin potassium) penicillin G sodium (benzylpenicillin sodium)

General
Brand names: Crystapen, Pfizerpen
Pharmacologic classification: natural penicillin
Therapeutic classification: antibacterial

Indications and dosage
• Moderate to severe systemic infections (including meningitis). *Adults:* 1.2 to 24 million units daily I.M. or I.V., divided into doses given q 4 hours.

Adverse reactions
Blood: hemolytic anemia, leukopenia, thrombocytopenia
CNS: arthralgia, neuropathy, *seizures*
CV: *CHF with high doses (sodium)*
Local: vein irritation, pain at injection site, thrombophlebitis
Other: hypersensitivity (chills, fever, edema, maculopapular rash, **exfoliative dermatitis**, urticaria, **anaphylaxis**), overgrowth of nonsusceptible organisms; hyperkalemia (potassium)

---

pergolide mesylate

General
Brand name: Permax
Pharmacologic classification: ergot derivative
Therapeutic classification: antiparkinsonian agent

Indications and dosage
• Adjunctive treatment to levodopa-carbidopa in the management of the symptoms associated with Parkinson's disease. Adults: initially, 0.05 mg P.O. daily for the first 2 days. Gradually increase dosage by 0.1 to 0.15 mg every third day over the next 12 days of therapy. Subsequent dosage can be increased by 0.25 mg every third day until optimum response is seen. The drug

---

Common adverse reactions in *italics;* life-threatening, in ***bold italics.***

is usually administered in divided doses t.i.d. Gradual reductions in levodopa-carbidopa dosage may be made during dosage titration.

Adverse reactions
CNS: asthenia, *dyskinesia, dizziness, hallucinations,* dystonia, confusion, *somnolence,* insomnia, depression, tremor, personality disorder, psychosis, abnormal gait, akathisia, extrapyramidal syndrome, incoordination, paresthesia, akinesia, hypertonia, neuralgia, speech disorder
CV: *orthostatic hypotension,* vasodilation, palpitations, hypotension, syncope, hypertension, *arrhythmias, myocardial infarction*
EENT: *rhinitis,* epistaxis, abnormal vision, diplopia, eye disorder
GI: abdominal pain, *nausea, constipation,* diarrhea, dyspepsia, anorexia, vomiting, dry mouth, taste alteration
GU: urinary frequency, urinary tract infection, hematuria
Skin: rash, sweating
Other: accident or injury; chest, neck, and back pain; flulike syndrome; chills; infection; facial, peripheral, or generalized edema; weight gain; arthralgia; bursitis; myalgia; twitching

phenacemide

General
Brand name: Phenurone
Pharmacologic classification: substituted acetylurea derivative, open-chain hydantoin
Therapeutic classification: anticonvulsant

Indications and dosage
• Refractory, complex-partial, generalized tonic-clonic, absence, and atypical absence seizures. *Adults:* 500 mg P.O. t.i.d. May increase by 500 mg weekly up to 5 g daily, p.r.n.

Adverse reactions
Blood: *aplastic anemia, agranulocytosis,* leukopenia

CNS: drowsiness, dizziness, insomnia, headaches, paresthesia, *depression, suicidal tendencies,* aggressiveness, acute psychoses
GI: anorexia, weight loss
GU: nephritis with marked albuminuria
Hepatic: hepatitis, jaundice
Skin: rashes

phenobarbital (phenobarbitone) phenobarbital sodium (phenobarbitone sodium)

General
Brand names: Barbita, Gardenal, Luminal
Controlled substance schedule: IV
Pharmacologic classification: barbiturate
Therapeutic classification: anticonvulsant, sedative-hypnotic

Indications and dosage
• All forms of epilepsy. *Adults:* 100 to 200 mg P.O. daily, divided t.i.d. or given as single dosage h.s. Adjust to a serum level of 10 to 40 mcg/ml.
• Status epilepticus. *Adults:* 10 mg/kg as I.V. infusion no faster than 50 mg/minute. May give up to 20 mg/kg total. Administer in acute care or emergency area only.

Adverse reactions
CNS: *drowsiness, lethargy, hangover,* paradoxical excitement in older patients, *coma*
GI: nausea, vomiting
Respiratory: *respiratory depression*
Skin: rash, *Stevens-Johnson syndrome,* urticaria
Local: pain, swelling, thrombophlebitis, necrosis, nerve injury
Other: *angioedema*

Common adverse reactions in *italics;* life-threatening, in ***bold italics.***

phenytoin
(diphenylhydantoin)
phenytoin sodium

General
Brand names: Dilantin, Diphenylan
Pharmacologic classification: hydantoin derivative
Therapeutic classification: anticonvulsant

Indications and dosage
• Generalized tonic-clonic seizures, status epilepticus, nonepileptic seizures (after head trauma). *Adults:* Loading dose is 900 mg to 1.5 g or 15 to 18 mg/kg I.V. at 50 mg/minute or P.O. divided t.i.d.; maintenance dosage is 300 mg P.O. daily (extended only) or divided t.i.d. (extended or prompt). Adjust dosage to achieve a total serum level of 10 to 20 mcg/ml or a free serum level of 1 to 2 mcg/ml.
• If patient has not received phenytoin previously or has no detectable blood level, use loading dose. *Adults:* 900 mg to 1.5 g I.V. divided t.i.d. at 50 mg/minute. Do not exceed 500 mg each dose.
• If patient has been receiving phenytoin but has missed one or more doses and has subtherapeutic levels. *Adults:* 100 to 300 mg I.V. at 50 mg/minute.
• Neuritic pain (migraine, trigeminal neuralgia, Bell's palsy). *Adults:* 200 to 400 mg P.O. daily.

Adverse reactions
Blood: *thrombocytopenia, leukopenia, agranulocytosis, pancytopenia,* macrocytosis, megaloblastic anemia
CNS: *ataxia, slurred speech, confusion,* dizziness, insomnia, nervousness, twitching, headache
CV: hypotension, *ventricular fibrillation*
EENT: nystagmus, diplopia, blurred vision
GI: nausea, vomiting, gingival hyperplasia (especially children)
Hepatic: *toxic hepatitis*
Skin: scarlatiniform or morbilliform rash; bullous, exfoliative, or purpuric dermatitis; Stevens-Johnson syndrome; hirsutism; toxic epidermal necrolysis; photosensitivity
Local: pain, necrosis, and inflammation at injection site; purple glove syndrome
Other: periarteritis nodosa, lymphadenopathy, hyperglycemia, osteomalacia, hypertrichosis, lupuslike syndrome

procyclidine hydrochloride

General
Brand names: Kemadrin, PMS Procyclidine, Procyclid
Pharmacologic classification: anticholinergic
Therapeutic classification: antiparkinsonian agent

Indications and dosage
• Parkinsonism, muscle rigidity. *Adults:* Initially, 2 to 2.5 mg P.O. t.i.d. dosage after meals. Increase gradually as needed. Usual dosage range is 20 to 30 mg/day, but some patients may require up to 60 mg daily.

Adverse reactions
CNS: disorientation, euphoria, restlessness, irritability, incoherence, dizziness, increased tremor, light-headedness, giddiness
EENT: blurred vision, mydriasis
GI: *constipation, dry mouth,* nausea, vomiting, epigastric distress
GU: urinary hesitancy, urine retention
Skin: rash
Other: muscle weakness

propranolol hydrochloride

General
Brand names: Apo-Propranolol, Deralin, Detensol, Inderal, Inderal LA
Pharmacologic classification: beta-adrenergic blocker
Therapeutic classification: adjunctive therapy for migraine

Indications and dosage

• Prevention of frequent, severe, uncontrollable, or disabling migraine or vascular headache. *Adults:* initially, 80 mg P.O. daily in divided doses or as a sustained-release capsule once daily. Usual maintenance dosage is 160 to 240 mg daily, divided t.i.d. or q.i.d. or as a sustained-release capsule.

Adverse reactions

CNS: *fatigue, lethargy,* vivid dreams, hallucinations, depression
CV: *bradycardia, hypotension, CHF,* peripheral vascular disease
GI: nausea, vomiting, diarrhea
Metabolic: hypoglycemia without tachycardia (in diabetic patients)
Skin: rash
Other: *increased airway resistance,* fever, arthralgia

---

pyridostigmine bromide

General

Brand names: Mestinon, Mestinon Supraspan, Mestinon Timespan
Pharmacologic classification: cholinesterase inhibitor
Therapeutic classification: muscle stimulant

Indications and dosage

• Myasthenia gravis. *Adults:* 60 to 120 mg P.O. q 3 or 4 hours. Usual daily dosage is 600 mg, but up to 1,500 mg may be needed. Give 1/30 of oral dose I.M. or very slow I.V. push. Large doses of parenteral pyridostigmine should be accompanied by 0.6 to 1.2 mg of atropine. Dosage must be adjusted for each patient, depending on response and adverse reactions. Alternatively, may give 180 to 540 mg of timed-release tablets (1 to 3 tablets) b.i.d., with at least 6 hours between doses.

Adverse reactions

CNS: headache (with high doses), dizziness, muscle weakness, incoordination, mental confusion, jitters, sweating, *seizures*
CV: bradycardia, hypotension

EENT: miosis, blurred vision
GI: abdominal cramps, nausea, vomiting, diarrhea, excessive salivation
GU: urinary frequency, incontinence
Skin: rash
Local: thrombophlebitis
Other: *bronchospasm, bronchoconstriction,* increased bronchial secretions, muscle cramps, muscle fasciculations, *respiratory paralysis*

---

secobarbital sodium

General

Brand names: Novosecobarb, Seconal Sodium
Controlled substance schedule: II
Pharmacologic classification: barbiturate
Therapeutic classification: sedative-hypnotic, anticonvulsant

Indications and dosage

• Acute tetanus seizure. *Adults:* 5.5 mg/kg I.M. or slow I.V., repeated q 3 to 4 hours, if needed; I.V. injection rate not to exceed 50 mg/15 seconds.
• Acute psychotic agitation. *Adults:* 50 mg/minute I.V. up to 250 mg I.V. initially; additional doses given cautiously after 5 minutes if desired response is not obtained. Not to exceed 500 mg total.
• Status epilepticus. *Adults:* 250 to 350 mg I.M. or I.V.

Adverse reactions

CNS: *drowsiness, lethargy, hangover,* paradoxical excitement (older patients)
GI: nausea, vomiting
Skin: rash, urticaria, *Stevens-Johnson syndrome*
Other: *angioedema,* exacerbation of porphyria

---

selegiline hydrochloride (L-deprenyl hydrochloride)

General

Brand name: Eldepryl
Pharmacologic classification: monoamine oxidase inhibitor

Therapeutic classification: antiparkinsonian agent

Indications and dosage
• Adjunct to levodopa-carbidopa in the management of symptoms associated with Parkinson's disease. *Adults:* 10 mg P.O. daily, taken as 5 mg at breakfast and 5 mg at lunch. After 2 or 3 days of therapy, begin gradual decrease of levodopa-carbidopa dosage.

Adverse reactions
CNS: *dizziness,* increased tremor, chorea, loss of balance, restlessness, blepharospasm, increased bradykinesia, facial grimace, stiff neck, dyskinesia, involuntary movements, increased apraxia, behavioral changes, tiredness, headache
CV: orthostatic hypotension, hypertension, hypotension, **arrhythmias,** palpitations, new or increased anginal pain, tachycardia, peripheral edema, syncope
GI: *nausea,* vomiting, constipation, weight loss, anorexia or poor appetite, dysphagia, diarrhea, heartburn, dry mouth, taste alteration
GU: slow urination, transient nocturia, prostatic hypertrophy, urinary hesitancy, urinary frequency, urine retention, sexual dysfunction
Skin: rash, hair loss, sweating
Other: malaise

sumatriptan succinate

General
Brand name: Imitrex
Pharmacologic classification: serotonin agonist
Therapeutic classification: antimigraine agent

Indications and dosage
• Acute migraine headache. *Adults:* 6 mg S.C. May repeat after a minimum of 1 hour. Maximum recommended dosage is two 6-mg injections daily.

Adverse reactions
CNS: *dizziness, vertigo,* paresthesia, drowsiness, headache, anxiety, malaise, fatigue, weakness
CV: *atrial or ventricular fibrillation, ventricular tachycardia, ECG changes such as ischemic ST-segment elevation* (rare)
Local: pain on injection
EENT: discomfort of the throat, nasal cavity, or sinus, mouth, jaw, or tongue; visual alterations
GI: abdominal discomfort, dysphagia
Other: *tingling, burning sensation, pressure in head,* cold sensation, pressure or tightness in chest, neck pain, myalgia, muscle cramps, sweating

ticlopidine hydrochloride

General
Brand name: Ticlid
Pharmacologic classification: antiplatelet agent
Therapeutic classification: antithrombotic

Indications and dosage
• Prevention of stroke in patients with a history of stroke who do not respond to or cannot tolerate aspirin. *Adults:* 250 mg P.O. b.i.d.

Adverse reactions
Blood: *neutropenia,* thrombocytopenia, *thrombotic thrombocytopenic purpura, pancytopenia, bleeding*
GI: diarrhea, nausea, vomiting, dyspepsia
Skin: rash

trihexyphenidyl hydrochloride

General
Brand names: Artane, Artane Sequels, Novohexidyl
Pharmacologic classification: anticholinergic
Therapeutic classification: antiparkinsonian agent

Common adverse reactions in *italics;* life-threatening, in **bold italics.**

Indications and dosage
• Drug-induced parkinsonism. *Adults:*
1 mg P.O. 1st day, 2 mg 2nd day, then
increase by 2 mg q 3 to 5 days until total of 6 to 10 mg is given daily. Usually
give t.i.d. with meals and, if needed,
q.i.d. (last dose should be before bedtime) or may switch to extended-release form b.i.d. Postencephalitic parkinsonism may require 12 to 15 mg total daily dosage.

Adverse reactions
Adverse reactions are dose related.
CNS: nervousness, dizziness, headache, restlessness, increased tremor,
agitation, irritability, hallucinations, euphoria, incoherence, delusion, amnesia, disorientation
EENT: blurred vision, mydriasis, increased intraocular pressure
GI: constipation, *dry mouth, nausea,
vomiting, epigastric distress*
GU: urinary hesitancy, urine retention

trimethadione

General
Brand name: Tridione
Pharmacologic classification: oxazo-
lidinedione derivative
Therapeutic classification: anticon-
vulsant

Indications and dosage
• Refractory absence seizures. *Adults:*
Initially, 300 mg P.O. t.i.d. May increase
by 300 mg weekly to 600 mg P.O. q.i.d.

Adverse reactions
Blood: *neutropenia, leukopenia,* eosinophilia, *thrombocytopenia, pancytopenia, agranulocytosis, hypoplas-
tic and aplastic anemia*
CNS: drowsiness, fatigue, malaise, insomnia, dizziness, headache, paresthesia, irritability
CV: hypertension, hypotension
EENT: hemeralopia, diplopia, photophobia, epistaxis, retinal hemorrhage
GI: nausea, vomiting, anorexia, abdominal pain, bleeding gums

GU: nephrosis, albuminuria, vaginal
bleeding
Hepatic: abnormal liver function tests,
hepatitis
Skin: acneiform and morbilliform rash,
*exfoliative dermatitis, erythema
multiforme,* petechiae, alopecia
Other: lymphadenopathy, lupus-like
syndrome, myasthenic symptoms

urea
(carbamide)

General
Brand name: Ureaphil
Pharmacologic classification: car-
bonic acid salt
Therapeutic classification: osmotic
diuretic

Indications and dosage
• Reduction of intracranial or intraocular pressure. *Adults:* 1 to 1.5 g/kg as a
30% solution by slow I.V. infusion over
1 to 2½ hours. Maximum adult daily
dosage is 120 g. To prepare 135 ml of
30% solution, mix contents of 40-g vial
of urea with 105 ml of dextrose 5% or
10% in water or 10% invert sugar in
water. Each milliliter of 30% solution
provides 300 mg urea.

Adverse reactions
CNS: *headache*
CV: tachycardia, *CHF,* pulmonary
edema
GI: *nausea, vomiting*
Metabolic: sodium and potassium
depletion
Local: irritation or necrotic sloughing
with extravasation

valproate sodium
valproic acid
divalproex sodium

General
Brand names: Depakene Syrup, Epi-
val
Pharmacologic classification: car-
boxylic acid derivative

Therapeutic classification: anticonvulsant

Indications and dosage
• Simple and complex absence seizures, mixed seizure types (including absence seizures), investigationally in generalized tonic-clonic seizures. *Adults:* Initially, 15 mg/kg P.O. daily divided b.i.d. or t.i.d.; then may increase by 5 to 10 mg/kg daily at weekly intervals up to maximum of 60 mg/kg daily, divided b.i.d. or t.i.d. Adjust dose to maintain serum levels between 50 and 100 mcg/ml.

Adverse reactions
Because drug is usually used in combination with other anticonvulsants, adverse reactions reported may not be caused by valproic acid alone.
Blood: inhibited platelet aggregation, thrombocytopenia, increased bleeding time
CNS: *sedation,* emotional upset, depression, psychosis, aggression, hyperactivity, behavioral deterioration, muscle weakness, tremor
EENT: stomatitis
GI: *nausea, vomiting,* indigestion, diarrhea, abdominal cramps, constipation, increased appetite and weight gain, *anorexia and weight loss,* **pancreatitis**
Hepatic: *elevated liver enzymes,* **toxic hepatitis**
Metabolic: *elevated serum ammonia*
Other: alopecia

---

vincristine sulfate

General
Brand names: Oncovin, Vincasar PFS
Pharmacologic classification: vinca alkaloid (cell cycle–specific phase, M phase)
Therapeutic classification: antineoplastic

Indications and dosage
• Brain medulloblastoma. *Adults:* 0.4 to 1.4 mg/m^2 I.V. weekly. Maximum single dose is 2 mg. Don't administer intrathecally.

Adverse reactions
Blood: rapidly reversible mild anemia and leukopenia
CNS: *peripheral neuropathy,* sensory loss, *loss of deep tendon reflexes, paresthesia, wristdrop and footdrop,* ataxia, cranial nerve dysfunction (headache, *jaw pain,* hoarseness, vocal cord paralysis, visual disturbances), *muscle weakness and cramps,* depression, agitation, insomnia
CV: hypotension, hypertension
EENT: diplopia, optic and extraocular neuropathy, ptosis
GI: diarrhea, *constipation, cramps,* ileus that mimics surgical abdomen, *nausea, vomiting,* anorexia, *stomatitis,* weight loss, dysphagia, **intestinal necrosis**
GU: urine retention, syndrome of inappropriate antidiuretic hormone
Local: severe local reaction when extravasated, *phlebitis,* cellulitis
Other: **acute bronchospasm,** reversible alopecia, fever, rash

---

warfarin sodium

General
Brand names: Coumadin, Panwarfin
Pharmacologic classification: coumarin derivative
Therapeutic classification: anticoagulant, antithrombotic

Indications and dosage
• Prevention of stroke after acute cardioembolic stroke. *Adults:* 1 to 15 mg P.O. daily adjusted to achieve an international normalized ratio of 2.0 to 3.0.

Adverse reactions
Blood: **hemorrhage from any site with excessive dosage**
GI: paralytic ileus, intestinal obstruction, diarrhea, nausea, vomiting, abdominal pain
GU: excessive uterine bleeding
Hepatic: elevated liver function tests
Skin: dermatitis, urticaria, *rash,* necrosis, gangrene, alopecia
Other: *fever,* hepatitis, jaundice

Common adverse reactions in *italics;* life-threatening, in **bold italics.**

Index

Fear as nursing diagnosis, 33
  epilepsy and, 290
  trigeminal neuralgia and, 300
Flaccid posturing, 17i
Fluid volume deficit, intracranial hemorrhage and, 113
Functional incontinence, spinal cord tumors and, 269

G

Gas exchange, impaired, Guillain-Barré syndrome and, 169, 170
Glasgow Coma Scale, level of consciousness assessment and, 6-7, 7t
Gram stain and culture, meningitis and, 147
Graphesthesia, testing for, 59
Guillain-Barré syndrome, 166-174
  assessing, 166-167, 169, 170
  causes of, 167
  classifying, 169
  complications of, 167
  discharge preparation for, 173
  evaluating patient's response to therapy for, 174
  implementing interventions for, 171-173
  incidence of, 167
  nerve degeneration in, 168i
  nursing diagnoses for, 169
  patient outcomes for, 169-171
  patient teaching for, 173
  phases of, 167
  prognosis for, 167
  risk factors for, 167
  treatment of, 171

H

Halo device, 140i, 313
Headache, 42, 276-285
  assessing, 42, 44-46, 276, 278-279
  causes of, 43-44, 276
  classifying, 277-278
  discharge preparation for, 285
  evaluating patient's response to therapy for, 282, 284-285
  implementing interventions for, 281-282
  nursing diagnoses for, 279
  patient outcomes for, 280-281
  patient teaching for, 282
  prevention diet for, 283-284
  treatment of, 281
Head injuries, 102-127
  confusion in, 77

Head trauma
  memory loss and, 68
  sensory disturbances in, 57
Health history, 2-4
Heel-to-toe walking, cerebellar function assessment and, 21i
Hemorrhage as cause of CVA, 185i
Hepatic encephalopathy, decreased LOC and, 72
Herniated disk, 127-134
  assessing, 127, 129-130
  back pain in, 49
  causes of, 127
  development of, 128-129i
  discharge preparation for, 133
  evaluating patient's response to therapy for, 133-134
  implementing interventions for, 130-133
  neck pain in, 47
  nursing diagnoses and, 130
  patient outcomes and, 130
  patient teaching for, 132, 133
  sensory disturbances in, 57
  treatment of, 131
  weakness and, 60
Herniated nucleus pulposus. See Herniated disk.
Hopelessness as nursing diagnosis, 33
Hypertensive encephalopathy, decreased LOC and, 72
Hypertensive-hypervolemic therapy, 202
Hyperthermia
  encephalitis and, 154
  meningitis and, 147, 149
Hypoglycemic encephalopathy, decreased LOC and, 72
Hypoxic encephalopathy, decreased LOC and, 72

I

ICP. See Intracranial pressure, increased, and Intracranial pressure monitoring.
ICP waveforms, interpreting, 93, 94-95i, 96
Implementation as nursing process step, 36-38
  reviewing, 39
Individual coping, ineffective, as nursing diagnosis, 33
  epilepsy and, 290
  Guillain-Barré syndrome and, 169, 170
  MS and, 245, 246
Infection
  as CBF monitoring complication, 98
  as ICP monitoring complication, 93
Infection, high risk for, as nursing diagnosis, 31
  brain laceration and, 122, 124

Injury, high risk for, as nursing diagnosis, 31
  Alzheimer's disease and, 212
  Bell's palsy and, 307, 308
  brain abscess and, 159, 162
  brain laceration and, 122, 124
  brain tumors and, 259
  cerebral aneurysm and, 200, 201
  cerebral contusion and, 107
  concussion and, 102, 103
  CVA and, 188
  epilepsy and, 290
  Guillain-Barré syndrome and, 169, 170
  meningitis and, 147, 149
  Parkinson's disease and, 222, 223
  skull fracture and, 118
  spinal cord injury and, 135
  spinal cord tumors and, 269
  TIAs and, 178
Interventions
  developing, 34, 36
  therapeutic, 37
Intracerebral hematoma, 112i
  treatment of, 114
Intracerebral hemorrhage
  decreased LOC and, 73
  headache in, 44
Intracranial abscess. See Brain abscess.
Intracranial hematomas, 110. See also Intracranial hemorrhage.
  treatment of, 114
  types of, 111-112i
Intracranial hemorrhage, 110-116
  assessing, 110, 111-112i, 112
  breathing patterns and, 110
  causes of, 110
  complications of, 110
  discharge preparation for, 115
  evaluating patient's response to therapy for, 115-116
  implementing interventions for, 113-115
  nursing diagnoses for, 113
  patient outcomes for, 113
  patient teaching for, 114-115
  treatment of, 114
Intracranial pressure, increased
  cerebral compliance and, 84-85i
  compensatory mechanisms and, 84-85i
  evaluating measurements of, 92t